Frontiers in Anti-Cancer Drug Discovery

Volume 3

Editor
Atta-ur-Rahman, *FRS*
Honorary Life Fellow
Kings College
University of Cambridge
UK

Co-Editor
M. Iqbal Choudhary
H.E.J. Research Institute of Chemistry
International Center for Chemical and Biological Sciences
University of Karachi
Pakistan

CONTENTS

CHAPTERS

Contd…..

PREFACE

Cancer is the leading cause of death and an enduring threat to human well being. No other disease has received so much of scientific and societal attention as cancers over the last several decades. However, effective treatment to various forms of cancer is still much sought for. It is therefore imperative to gain knowledge and develop a deeper understanding about the causes of cancer, and the appropriate interventions to prevent and manage the disease. It is necessary to develop scientific strategies for cancer prevention and control, and to disseminate existing knowledge to assist the development of evidence-based approaches towards cancer diagnosis and treatment.

Volume 3 of the eBook series "**Frontiers in Anti-Cancer Drug Discovery**" is a compilation of eight excellent reviews on various, approaches, concerns and issues related to cancer prevention, diagnosis, and treatment.

Understanding carcinogenesis at the molecular level is possible by employing modern molecular biological techniques. The review contributed by Raza *et al.* describes the role of topoisomerase inhibitors in cancer treatment. DNA Topoisomerases are important targets in the development of cancer therapeutics. Inhibitors of topoisomerases cause DNA strand breakages that can ultimately lead to cancer cell death. The authors have also reviewed various classes of inhibitors including catalytic and dual inhibitors with fewer side effects.

Chapter 2, contributed by Vladan P. Čokić and Juan F. Santibáñez, discusses new approaches to the understanding of molecular pathomechanism of myeloprolife-rative neoplasms (MPNs), new innovative JAK (Janus kinase 2) inhibiting drugs and potential therapeutic strategies for the treatment of BCR/ABL-negative myeloproliferative neoplasms. This review highlights the role of TGF-β, JAK2 and others factors that is a challenge to exploit the combinatory therapeutic targets for future treatment of MPNs.

Drug resistance in cancerous cells is a key challenge in the treatment of cancer. Chapter 3 by Pesic *et al.* highlights the importance of ABCB1 therapy as an important step in cancer treatment. The ABCB1 is over-expressed in multi-drug resistance cells mainly due to its remarkable spectrum of substrates. This review also presents an overview of new anti-cancer therapeutic strategies and discusses their benefits and limitations.

Chapter 4 by de Souza *et al.* describes the cancer cell metabolism in great detail. This review also compares the functions and regulation of cancer cells with those of non-cancerous cells. They also discuss the challenges and prospects of targeting cancer cell metabolism for cancer treatment.

The resistance of tumors to cytotoxic treatments has been a major barrier in the chemotherapeutic management of cancer. In view of the involvement of nitric oxide in anticancer mechanism, Kenote *et al.* in chapter 5 discuss its role as a potential adjuvant therapeutic in cancer therapy.

There are many genetic and molecular factors underlying carcinogenesis and that can potentially serve as targets for therapeutic interventions. In chapter 6, Kumar and Shah focus on the key molecular mechanisms for various types of human cancers such as lung cancer, genitourinary cancer, breast cancer, gynecological cancer, gastrointestinal tumors, etc.

Nanotechnology is the science which can be employed for manipulating substances at the cellular and molecular levels. This technology is being applied to stimulate the research in cancer biology that could lead to early diagnosis and enhanced clinical management. Considering the importance of nanotechnology in cancer Yadav *et al.* in chapter 7 summarize the appropriate drug delivery systems that deliver the chemotherapeutic agents to cancerous tissues without harming non-cancerous tissues.

Last but not the least, Akhter *et al.* in chapter 8 describes the role of theranostic metallic nanomedicines as chemotherapeutic agents for cancer treatment.

This delightful feast of well written scientific articles on a topics of general relevance makes this eBook a *"must to read"* for practitioners, scientists, and students. We must thank the contributing scholars for making this volume an important treatise of scientific knowledge. We are also profoundly grateful to the editorial staff, particularly Mr. Mahmood Alam (Director Publication) and Ms. Fariya Zulfiqar (Assistant Manager) for their hard work and persistent efforts.

Prof. Atta-ur-Rahman, *FRS*
Honorary Life Fellow
Kings College
University of Cambridge
UK

Prof. M. Iqbal Choudhary
H.E.J. Research Institute of Chemistry
International Center for Chemical and Biological Sciences
University of Karachi
Pakistan

LIST OF CONTRIBUTORS

Ahmad Raza
University of Minnesota Medical School, Division of Hematology, Oncology and Transplantation, University of Minnesota, Minneapolis, MN 55455, USA

Alexandre Donizeti Martins Cavagis
Department of Physics, Chemistry and Mathematics. Federal University of São Carlos (UFSCar), Campus Sorocaba, Rodovia João Leme dos Santos, Km 110, CEP 18052-780, Sorocaba, SP, Brazil

Ana Carolina Santos de Souza
Center of Natural Sciences and Humanities, Federal University of ABC, Rua Santa Adélia, 166, 09210-170, Santo André, SP, Brazil

Blake A. Jacobson
University of Minnesota Medical School, Division of Hematology, Oncology and Transplantation, University of Minnesota, Minneapolis, MN 55455, USA

Carmen Veríssima Ferreira
Laboratory of Bioassays and Signal Transduction, Institute of Biology, State University of Campinas, Cidade Universitária Zeferino Vaz, s/n, CP 6109, 13083-970, Campinas, SP, Brazil

Dana M. Jarigese
Department of Animal Sciences, Colorado State University, Fort Collins, CO, USA

Deepak Yadav
Department of Ilmul-Advia (Pharmacology), Faculty of Medicine, Jamia Hamdard, New Delhi-110062, India

Farhan Jalees Ahmad
Nanomedicine Research Lab, Department of Pharmaceutics, Faculty of Pharmacy, Jamia Hamdard, New Delhi 110062, India

Farshad Ramazani
Department of Pharmaceutics, Department of Pharmaceutical Sciences, Utrecht University, Universiteitsweg 99, 3584 CG, Utrecht, The Netherlands

Giselle Zenker Justo
Department of Biochemistry (Campus São Paulo) and Department of Biological Sciences (Campus Diadema), Federal University of São Paulo, 3 de Maio, 100, 04044-020, São Paulo, SP, Brazil

Hemant Kardum
Department of Botany, Faculty of Science, Jamia Hamdard, New Delhi-110062, India

Iqbal Ahmad
Nanomedicine Research Lab, Department of Pharmaceutics, Faculty of Pharmacy, Jamia Hamdard, New Delhi 110062, India

Jasna Bankovic
Institute for Biological Research "Sinisa Stankovic", University of Belgrade, Belgrade, Serbia

Javed Ahmad
Nanomedicine Research Lab, Department of Pharmaceutics, Faculty of Pharmacy, Jamia Hamdard, New Delhi 110062, India

Juan F. Santibáñez
Laboratory for Experimental Hematology, Institute for Medical Research, University of Belgrade, Belgrade, Serbia

Manju Belwal
Department of Pharmaceutics, B. S. Anangpuria Institute of Pharmacy, Faridabad, India

Mark A. Brown
Cell and Molecular Biology Program, Colorado State University, Fort Collins, CO, USA; Department of Clinical Sciences, Colorado State University, Fort Collins, CO, USA; Department of Ethnic Studies, Colorado State University, Fort Collins, CO, USA; Colorado School of Public Health, Fort Collins, CO, USA

Melissa A. Edwards
Cell and Molecular Biology Program, Colorado State University, Fort Collins, CO, USA

Milica Pesic
Institute for Biological Research "Sinisa Stankovic", University of Belgrade, Belgrade, Serbia

Mira M. Shah
Department of Radiation Oncology, Henry Ford Hospital, Detroit MI 48202, USA

Mohammad F. Anwar
Department of Chemistry, Faculty of Science, Jamia Hamdard, New Delhi-110062, India

Mohammad Zaki Ahmad
Department of Pharmaceutics, College of Pharmacy, Najran University, Kingdom of Saudi Arabia

Mohd Asif
Department of Ilmul-Advia (Pharmacology), Faculty of Medicine, Jamia Hamdard, New Delhi-110062, India

Nicole J. Kenote
Department of Environmental and Radiological Health Sciences, Colorado State University, Fort Collins, CO, USA

Nikola Tanic
Institute for Biological Research "Sinisa Stankovic", University of Belgrade, Belgrade, Serbia

Robert A. Kratzke
University of Minnesota Medical School, Division of Hematology, Oncology and Transplantation, University of Minnesota, Minneapolis, MN 55455, USA

Ryan Etchison
University of Minnesota Medical School, Division of Hematology, Oncology and Transplantation, University of Minnesota, Minneapolis, MN 55455, USA

Saima Amin
Nanomedicine Research Lab, Department of Pharmaceutics, Faculty of Pharmacy, Jamia Hamdard, New Delhi 110062, India

Sanath Kumar
Department of Radiation Oncology, Henry Ford Hospital, Detroit MI 48202, USA

Sohail Akhter
Department of Pharmaceutics, Department of Pharmaceutical Sciences, Utrecht University, Universiteitsweg 99, 3584 CG, Utrecht, The Netherlands; Nanomedicine Research Lab, Department of Pharmaceutics, Faculty of Pharmacy, Jamia Hamdard, New Delhi 110062, India

Sunanda Singh
Department of Biotechnology, Banasthali University, Banasthali, Rajasthan, India

Suruchi Suri
Department of Chemistry, Faculty of Science, Jamia Hamdard, New Delhi-110062, India

Tysha N. Medeiros
Department of Biochemistry and Molecular Biology, Colorado State University, Fort Collins, CO, USA

Veena Garg
Department of Biotechnology, Banasthali University, Banasthali, Rajasthan, India

Vladan P. Čokić
Laboratory for Experimental Hematology, Institute for Medical Research, University of Belgrade, Belgrade, Serbia

Ziyaur Rahman
Irma Lerma Rangel College of Pharmacy, Texas A&M Health Science Center, Kingsville, Texas, USA

Send Orders for Reprints to reprints@benthamscience.net

Frontiers in Anti-Cancer Drug Discovery, 2014, *3*, 3-31

CHAPTER 1

Innovative Therapeutics Targeting Topoisomerases in Cancer

Ahmad Raza, Ryan Etchison, Blake A. Jacobson and Robert A. Kratzke[*]

University of Minnesota Medical School, Division of Hematology, Oncology and Transplantation, University of Minnesota, Minneapolis, MN 55455, USA

Abstract: DNA topoisomerases are promising targets in the development of cancer therapeutics. They are comprised of a large number of structurally diverse compounds and function by trapping the DNA-enzyme covalent complex, resulting in DNA strand breaks that can ultimately lead to cancer cell death. Topoisomerases are broadly classified as type I and type II. Type I enzyme (hTopoI) transiently breaks the DNA strands one at a time, while type II enzyme (hTopoII) forms a dimeric enzyme molecule that transiently breaks both DNA strands in the double helix in concert. Camptothecin was first isolated from a tree *Camptotheca acuminate*, which showed evidence of hTopI poisoning. Irinotecan and topotecan, two camptothecin analogs designed to be soluble, are widely used in clinical practice. Because of the instability of these analogs, however, other hTopoI inhibitors are being introduced that are more potent and stable. Drugs that interfere with hTopoII are typically classified by their mechanism of action. Poisons (including etoposide and doxorubicin) stabilize the covalent TopoII-5′ phosphotyrosyl DNA intermediate or cleavable complex. hTopoII catalytic inhibitors inhibit the enzymatic activity of hTopoII by disrupting the enzymatic recognition of DNA without causing DNA breaks. Recently described hTopoII catalytic inhibitors include aclarubicine, which is successfully used in clinical oncology practice. A series of 9-aminoacridine compounds with hTopoII inhibitor activity have shown promise in inhibiting pancreatic cancer cell proliferation *in vivo* and have been shown to induce apoptosis. On the basis of the hypothesis that targeting both hTopoI and hTopoII might increase overall anti-tumor activity and overcome resistance, compounds with dual inhibitor activity have been described and are under investigation. In conclusion, the area of topoisomerase inhibitors in cancer therapeutics is evolving and development of dual inhibitors, catalytic inhibitors of hTopoII, and specific inhibitors of hTopoII α isoforms will help to identify more potent compounds with fewer side effects.

Keywords: Apoptosis, cancer, catalytic inhibitors, DNA strand breaks, DNA topoisomerase, hTopoI, hTopoII, topoisomerase poisons.

*Address correspondence to Robert Arthur Kratzke: University of Minnesota Medical School, Division of Hematology, Oncology and Transplantation, University of Minnesota, Minneapolis, MN 55455, USA; Tel: 612-626-0400; Fax: 612-625-6919; E-mail: kratz003@umn.edu

INTRODUCTION

DNA topoisomerase inhibitors are comprised of a large number of structurally diverse compounds, which act to block the action of the topoisomerase class of proteins through various mechanisms. These compounds have a long history in the treatment of human cancers dating back to the 1960s. The first identified topoisomerase inhibitors were doxorubicin and daunomycin, which were isolated from a strain of bacteria in the genus *Streptomyces*. Despite their age, they are still amongst the most prescribed and effective drugs currently used in the treatment of cancer today, thus underscoring the usefulness of topoisomerase inhibitors as effective anticancer agents. Since their discovery, the library of topoisomerase inhibitors has expanded greatly to include many diverse compounds with varying mechanisms of action. This chapter outlines the major classes of topoisomerase inhibitors and discusses their role in the treatment of human cancers.

TOPOISOMERASE: FUNCTION AND MECHANISM

The topoisomerases are a class of proteins, which are responsible for altering and maintaining the topology of DNA in cells by relieving torsion and super helical coils of DNA. These enzymes function primarily in the S, G2, and M phases of the cell cycle and are responsible for relaxing and untangling DNA during replication, transcription, and decantenation [1]. This function is considered essential to maintaining cell viability and allowing progression through the cell cycle of actively proliferating cells. Failure of the topoisomerases to relax DNA either through active inhibition or structural defect of the enzymes most often leads to cell cycle arrest or programmed cell death.

The existence of the topoisomerase class of proteins was originally hypothesized by Watson and Crick as being necessary for the maintenance of relaxed DNA. However, it was not until the early 1970s that topoisomerase was first characterized as a unique enzyme in the bacterium *Escherichia coli* [2]. Topoisomerase enzymes and their homologues exist in both prokaryotic and eukaryotic cells alike. The human genome alone encodes six topoisomerase enzymes; the functional human topoisomerase I (hTopoI) gene is located on chromosome 20q11.2-13.1, and both isoforms of the functional human topoisomerase II (hTopoII) gene are located on chromosome 17q21-22 [3, 4]. Topoisomerases can be classified as either type I or type II topoisomerases, despite differences in their structure and specific function in prokaryotic and eukaryotic cells.

Type I topoisomerases are able to modify the topology of DNA by breaking a single strand of duplex DNA and forming a covalent link between the catalytic tyrosyl residue of the hTopoI enzyme to the 3' end of the broken DNA. This allows the "controlled rotation" of the DNA and reduces torsion present within the DNA generated through such processes as DNA replication [5]. This enzymatic process has been described as a DNA swivel that is transiently produced to allow the DNA strands to rotate around each other in a processive and restrained manner, thus removing supercoiling stress [6]. This process is relatively error free, allowing the cell to freely alter DNA topology without causing dsDNA breaks. hTopoI functions in an ATP-independent manner driven instead by the torque present in the DNA and proceeding energetically downhill. As a result, DNA unwinding due to the activity of hTopoI proceeds in an uncontrolled manner until religation occurs; that is, there is no mechanism in place which religates the DNA after a specific number of supercoils are removed. Thus, DNA unwinding proceeds until the DNA is sufficiently relaxed to allow the religation of the nicked DNA to spontaneously occur.

Type II topoisomerases remove a single DNA supercoil through the cleavage and translocation of duplex DNA. The DNA supercoil is unwound through a DNA gate *via* the transient formation of a covalent cleavage complex with two duplex DNA strands [2, 7]. This process also has high fidelity and rarely results in genetic mutation because of the dsDNA breaks induced by topoII. Unlike hTopoI, hTopoII is ATP-dependent and requires two ATP molecules to remove a single DNA supercoil during one catalytic cycle. Whereas hTopoI proceeds in a manner that returns DNA to an equilibrium state, recent evidence suggests that hTopoII does not merely randomly catalyze passage of duplex DNA but rather globally controls the topology of DNA, simplifying the topology of DNA below that of thermodynamic equilibrium [8].

The molecular mechanisms by which the hTopoI and hTopoII function are similar to each other. In the strand-breakage reaction by a DNA topoisomerase, the tyrosyl oxygen of the catalytic tyrosine attacks a phosphorus atom in the DNA backbone, forming a transient covalent phosphotyrosine intermediate and breaking a DNA phosphodiester bond *via* a transesterification reaction. The product of this reaction is the creation of a transient enzyme-mediated gate in the DNA that allows passage of another ssDNA strand or double helix through it [9]. After this passage event, the oxygen of the DNA hydroxyl group that is generated in the first reaction attacks the phosphorus atom in the phosphotyrosine link, breaking the covalent bond between the enzyme and DNA, thus reforming the DNA backbone *via* a second transesterification reaction. This reaction alone is ATP-independent as no phosphate groups are displaced and occurs spontaneously in topoisomerases; however, whereas hTopoI accomplishes its function without the hydrolysis of ATP, hTopoII requires the hydrolysis of two ATP molecules to induce the necessary conformational changes in the enzyme to translocate the second duplex DNA through the first [7, 10].

TOPOISOMERASE I INHIBITORS

The regulation of hTopoI is altered in neoplastic cells. Evidence has indicated that human tumors have increased levels of Top1 mRNA and protein [11]. For this reason, along with the critical roles that topoismerase plays in DNA replication and transcription, topoisomerase was identified as an effective anti-cancer target. Although the transport of hTopoI inhibitors into cells occurs freely *via* passive diffusion across the cell membrane into the cytosol, the intracellular concentration of hTopoI inhibitors is primarily controlled or reduced by the action of efflux pumps located in the cellular membrane of many tissues. Multi-drug resistance (MDR) can develop in cancer cells. Cancer cells can become resistant to the clinically approved Topo I inhibitors by over-expressing the drug efflux activity by the ATP-binding cassette (ABC) transporter P-glycoprotein (P-GP) located in the cellular membrane. As a result, the reversal of drug resistance and the reduction of toxicity of hTopoI inhibitors remain major issues in the development of these compounds [9]. Therefore, new formulations and analogs of current research compounds are continuously being developed and tested to achieve these goals (Table **1**).

Table 1:   Topoisomerase I Inhibitors

Topoisomerase I Inhibitors			
Compound	**Class**	**Compound**	**Class**
Irinotecan	Camptothecin	CRLX101	Camptothecin Conjugate
Topotecan	Camptothecin	CT2106	Camptothecin Conjugate
Gimatecan	Camptothecin Analog	Pegamotecan	Camptothecin Conjugate
Belotecan	Camptothecin Analog	NKTR-102	Camptothecin Conjugate
Lurtotecan	Camptothecin Analog	NSC727357	Non Camptothecin
Exatecan	Camptothecin Analog	LMP400	Non Camptothecin
Diflomotecan	Camptothecin Analog	LMP776	Non Camptothecin
S38809	Camptothecin Analog	ARC11	Non Camptothecin
S39625	Camptothecin Analog	Genz644282	Non Camptothecin

hTopoI primarily functions during the S phase of the cell cycle; thus, hTopoI inhibitors primarily exhibit S-phase cytotoxicity and G2-M checkpoint cell cycle arrest. hTopoI inhibitors primarily act to trap or lock the hTopoI-DNA cleavage complex following breakage of the phosphodiester backbone and creation of the phosphotyrosyl bond. The cytotoxicity of these compounds results from the collision of an advancing replication fork with an inhibitor-trapped cleavage complex triggering replication fork arrest and breakage of the DNA at the site of the complex, generating a dsDNA break [12]. Repetition of this process leads to multiple dsDNA breaks that are interpreted by the cell as DNA damage, thus preventing the cell from progressing from S-phase into G2 phase or passed the G2-M phase checkpoint, ultimately resulting in cell death [12].

Camptothecin

Camptothecin is the prototype hTopoI inhibitor from which a vast array of derivatives, analogs, and conjugates have been synthesized and characterized. Camptothecin was originally isolated in 1966 from the bark of *Camptotheca acuminate*, a tree native to China which was used as a cancer treatment in traditional Chinese medicine, during a large screening process of natural products for anticancer activity [13]. Camptothecin is a quinoline alkaloid that forms a reversible ternary complex with the hTopoI-DNA cleavage complex. For camptothecin-like drugs to achieve maximum inhibitory activity, they must selectively stabilize the hTopoI-DNA cleavage complex during DNA replication and transcription.

Camptothecin exists in a number of different forms, and malignant cells have been shown to be sensitive to the effects of camptothecin. Sodium camptothecin displayed marked preclinical activity and proved an effective anticancer agent in patients with advanced disseminated melanoma or gastrointestinal malignancies. Despite this success, sodium camptothecin elicited severe toxicity including myelosuppression, vomiting, diarrhea, and hemorrhagic cystitis, which resulted in the discontinuation of the clinical trial [14, 15].

Camptothecin also exists in a lactone (closed E-ring) and carboxylate (open E-ring) form. Lactone camptothecin is the active form and binds to DNA with a ten-times greater affinity than the carboxylate form. At human physiologic pH, lactone camptothecin is converted to carboxylate camptothecin. This carboxylate form displays a high affinity for serum albumin that preferentially binds to the carboxylate form over the lactone form [16, 17]. Despite success as anticancer agents in preliminary trials, camptothecin and its early semi-synthetic analogs were shown to be poorly water soluble, which created problems for drug delivery. Thus, further research and synthetic alteration was conducted that resulted in the creation of two analogs that display increased solubility and are currently approved by the FDA for use in cancer therapy: irinotecan (CPT-11) and topotecan.

Irinotecan (CPT-11) is FDA approved for the treatment of metastatic colorectal cancer and esophageal cancer in combination with other chemotherapy agents. There also exists some evidence for its use in a variety of other malignancies. The lactone ring is the active form of irinotecan and comprises approximately 30-40% of the total irinotecan concentration in plasma after treatment. Irinotecan, a prodrug, is activated in the body by hydrolysis into SN-38 (7-ethyl-10-hydroxy-camptothecin), an inhibitor of hTopoI that inhibits both replication and transcription in the cell. SN-38 is then inactivated *via* glucuronidation by uridine diphosphate glucoronosyltransferase 1A1 (UGT1A1) in the liver [18]. A variant of the UGT1A1 enzyme exists called the "*28 variant," which has a 7-TA repeat sequence located in the promoter region of the gene coding UGT1A1 and lowers expression of the enzyme in these individuals. Individuals with this genotype are unable to deactivate SN-38 as efficiently as those with normal UGT1A1, thus resulting in a dramatic increase in toxicity to the individual [19]. As a result, irinotecan was reevaluated by the FDA and became one of the first chemotherapy drugs to be dosed according to the patient's genotype [20].

Topotecan is the second FDA-approved semi-synthetic analog of camptothecin with established activity in the systemic treatment of small cell and non-small cell lung cancer (SCLC and NSCLC, respectively) [21]. It is a 10-hydroxy camptothecin with a positively charged dimethylaminomethyl group at position 9 [22]. Topotecan functions as a DNA intercalator and inhibits the progression of DNA replication and transcription *via* a distortion of the double helix. Topotecan is metabolized by the monooxygenase CYP3A into N-desmethyl topotecan (which is markedly less active than topotecan) before being secreted primarily by the kidneys [23]. Topotecan is available in both an oral and intravenous formulation, with both forms having similar efficacy in relapsed SCLC [24]. It was the first FDA-approved hTopoI inhibitor available in oral form.

Camptothecin Analogs

There has been a constant effort to improve the efficacy and toxicity profile of camptothecin by producing water-soluble variants that maintain the intact lactone (closed E-ring). Currently, all derivatives contain at least a pentacyclic ring system of camptothecin and an intact α -hydroxylactone group in the E-ring. Additional modifications to the A- and B-rings also exist that are well tolerated and, in many cases, enhance the drug's potency [25]. These modifications have resulted in the synthesis of a variety of different camptothecin derivatives that display varying levels of usefulness as anticancer agents.

Gimatecan is an orally active compound that is a seven-position modified lipophilic camptothecin derivative and potent inhibitor of hTopoI. Gimatecan displays rapid uptake and enhanced accumulation in cells that results in prolonged stabilization of the hTopoI-DNA-drug ternary complex when compared to the conventional camptothecins alone. It also exerts a stronger and more persistent

DNA cleavage function than the other members of the camptothecin family. Gimatecan is highly active in ovarian cancer models and has attained a level of success in clinical trials. This agent has been tested in a phase II clinical trial and was found to be active in patients with recurrent epithelial ovarian, fallopian tube, or peritoneal cancer that had been previously treated with platinum and taxane compounds [26-28].

Belotecan, a camptothecin derivative with modifications to the B- and E-rings, has increased water solubility and activity. Preclinical studies involving belotecan show it to be a more potent hTopoI inhibitor than both topotecan and camptothecin [29]. A phase II clinical trial was conducted with belotecan that showed it to have a high level of activity and success in the treatment of SCLC [30].

Lurtotecan, a derivative of camptothecin with similar or superior *in vivo* potency to topotecan, has demonstrated potent antitumor activity in several xenograft models. Delivery of lurtotecan into tumors occurs *via* liposome encapsulation, which improves penetration and delivery to tumors while reducing systemic side effects. In a phase II study liposome-encapsulated lurtotecan demonstrated moderate hematologic toxicity and no evidence of clinical activity in a group of heavily pretreated women previously exposed to the hTopoI inhibitor topotecan [31]. It was also evaluated in metastatic or loco-regional recurrent squamous cell carcinoma of the head and neck but failed to demonstrate any clinical activity [32].

Exatecan mesylate is a water-soluble hexacyclic analog of camptothecin that does not require enzymatic activation. Exatecan mesylate inhibits hTopoI by stabilizing the hTopoI-DNA transient cleavage complex and has been shown to be a more potent inhibitor than camptothecin, topotecan, or SN-38 against various human cancer cell lines [33, 34]. In particular, it has demonstrated substantial antitumor activity against both pancreatic and metastatic breast carcinomas. Exatecan mesylate is not a substrate for the multidrug transporter P-GP, which is responsible for the development of MDR in cells, a characteristic that makes exatecan mesylate unique among all other camptothecin analogs [35].

Diflomotecan is a member of the homocamptothecin family and was developed by modifying the camptothecin lactone ring from a six-membered α - hydroxylactone to a seven-membered β-hydroxylactone ring [36]. Diflomotecan is a 10,11-difluoro-homocamptothecin that exhibits greatly enhanced plasma stability and superior preclinical antitumor activity compared to the two current FDA-approved camptothecin derivatives, irinotecan and topotecan. Recent evidence suggests that hTopoI-DNA cleavage complexes formed in the presence of synthetic E-ring-modified camptothecin analogs are more stable; thus, these compounds can potentially demonstrate a higher level of anticancer activity than analogs with unmodified E-rings [37]. This agent has already been tested in a phase I pharmacological and bioavailability study and has shown high levels of oral bioavailability. The toxicity is primarily hematological, and neutropenia is the major dose-limiting toxicity [38]. It should also be noted that diflomotecan does not demonstrate severe gastrointestinal toxicity as many other hTopoI inhibitors do. A phase II clinical trial is currently underway (clinicaltrials.gov NCT00080015).

E-ring camptothecin keto analogs have five-membered E-ring structures that are missing the lactone ring oxygen. hTopoI-DNA cleavage complexes produced by these compounds have been shown to be relatively stable. These compounds do not serve as substrates for either the ABCB1 (multidrug resistance-1/P-GP) or ABCG2 (mitoxantrone resistance/breast cancer resistance protein) efflux transporters, thus increasing their intracellular concentration and preventing their rapid removal from cells and the incidence of MDR [39]. In preclinical studies compounds S38809 and S39625 have demonstrated selective hTopoI inhibitor activity and have superior cytotoxicity toward colon, breast, and prostate cancers, as well as leukemia, in comparison to camptothecin. S39625 is currently undergoing advanced preclinical development on the basis of its promising activity in tumor models [40].

Camptothecin Conjugates

Camptothecin conjugates have seen an increase in development and use in clinical trials in recent years. These compounds are fusion molecules created by joining camptothecin or one of its derivatives/analogs to a drug delivery molecule. One of the most studied camptothecin conjugates is CRLX101, a nanoparticle conjugate that consists of a cyclodextrin-based polymer (CDP, a drug delivery agent) joined to camptothecin. This compound has demonstrated marked antitumor effects against human colon carcinoma xenografts and irinotecan-resistant tumors. It also exhibits higher plasma concentration and plasma half-life ranges than irinotecan. After injection, active camptothecin is slowly released as the bond between it and CDP is hydrolyzed, thus facilitating the slow release of the compound and the prolonged plasma concentration. CRLX101 is currently undergoing a series of phase II trials including one for patients with refractory NSCLC (NCT01380769) and one for patients with advanced or metastatic stomach, gastroesophageal, or esophageal cancer (NTC01612546) [41, 42].

A number of other notable camptothecin conjugates are worth mentioning as well. CT2106 is a conjugate that is more water soluble than camptothecin and has shown promising results in a phase I trial [43]. Pegamotecan, a pegylated camptothecin, has demonstrated activity against gastric cancer in a phase II trial [44]. Finally, NKTR-102 is an irinotecan polymer conjugate that is currently undergoing a phase III clinical trial for refractory breast cancer and a phase II trial for metastatic colorectal cancer. NKTR-102 has previously demonstrated activity in metastatic breast cancer and ovarian cancer [27, 45, 46].

Non-Camptothecin hTopoI Inhibitors

Non-camptothecin hTopoI inhibitors, such as the indenoisoquinolines and dibenzonaphthyridinones, were introduced because of instabilities present in a number of the camptothecin derivatives and analogs. These inhibitors are currently under development and promise to be more potent and stable hTopoI inhibitors than the camptothecins [40, 47].

The indenoisoquinolines are chemically stable compounds that lack the hydroxylactone E-ring, which is ubiquitous across all the camptothecin analogs. They also target different DNA sequences in the formation of hTopoI-DNA cleavable complexes and produce dramatically more stable complexes than those formed by camptothecin and its analogs [48]. Examples of the indenoisoquinolines include NSC314622, which inhibits hTopoI-mediated DNA supercoil relaxation without intercalation into DNA, NSC727357 (a bisindenoisoquinoline), which has demonstrated activity against melanoma in a xenograft model, and LMP400 and LMP776, which are currently undergoing a phase I study in relapsed solid tumors and lymphomas [49].

The dibenzonaphthyridinones are hTopoI inhibitors that are structurally related to camptothecin and stimulate more TopoI-mediated DNA cleavage more effectively than the camptothecins [50]. One of the most studied of these agents is ARC-111, which has been shown to induce reversible hTopoI cleavage complexes in tumor cells as evidenced by specific reduction of the hTopoI immunoreactive band in a band depletion assay. ARC-111 also does not function as a substrate for the ABCG2 transporter [51]. Another dibenzonaphthyridione, Genz-644282, has shown an improved therapeutic index in comparison to topotecan and SN-38 in a preclinical setting and is currently in clinical trials [52].

TOPOISOMERASE II INHIBITORS

hTopoII functions primarily in the cellular processes of DNA replication, transcription, and decantenation. hTopoII is most active in the S phase of the cell cycle where it is associated with the replication fork protein complex and is responsible for removing both positive and negative DNA supercoils resulting from the progression of the replication fork along DNA. hTopoII also functions during the M phase of the cell cycle and is necessary for proper chromosome condensation and segregation. Interference at any point within the catalytic cycle of hTopoII by an inhibitor will halt these cellular processes and lead to a crisis for the cell. The inhibition of hTopoII during the S phase most often leads to ssDNA or dsDNA breaks that signal the cell to activate the DNA damage and repair pathways. Failure of these pathways to repair the DNA is lethal to cells and leads to cell cycle arrest and most often to programmed cell death. Similarly, inhibition of hTopoII during the M phase prevents proper chromosome segregation from occurring leading to cell cycle arrest and apoptosis.

All vertebrates have two isoforms of TopoII, TopoIIα and TopoIIβ, that display similar catalytic features but execute separate cellular functions [53]. TopoIIα is expressed abundantly in propagating cells principally in late S and G2/M phases of the cell cycle and is vital for chromosome segregation; TopIIβ is distinguished for its role in controlling gene expression and is linked with developmental and differentiation events [54]. The hTopoII targeting drugs used in the clinic target both hTopoIIα and hTopoIIβ isoforms. Evidence suggests that targeting hTopoIIβ leads to unwanted consequences such as stimulation of cardiotoxicity and introduction of secondary malignancies [53]. Further, because hTopoIIα expression is elevated in cancer cells, it is an attractive target for anticancer drugs [6]. Therefore, more effort in drug development specific to inhibition of hTopoIIα may be useful for greater antitumor efficacy and diminished toxicity while reducing therapy-related malignancies.

hTopoII inhibitors are commonly classified by their mechanism of action (Table **2**). There are two commonly accepted classes of inhibitor: the poisons and the catalytic inhibitors. The hTopoII poisons act to stabilize the hTopoII-DNA transient covalent cleavage complex after DNA cleavage, preventing the religation of duplex DNA and leading to an accumulation of cleavage complexes with covalently bound dsDNA breaks [1, 55]. This causes extensive damage and fracturing of the genome within a cell and leads to activation of the repair and

Table 2:   **Topoisomerase II Inhibitors and Dual Inhibitors of Topoisomerase I and II**

Topoisomerase II Poisons			
Compound	**Class**	**Compound**	**Class**
Anthracyclines	Intercalating Poisons	TOP53	Non Intercalating Poisons
Mitoxantrone	Intercalating Poisons	Amonafide	Intercalating Poisons
Etoposide	Non Intercalating Poisons	Elinafide	Intercalating Poisons
F11782	Non Intercalating Poisons	Amsacrine	Intercalating Poisons
GL331	Non Intercalating Poisons		
Topoisomerase Catalytic Inhibitors			
Aclarubicin	Sumarin	Merbarone	ICRF-154
ICRF-193	Fostriecin	Aminoacridines	QAP-1
Topoisomerase I and II Dual Inhibitors			
Quinone Derivatives	Homocamptothecins	Taspine	Tafluposide
Batracycline	Phenazine		

recombination pathways. These pathways, despite their effectiveness, are often unable to reverse the hTopoII-5' phosphotyrosyl DNA covalent bonds and ultimately trigger programmed cell death pathways.

The catalytic inhibitors act on hTopoII to disrupt the enzymatic recognition of DNA, stabilize noncovalent hTopoII-DNA complexes, or inhibit ATP binding to and hydrolysis by hTopoII, all without introducing dsDNA breaks into the genome [55, 56]. In doing so they accomplish the same result as the poisons, namely forcing cancer cells to undergo programmed cell death, but with reduced cytotoxicity and genotoxicity to the patient. As a result of this, focus has begun to shift from research on the poisons to the development of new catalytic inhibitors for use in a clinical setting.

Topoisomerase II Poisons

hTopoII poisons act directly to increase the level of hTopoII-DNA transient covalent cleavage complexes within a cell and generate dsDNA breaks. The poisons are the most clinically aggressive agents and include compounds such as etoposide, doxorubicin, and mitoxantrone, three of the most prescribed chemotherapy agents in medical history. Although the exact mechanism of action for hTopoII poisons remains unclear, several postulations have been proposed for how hTopoII poisons interact with the enzyme/DNA to inhibit hTopoII activity. Interfacial inhibition is one of the proposed mechanisms where the drug interacts with the interface between the enzyme and the DNA, leading to a strong association of the enzyme for the DNA that cannot be broken by the DNA repair mechanisms [57]. Another mechanism is redox-dependent hTopoII inhibition where redox activity is required for inhibition of the enzyme, a poorly understood process that can lead to conformational changes in the enzyme that inhibit its catalytic process [58].

There are many different sub-classes of hTopoII poisons currently used in the clinical setting today and that function through a variety of different mechanisms. These compounds are among the most highly prescribed drugs because of their proven effectiveness at combating cancer. Despite this, they all have one commonality: they are highly toxic to patients and can cause chemotherapy-induced secondary malignancies as well as other serious adverse side effects. For example, the anthracycline class of hTopoII poisons generates free radicals that can damage DNA and other cellular structures leading to severe cardiotoxicity, while etoposide-treated patients develop treatment-related acute myelocytic leukemia and myelodysplastic syndromes. The use of the hTopoII poisons then is a balance between their superior anticancer activity as compared to catalytic inhibitors and their deleterious side effects.

Among the first hTopoII poisons to be widely used in the treatment of cancer were the anthracyclines. Anthracyclines have been used for more than 30 years in the clinical setting and include doxorubicin, daunomycin, idarubicin, and aclarubicin. These compounds are used most commonly for the treatment of solid tumors such as those arising in the breast, bile ducts, endometrial tissue, esophagus, and liver. They are also used to treat osteosarcomas, soft-tissue sarcomas, non-Hodgkin's lymphoma, and acute myeloid leukemia. The first of these to be discovered, doxorubicin, was first approved by the FDA in 1974 and is still actively prescribed today. There has been considerable controversy about their exact mechanism of action. The initially proposed mechanism of action included intercalation into DNA with consequent inhibition of macromolecular synthesis; however, other proposed mechanisms include free radical formation with consequent induction of DNA damage or lipid peroxidation and DNA binding and alkylation. The currently accepted MOA for these agents is DNA damage *via* the inhibition of hTopoII, resulting in apoptotic cell death [59].

A recent advancement in doxorubicin therapy involves a novel formulation that is aimed to improve delivery of this cytotoxic agent. Pegylated liposomal doxorubicin (PDL) was designed to incorporate the features of liposomal drug delivery along with the qualities associated with the hydrophilic polymer poly-ethylene-glycol (PEG). PLD is a unique formulation in which doxorubicin is encapsulated in the inner water phase of lipid vesicles with a PEG coating of the liposomal shell. PEG adds to the steric stabilization of the liposomal vesicles and imparts protection from clearance by the hepatic reticulo-endothelial system. The passive targeting approach from the encapsulation in liposomes diminishes toxicity and improves the effectiveness of doxorubicin. Combining advances of liposome design with pegylation results in improvements in pharmacokinetics and pharmacodynamics over the established administration of doxorubicin [60].

Etoposide is another commonly used hTopoII poison. First synthesized in 1966, etoposide is a derivative of podophyllotoxin, a natural antimitotic product found in the American Mayapple plant. Initial studies of podophyllotoxin showed it to be a potent inhibitor of cell growth and further research resulted in the creation of etoposide and teniposide. Etoposide was approved by the FDA in 1983 for chemotherapy use in the clinic and has since become the most widely prescribed anticancer drug [61]. Etoposide is commonly given in its prodrug form, etoposide phosphate, which is metabolized in the body into its active form. Etoposide does not bind to DNA but rather to hTopoII *via* its polycyclic core [62]. Although the exact MOA is unknown, etoposide works to inhibit the ligation activity of hTopoII. Evidence suggests that this compound achieves this function through interfererence with non-covalent interactions between hTopoII and the DNA or by altering DNA termini location, inserting between termini and preventing religation of the phosphate backbone [63-65].

Etoposide, despite its widespread success, has been known to induce treatment-related acute myeloid leukemia in a small population of patients. The most likely mechanism by which this occurs is through the balanced translocation of DNA involving chromosome bands 11q23 or 21q22 with subsequent activation of the mixed-lineage leukemia (MLL) gene [66, 67]. The exact mechanism by which the hTopoII cleavage complex induces these chromosomal translocations is not fully understood [68, 69].

Epipodophyllotoxin derivatives are non-intercalating hTopoII poisons. F11782 is a member of this class of compounds, which appears to have a dual mechanism of action. It has been shown to inhibit the DNA nucleotide excision repair (NER) pathway F 11782 and was also found to induce a non-covalent salt-stable complex of human topoisomerase II with DNA [70]. Despite this, F11782 has anticancer activity in the preclinical setting. Another agent, GL-331, has shown activity against lymphoma cell lines and a greatly expanded *in vitro* activity compared to etoposide [71]. This agent is currently undergoing clinical trials. Finally TOP-53 has displayed high activity against NSCLC in animal tumor models. TOP-53 was able to retain its activity in cell lines that had developed resistance to etoposide, indicating that substituents on the etoposide C-ring are important for hTopoII-drug interactions to occur [72].

Naphthalimides are DNA intercalators that have shown enhanced anticancer activity against human cancer cell lines. One early representative of this class of compounds, amonafide, was evaluated in clinical trials as a potential anti-cancer agent but failed to pass phase III trials owing to dose-limiting bone marrow toxicity. Elinafide has improved therapeutic properties compared to amonafide and is a bis-intercalating agent. It has marked *in vitro* and *in vivo* activity and has been evaluated in clinical trials targeting solid tumors. Additionally, derivatives of a structurally related group to the naphthalimides, the azonafides, have shown substantial activity against various cancers, especially leukemias, breast cancer, and melanoma [73].

Quinolone derivatives used in chemotherapy treatments are intercalating agents as opposed to antibacterial quinolones that function *via* a different mechanism. Voreloxin is a quinolone derivative with a naphthyridine structure. It has been shown to induce dsDNA breaks, irreversible G2 arrest, and the rapid onset of apoptosis [74]. It has shown marked activity against human tumor cell lines and xenografts, particularly in drug-resistant tumors [75]. This agent is currently in clinical trials and has shown activity against SCLC [76].

Mitoxantrone is an anthracenedione and a potent intercalating agent. It has been approved for use in patients with leukemias and advanced hormone refractory prostate cancer. However, severe cardiotoxicity has been associated with its use in patients [77].

Aminoacridines are a class of hTopoII poisons that contain a tricyclic core that is capable of DNA intercalation. Acridine-based agents have been in use for decades as antibacterial and antiprotozoal agents because of their ability to effectively inhibit cellular proliferation. It was later learned that these agents inhibit the topoisomerase class of proteins and focus shifted from their antibacterial properties to their use as anticancer agents. Amsacrine, the first compound to be shown to be a hTopoII poison, is an example of an early acridine-based chemotherapy agent. It has limited activity except in relapsed acute myeloid leukemias [78].

Aminoacridine derivatives were studied for topoisomerase inhibition, a few of which displayed dual hTopoI and hTopoII inhibition properties, though none of these are currently in clinical development. Substituted aminoacridine derivatives, however, have been shown to inhibit topoisomerase. These substituted derivatives with hTopoI inhibitory functions have similar potency as camptothecin, while derivatives with hTopoII inhibitor functions have similar potency to teniposide (VM-26). However, they possess only modest cytotoxic activity [79]. Further development of these substituted aminoacridine derivatives have resulted in agents that have catalytic inhibitory activity in hTopoII [80].

Topoisomerase II Catalytic Inhibitors

Catalytic inhibitors of hTopoII do not cause an increase in the levels of hTopoII-DNA covalent cleavage complexes in the cell and are thought to kill cells through the elimination of the essential enzymatic activity of hTopoII. The catalytic inhibitors work by halting the catalytic cycle of hTopoII in any location along its catalytic pathway other than when the DNA is cleaved; that is, they inhibit hTopoII either before it breaks the phosphodiester backbone of the DNA or once it has rejoined it. In this way, catalytic inhibitors do not introduce ssDNA or dsDNA breaks in the genome and thus exhibit greatly reduced genotoxicity to the cell and the patient.

The catalytic inhibitors are a heterogeneous group of compounds that act by either interfering with the binding between DNA and hTopoII, by stabilizing non-covalent hTopoII-DNA complexes, or by inhibiting ATP binding [55, 62]. One common MOA by which many catalytic inhibitors function is to block the catalytic cycle after hydrolysis of the first ATP and strand passage but prior to hydrolysis of the second ATP. Thus, in this case, the catalytic inhibitor blocks the conformational change that allows release of the passaged strand. At this point in the reaction cycle, hTopoII encircles the strand that the enzyme has cleaved. By locking hTopoII in this conformation, the enzyme is unable to dissociate from DNA and its essential enzymatic activity is hindered. This is also the point in the reaction cycle at which hTopoII is blocked by non-hydrolysable ATP analogs [53].

Perhaps the greatest potential advantage of the catalytic inhibitors over the poisons is their ability to inhibit hTopoII to much the same effect as the poisons but with greatly reduced cytotoxicity and genotoxicity. This advantage is a direct result of their ability to block the catalytic cycle of hTopoII other than when the enzyme is covalently bound to cleavage complex; thus, dsDNA breaks are not introduced into the genome. The cell reacts similarly to both poisons and catalytic inhibitors by activating the repair and recombination pathways in an attempt to rectify the problem, but whereas poisons generate dsDNA breaks that can be incorrectly recombined or remain broken and cause further damage to the genome, catalytic inhibitors do not generate these breaks and thus prevent collateral genome damage from occurring. In either case, the programmed cell death pathways are activated and the cancerous cells are killed. Despite this achievement the catalytic inhibitors thus far elucidated have proven largely ineffective as viable chemotherapy agents. Although they function adequately as anticancer agents, most suffer from either high toxicity or possess an active concentration range outside that achievable in a physiological setting [81].

Aclarubicin is an anthracycline anticancer agent derived from *Streptomyces galilaeus* and is used clinically in the treatment of acute myelocytic leukemia. It does not enhance levels of hTopoII-mediated cleavage complexes but is a potent inhibitor of both the hTopoII-mediated cleavage reaction and hTopoII catalytic activity [82]. Interestingly, aclarubicin has also been shown to inhibit hTopoI in a concentration-dependent manner with high concentrations of aclarubicin stimulating the formation of covalent hTopoI-DNA complexes [83].

Suramin is a polysulfonated naphthylurea compound that is used primarily for its antitrypanosomal and antifilarial properties. Lower doses of suramin inhibit hTopoI and certain growth factor receptors within the cell. In addition to inhibition of hTopoII, suramin acts to inhibit the binding of several polypeptide growth factors like platelet-derived growth factor, basic fibroblast growth factor, epidermal growth factor, and insulin-like growth factor. It has concentration-dependent antiproliferative activity against a variety of human tumor cell lines

[84]. Also, a phase I trial provides evidence of antitumor activity when suramin is used in combination with docetaxel or gemcitabine in NSCLC [85].

Merbarone (NSC336628) is a conjugate of thiobarbituric acid and aniline joined together *via* an amide linkage. This compound inhibits the catalytic activity of hTopoII with some selectivity toward the hTopoIIα isoform (the α isoform is the primary target of most anticancer agents). Inhibition by merbarone leads to the formation of dsDNA breaks, S phase retardation, and G2 arrest [86]. Owing to merbarone-mediated chromosome and DNA damage, the MOA for merbarone is in question. In a recent study, merbarone exhibited both cytotoxic as well as genotoxic qualities, but also inhibited topo II catalytic activity and induced endoreduplication. Additionally, the mechanism of action for merbarone is purported to occur principally by blocking hTopoII-mediated cleavage and preventing cleavage complexes of DNA-enzyme formation. Further, merbarone-induced DNA damage was reliant upon continuing DNA synthesis [87]. Merbarone appears to have characteristics of both an hTopoII catalytic inhibitor and poison. Also, merbarone exhibits activity against L1210 leukemia and some murine tumor models; however, this agent has weak antitumor activity and has associated nephrotoxicity [88].

The bisdioxopiperazine derivatives (primarily bis-2,6-dioxopiperazine) are a large class of compounds that were originally synthesized as membrane permeable analogs of the metal chelator ethylenediaminetetraacetic acid (EDTA) [89]. Multiple bisdioxopiperazine derivatives have been studied for anticancer activity. ICRF-154 is a compound with antitumor activity from which numerous derivatives have been synthesized with enhanced activity. ICRF-159 (Razoxane) is a monomethyl derivative of ICRF-154 with comparable antitumor activity revealed in laboratory studies. ICRF-187 is also a derivative of ICRF-154 and is used clinically to reduce doxorubicin-induced cardiotoxicity in patients [55]. ICRF-193 is a dimethyl derivative of ICRF-154 and is the most potent bisdioxopiperazine derivative to act as a hTopoII inhibitor. Interestingly, there is evidence to suggest that ICRF-193 is in fact a very significant hTopoII poison instead of a catalytic inhibitor [90]. A more recent study demonstrates that ICRF-193 requires the strand passage activity of hTopoII for enzyme inhibition and not hTopoII DNA cleavage, revealing that ICRF-193 is a hTopoII catalytic inhibitor

[91]. Further, evidence was presented that indicated that inhibition by ICRF-193 is most likely the result of the stable, concurrent interaction of TopoII with both DNA segments.

Fostriecin (CI-920) is a structurally novel phosphorus-containing antibiotic that was discovered during beer fermentation employing a previously unknown subspecies of *Streptomyces pulveraceus*. It was detected as a component from a complex of similar compounds that were cytotoxic to L1210 leukemia cells [92]. It has been shown to inhibit hTopoII catalytically as well as inhibit a variety of different phosphatase enzymes within the cell. It functions to induce premature mitosis and to abrogate established S or G2 arrest in clear contrast to other topoisomerase inhibitors that induce cell cycle arrest in S and G2 phases [55]. A phase I study of fostriecin targeting SCLC did not exhibit tumor responses in any patients [93].

Acridine-based agents have previously been reported to show activity as hTopoII poisons; however, recent work with aminoacridine derivatives has uncovered a series of compounds that function instead as catalytic inhibitors of hTopoII [80]. These compounds have been shown to intercalate into DNA and to cause a bulge in the structure of the DNA double helix, distorting the proportions of the major and minor grooves [94]. They also possess side chain substitutions that extend into the major and minor groves of DNA and prevent the docking of hTopoII with DNA, thus inhibiting its enzymatic function. These compounds demonstrated activity comparable to that of amsacrine in hTopoII relaxation assays, but did not show activity in trapping hTopoII on DNA as a cleavage complex in an hTopoII cleavage assay [94, 95]. These substituted 9-aminoacridine derivatives suppressed pancreatic cancer cell proliferation both *in vitro* and *in vivo* [95]. In another investigation these same substituted 9-aminoacridine derivatives have shown success *in vitro* as anticancer agents in NSCLC (manuscript in preparation), SCLC lung cancer [96], and malignant mesothelioma [97]. A more recent study of 2 of these substituted 9-aminoacridine derivatives [compound **1** [{9-[2-(1*H*-Indol-3-yl)-ethylamino]-acridin-4-yl}-(4-methyl-piperazin-1-yl)-methanone   and   **2** compound   [9-(1-Benzyl-piperidin-4-ylamino)-acridin-3-yl]-(4-methyl-piperazin-1-yl)-methanone] targeting malignant glioma revealed efficacy both *in vitro* and *in vivo* [98]. A previous study demonstrated that acridine antitumor drugs could penetrate the blood-brain barrier, and this finding propelled the malignant glioma investigation [99]. It was compound **2** that significantly extended the median survival of mice in an orthotopic glioblastoma model.

ATP-competitive purine analogs have been shown to have potent and selective catalytic inhibitor activity against hTopoII. QAP 1 (quinoline aminopurine compound 1) can target both topoisomerase II alpha and beta. Another group of compounds, which are H-purine-2, 6-diamine derivates, were found to have potent activity against human topoisomerase II and are in further development [100].

TopoIIα has been thought to be the main target of topoisomerase poisons such as etoposide and doxorubicin, but there is evidence suggesting that etoposide-induced DNA sequence rearrangements and double strand breaks are TopoIIβ dependent [69, 101]. Recently, it was described that cardiomyocyte-specific deletion of topoisomerase II beta gene protected cardiomyocytes from doxorubicin-induced DNA double strand breaks [102]. NK314, a topoisomerase II poison, has been described as a TopoIIα-specific agent with *in vitro* activity against non-small cell cancer, colorectal cancer, and human cervical cancer cells [103]. Thus, development of TopoIIα-specific topoisomerase catalytic inhibitors can potentially reduce the toxicities and risk of secondary malignancies. Several TopoIIα-specific poisons and catalytic inhibitors are under development in modern era. Catalytic inhibitors of TopoIIα have varied mechanisms of actions and also include natural products [104]. Likewise, several TopoIIα-specific poisons are under development which include various bioflavonoids and natural products [105].

Topoisomerase I and II Dual Inhibitors

The concept of dual hTopoI and hTopoII inhibitors is based on the hypothesis that targeting both enzymes might increase the overall antitumor activity and overcome any drug-related resistance that might occur. This strategy might provide an advantage by improving the topoisomerase inhibitory activity of current and future compounds to the point of providing a clinically viable dual inhibitor with potentially reduced toxicity and side effects. Compounds with dual inhibitor activity have been elucidated and are currently under investigation. In particular, quinone derivatives and homocamptothecins have been the focus of research interest due to their dual inhibitory characteristics that arc a natural component of their structure. Also, taspine (or thaspine), an alkaloid isolated from cortex of the South American tree *Croton lechleri,* has shown dual topoisomerase I and II inhibitor function [106]. Thaspine was especially effective in cells overexpressing drug efflux transporters (P-GP) and in inducing apoptosis. In addition, the activity of tafluposide, batracylin, and phenazine derivatives have been investigated extensively and have undergone phase I and II clinical trials but have yet to produce a viable compound for clinical use [107].

CONCLUSION

The topoisomerases continue to be an important target in the treatment of cancer. Inhibitors of these enzymes have proven to be very effective in their anticancer properties and function and can be successfully combined with a wide variety of other agents to enhance their function. However, their role in cancer therapeutics is evolving. With the development of novel dual hTopoI/hTopoII inhibitors, catalytic inhibitors of hTopoII, and inhibitors specific to the hTopoIIα isoforms, new therapeutic approaches and strategies will need to be developed to incorporate them into the clinical setting. This research will help to identify new compounds that exhibit significantly increased and enhanced anticancer properties with lower toxicity and fewer side effects.

Novel topoisomerase inhibitors are already beginning the process of clinical trials now and the development of isoform specific inhibitors in the future should eliminate the occurrence of secondary malignancies that plague the current regimen of drugs. Additionally, further research into MDR proteins and systems in place within cells, such as the P-GP and BCRP transporters, will aid in the creation of compounds that can bypass or counter the activity of these systems in order to improve treatment outcomes. The future of topoisomerase inhibition is a bright one and, with the continued cooperation and effort of researchers the world round, may one day produce a cure.

ACKNOWLEDGEMENTS

Authors of this chapter would like to thank Michael J. Franklin for editorial support.

CONFLICT OF INTEREST

The authors confirm that this chapter contents have no conflict of interest.

REFERENCES

[1]   Walker JV, Nitiss JL. DNA topoisomerase II as a target for cancer chemotherapy. Cancer Invest 2002; 20(4): 570-89.

[2]   Wang JC. Interaction between DNA and an Escherichia coli protein omega. J Mol Biol 1971; 55: 523-33.

[3]   Tsai-Pflugfelder M, Liu LF, Liu AA, *et al.* Cloning and sequencing of cDNA encoding human DNA topoisomerase II and localization of the gene to chromosome region 17q21-22. Proc Natl Acad Sci U S A 1988 Oct; 85(19): 7177-81.

[4]   Kunze N, Yang GC, Dolberg M, *et al.* Structure of the human type I DNA topoisomerase gene. J Biol Chem 1991 May 25; 266(15): 9610-6.

[5]   Bodard AG, Racadot S, Salino S, *et al.* A new, simple maxillary-sparing tongue depressor for external mandibular radiotherapy: a case report. Head Neck 2009 Nov; 31(11): 1528-30.

[6]   Chen SH, Chan NL, Hsieh TS. New mechanistic and functional insights into DNA topoisomerases. Annual review of biochemistry 2013; 82: 139-70.

[7]   Graille M, Cladiere L, Durand D, *et al.* Crystal structure of an intact type II DNA topoisomerase: insights into DNA transfer mechanisms. Structure 2008 Mar; 16(3): 360-70.

[8]   Rybenkov VV, Ullsperger C, Vologodskii AV, Cozzarelli NR. Simplification of DNA topology below equilibrium values by type II topoisomerases. Science 1997 Aug 1; 277(5326): 690-3.

[9]   Brangi M, Litman T, Ciotti M, *et al.* Camptothecin resistance: role of the ATP-binding cassette (ABC), mitoxantrone-resistance half-transporter (MXR), and potential for glucuronidation in MXR-expressing cells. Cancer Res 1999 Dec 1; 59(23): 5938-46.

[10]   Wang JC. Cellular roles of DNA topoisomerases: a molecular perspective. Nat Rev Mol Cell Biol 2002 Jun; 3(6): 430-40.

[11]   Tsavaris N, Lazaris A, Kosmas C, *et al.* Topoisomerase I and IIalpha protein expression in primary colorectal cancer and recurrences following 5-fluorouracil-based adjuvant chemotherapy. Cancer Chemother Pharmacol 2009 Jul; 64(2): 391-8.

[12]   D'Arpa P, Beardmore C, Liu LF. Involvement of nucleic acid synthesis in cell killing mechanisms of topoisomerase poisons. Cancer Res 1990 Nov 1; 50(21): 6919-24.

[13]   Efferth T, Fu YJ, Zu YG, *et al.* Molecular target-guided tumor therapy with natural products derived from traditional Chinese medicine. Curr Med Chem 2007; 14(19): 2024-32.

[14]   Gottlieb JA, Guarino AM, Call JB, Oliverio VT, Block JB. Preliminary pharmacologic and clinical evaluation of camptothecin sodium (NSC-100880). Cancer Chemother Rep 1970 Dec; 54(6): 461-70.

[15]   Gallo RC, Whang-Peng J, Adamson RH. Studies on the antitumor activity, mechanism of action, and cell cycle effects of camptothecin. J Natl Cancer Inst 1971 Apr; 46(4): 789-95.

[16] Moukharskaya J, Verschraegen C. Topoisomerase 1 inhibitors and cancer therapy. Hematol Oncol Clin North Am 2012 Jun; 26(3): 507-25, vii.

[17] Verschraegen CF, Gupta E, Loyer E, *et al.* A phase II clinical and pharmacological study of oral 9-nitrocamptothecin in patients with refractory epithelial ovarian, tubal or peritoneal cancer. Anticancer Drugs 1999 Apr; 10(4): 375-83.

[18] Mathijssen RH, van Alphen RJ, Verweij J, *et al.* Clinical pharmacokinetics and metabolism of irinotecan (CPT-11). Clin Cancer Res 2001 Aug; 7(8): 2182-94.

[19] Ando Y, Saka H, Ando M, *et al.* Polymorphisms of UDP-glucuronosyltransferase gene and irinotecan toxicity: a pharmacogenetic analysis. Cancer Res 2000 Dec 15; 60(24): 6921-6.

[20] O'Dwyer PJ, Catalano RB. Uridine diphosphate glucuronosyltransferase (UGT) 1A1 and irinotecan: practical pharmacogenomics arrives in cancer therapy. J Clin Oncol 2006 Oct 1; 24(28): 4534-8.

[21] Neuhaus T, Ko Y, Muller RP, *et al.* A phase III trial of topotecan and whole brain radiation therapy for patients with CNS-metastases due to lung cancer. Br J Cancer 2009 Jan 27; 100(2): 291-7.

[22] Underberg WJ, Goossen RM, Smith BR, Beijnen JH. Equilibrium kinetics of the new experimental anti-tumour compound SK&F 104864-A in aqueous solution. J Pharm Biomed Anal 1990; 8(8-12): 681-3.

[23] Mathijssen RH, Loos WJ, Verweij J, Sparreboom A. Pharmacology of topoisomerase I inhibitors irinotecan (CPT-11) and topotecan. Curr Cancer Drug Targets 2002 Jun; 2(2): 103-23.

[24] Riemsma R, Simons JP, Bashir Z, Gooch CL, Kleijnen J. Systematic Review of topotecan (Hycamtin) in relapsed small cell lung cancer. BMC Cancer 2010; 10: 436.

[25] Basili S, Moro S. Novel camptothecin derivatives as topoisomerase I inhibitors. Expert Opin Ther Pat 2009 May; 19(5): 555-74.

[26] Perego P, Ciusani E, Gatti L, *et al.* Sensitization to gimatecan-induced apoptosis by tumor necrosis factor-related apoptosis inducing ligand in prostate carcinoma cells. Biochem Pharmacol 2006 Mar 14; 71(6): 791-8.

[27] Pecorelli S, Ray-Coquard I, Tredan O, *et al.* Phase II of oral gimatecan in patients with recurrent epithelial ovarian, fallopian tube or peritoneal cancer, previously treated with platinum and taxanes. Ann Oncol 2010 Apr; 21(4): 759-65.

[28] Sessa C, Cresta S, Cerny T, *et al.* Concerted escalation of dose and dosing duration in a phase I study of the oral camptothecin gimatecan (ST1481) in patients with advanced solid tumors. Ann Oncol 2007 Mar; 18(3): 561-8.

[29] Hong J, Jung M, Kim YJ, *et al.* Phase II study of combined belotecan and cisplatin as first-line chemotherapy in patients with extensive disease of small cell lung cancer. Cancer Chemother Pharmacol 2012 Jan; 69(1): 215-20.

[30] Rhee CK, Lee SH, Kim JS, *et al.* A multicenter phase II study of belotecan, a new camptothecin analogue, as a second-line therapy in patients with small cell lung cancer. Lung Cancer 2011 Apr; 72(1): 64-7.

[31] Seiden MV, Muggia F, Astrow A, *et al.* A phase II study of liposomal lurtotecan (OSI-211) in patients with topotecan resistant ovarian cancer. Gynecol Oncol 2004 Apr; 93(1): 229-32.

[32] Duffaud F, Borner M, Chollet P, *et al.* Phase II study of OSI-211 (liposomal lurtotecan) in patients with metastatic or loco-regional recurrent squamous cell carcinoma of the head and

neck. An EORTC New Drug Development Group study. Eur J Cancer 2004 Dec; 40(18): 2748-52.

[33]   Braybrooke JP, Boven E, Bates NP, *et al.* Phase I and pharmacokinetic study of the topoisomerase I inhibitor, exatecan mesylate (DX-8951f), using a weekly 30-minute intravenous infusion, in patients with advanced solid malignancies. Ann Oncol 2003 Jun; 14(6): 913-21.

[34]   Mitsui I, Kumazawa E, Hirota Y, *et al.* A new water-soluble camptothecin derivative, DX-8951f, exhibits potent antitumor activity against human tumors *in vitro* and *in vivo*. Jpn J Cancer Res 1995 Aug; 86(8): 776-82.

[35]   Ishii M, Iwahana M, Mitsui I, *et al.* Growth inhibitory effect of a new camptothecin analog, DX-8951f, on various drug-resistant sublines including BCRP-mediated camptothecin derivative-resistant variants derived from the human lung cancer cell line PC-6. Anticancer Drugs 2000 Jun; 11(5): 353-62.

[36]   Lesueur-Ginot L, Demarquay D, Kiss R, *et al.* Homocamptothecin, an E-ring modified camptothecin with enhanced lactone stability, retains topoisomerase I-targeted activity and antitumor properties. Cancer Res 1999 Jun 15; 59(12): 2939-43.

[37]   Miao Z, Zhang J, You L, *et al.* Phosphate ester derivatives of homocamptothecin: synthesis, solution stabilities and antitumor activities. Bioorg Med Chem 2010 May 1; 18(9): 3140-6.

[38]   Gelderblom H, Salazar R, Verweij J, *et al.* Phase I pharmacological and bioavailability study of oral diflomotecan (BN80915), a novel E-ring-modified camptothecin analogue in adults with solid tumors. Clin Cancer Res 2003 Sep 15; 9(11): 4101-7.

[39]   Hautefaye P, Cimetiere B, Pierre A, *et al.* Synthesis and pharmacological evaluation of novel non-lactone analogues of camptothecin. Bioorg Med Chem Lett 2003 Aug 18; 13(16): 2731-5.

[40]   Takagi K, Dexheimer TS, Redon C, *et al.* Novel E-ring camptothecin keto analogues (S38809 and S39625) are stable, potent, and selective topoisomerase I inhibitors without being substrates of drug efflux transporters. Mol Cancer Ther 2007 Dec; 6(12 Pt 1): 3229-38.

[41]   Schluep T, Cheng J, Khin KT, Davis ME. Pharmacokinetics and biodistribution of the camptothecin-polymer conjugate IT-101 in rats and tumor-bearing mice. Cancer Chemother Pharmacol 2006 May; 57(5): 654-62.

[42]   Schluep T, Hwang J, Cheng J, *et al.* Preclinical efficacy of the camptothecin-polymer conjugate IT-101 in multiple cancer models. Clin Cancer Res 2006 Mar 1; 12(5): 1606-14.

[43]   Homsi J, Simon GR, Garrett CR, *et al.* Phase I trial of poly-L-glutamate camptothecin (CT-2106) administered weekly in patients with advanced solid malignancies. Clin Cancer Res 2007 Oct 1; 13(19): 5855-61.

[44]   Scott LC, Yao JC, Benson AB, 3rd, *et al.* A phase II study of pegylated-camptothecin (pegamotecan) in the treatment of locally advanced and metastatic gastric and gastro-oesophageal junction adenocarcinoma. Cancer Chemother Pharmacol 2009 Jan; 63(2): 363-70.

[45]   Choi CH, Lee YY, Song TJ, *et al.* Phase II study of belotecan, a camptothecin analogue, in combination with carboplatin for the treatment of recurrent ovarian cancer. Cancer 2011 May 15; 117(10): 2104-11.

[46]   Dark GG, Calvert AH, Grimshaw R, *et al.* Randomized trial of two intravenous schedules of the topoisomerase I inhibitor liposomal lurtotecan in women with relapsed epithelial

ovarian cancer: a trial of the national cancer institute of Canada clinical trials group. J Clin Oncol 2005 Mar 20; 23(9): 1859-66.

[47]   Pommier Y, Cushman M. The indenoisoquinoline noncamptothecin topoisomerase I inhibitors: update and perspectives. Mol Cancer Ther 2009 May; 8(5): 1008-14.

[48]   Pommier Y. Topoisomerase I inhibitors: camptothecins and beyond. Nat Rev Cancer 2006 Oct; 6(10): 789-802.

[49]   Antony S, Agama KK, Miao ZH, *et al.* Bisindenoisoquinoline bis-1,3-{(5,6-dihydro-5,11-diketo-11H-indeno[1,2-c]isoquinoline)-6-propylamino}pr opane bis(trifluoroacetate) (NSC 727357), a DNA intercalator and topoisomerase inhibitor with antitumor activity. Mol Pharmacol 2006 Sep; 70(3): 1109-20.

[50]   Teicher BA. Next generation topoisomerase I inhibitors: Rationale and biomarker strategies. Biochemical pharmacology 2008 Mar 15; 75(6): 1262-71.

[51]   Li TK, Houghton PJ, Desai SD, *et al.* Characterization of ARC-111 as a novel topoisomerase I-targeting anticancer drug. Cancer Res 2003 Dec 1; 63(23): 8400-7.

[52]   Kurtzberg LS, Roth S, Krumbholz R, *et al.* Genz-644282, a novel non-camptothecin topoisomerase I inhibitor for cancer treatment. Clin Cancer Res 2011 May 1; 17(9): 2777-87.

[53]   Nitiss JL. Targeting DNA topoisomerase II in cancer chemotherapy. Nature reviews Cancer 2009 May; 9(5): 338-50.

[54]   Lyu YL, Kerrigan JE, Lin CP, *et al.* Topoisomerase IIbeta mediated DNA double-strand breaks: implications in doxorubicin cardiotoxicity and prevention by dexrazoxane. Cancer research 2007 Sep 15; 67(18): 8839-46.

[55]   Larsen AK, Escargueil AE, Skladanowski A. Catalytic topoisomerase II inhibitors in cancer therapy. Pharmacol Ther 2003 Aug; 99(2): 167-81.

[56]   Sadiq AA, Patel MR, Jacobson BA, *et al.* Anti-proliferative effects of simocyclinone D8 (SD8), a novel catalytic inhibitor of topoisomerase II. Invest New Drugs 2010 Feb; 28(1): 20-5.

[57]   Pommier Y, Cherfils J. Interfacial inhibition of macromolecular interactions: nature's paradigm for drug discovery. Trends Pharmacol Sci 2005 Mar; 26(3): 138-45.

[58]   Bender RP, Lehmler HJ, Robertson LW, Ludewig G, Osheroff N. Polychlorinated biphenyl quinone metabolites poison human topoisomerase IIalpha: altering enzyme function by blocking the N-terminal protein gate. Biochemistry 2006 Aug 22; 45(33): 10140-52.

[59]   Gewirtz DA. A critical evaluation of the mechanisms of action proposed for the antitumor effects of the anthracycline antibiotics adriamycin and daunorubicin. Biochem Pharmacol 1999 Apr 1; 57(7): 727-41.

[60]   Gabizon A, Shmeeda H, Grenader T. Pharmacological basis of pegylated liposomal doxorubicin: impact on cancer therapy. European journal of pharmaceutical sciences : official journal of the European Federation for Pharmaceutical Sciences 2012 Mar 12; 45(4): 388-98.

[61]   Hande KR. Etoposide: four decades of development of a topoisomerase II inhibitor. Eur J Cancer 1998 Sep; 34(10): 1514-21.

[62]   Hu T, Sage H, Hsieh TS. ATPase domain of eukaryotic DNA topoisomerase II. Inhibition of ATPase activity by the anti-cancer drug bisdioxopiperazine and ATP/ADP-induced dimerization. J Biol Chem 2002 Feb 22; 277(8): 5944-51.

[63]   Wilstermann AM, Osheroff N. Stabilization of eukaryotic topoisomerase II-DNA cleavage complexes. Curr Top Med Chem 2003; 3(3): 321-38.

[64]   Osheroff N. Effect of antineoplastic agents on the DNA cleavage/religation reaction of eukaryotic topoisomerase II: inhibition of DNA religation by etoposide. Biochemistry 1989 Jul 25; 28(15): 6157-60.

[65]   Wilstermann AM, Osheroff N. Positioning the 3'-DNA terminus for topoisomerase II-mediated religation. J Biol Chem 2001 May 25; 276(21): 17727-31.

[66]   Berger NA, Chatterjee S, Schmotzer JA, Helms SR. Etoposide (VP-16-213)-induced gene alterations: potential contribution to cell death. Proc Natl Acad Sci U S A 1991 Oct 1; 88(19): 8740-3.

[67]   Kudo K, Yoshida H, Kiyoi H, *et al.* Etoposide-related acute promyelocytic leukemia. Leukemia 1998 Aug; 12(8): 1171-5.

[68]   Pommier Y, Leo E, Zhang H, Marchand C. DNA topoisomerases and their poisoning by anticancer and antibacterial drugs. Chem Biol 2010 May 28; 17(5): 421-33.

[69]   Azarova AM, Lyu YL, Lin CP, *et al.* Roles of DNA topoisomerase II isozymes in chemotherapy and secondary malignancies. Proc Natl Acad Sci U S A 2007 Jun 26; 104(26): 11014-9.

[70]   Jensen LH, Renodon-Corniere A, Nitiss KC, *et al.* A dual mechanism of action of the anticancer agent F 11782 on human topoisomerase II alpha. Biochemical pharmacology 2003 Aug 15; 66(4): 623-31.

[71]   Huang TS, Lee CC, Chao Y, *et al.* A novel podophyllotoxin-derived compound GL331 is more potent than its congener VP-16 in killing refractory cancer cells. Pharm Res 1999 Jul; 16(7): 997-1002.

[72]   Byl JA, Cline SD, Utsugi T, *et al.* DNA topoisomerase II as the target for the anticancer drug TOP-53: mechanistic basis for drug action. Biochemistry 2001 Jan 23; 40(3): 712-8.

[73]   Ingrassia L, Lefranc F, Kiss R, Mijatovic T. Naphthalimides and azonafides as promising anti-cancer agents. Curr Med Chem 2009; 16(10): 1192-213.

[74]   Hawtin RE, Stockett DE, Byl JA, *et al.* Voreloxin is an anticancer quinolone derivative that intercalates DNA and poisons topoisomerase II. PLoS One 2010; 5(4): e10186.

[75]   Hoch U, Lynch J, Sato Y, *et al.* Voreloxin, formerly SNS-595, has potent activity against a broad panel of cancer cell lines and *in vivo* tumor models. Cancer Chemother Pharmacol 2009 Jun; 64(1): 53-65.

[76]   Krug LM, Crawford J, Ettinger DS, *et al.* Phase II multicenter trial of voreloxin as second-line therapy in chemotherapy-sensitive or refractory small cell lung cancer. J Thorac Oncol 2011 Feb; 6(2): 384-6.

[77]   de Forni M, Armand JP. Cardiotoxicity of chemotherapy. Curr Opin Oncol 1994 Jul; 6(4): 340-4.

[78]   Arlin ZA. Mitoxantrone and amsacrine: two important agents for the treatment of acute myelogenous leukemia (AML) and acute lymphoblastic leukemia (ALL). Bone Marrow Transplant 1989 Jan; 4 Suppl 1: 57-9.

[79]   Makhey D, Yu C, Liu A, Liu LF, LaVoie EJ. Substituted benz[a]acridines and benz[c]acridines as mammalian topoisomerase poisons. Bioorg Med Chem 2000 May; 8(5): 1171-82.

[80]   Goodell JR, Madhok AA, Hiasa H, Ferguson DM. Synthesis and evaluation of acridine- and acridone-based anti-herpes agents with topoisomerase activity. Bioorg Med Chem 2006 Aug 15; 14(16): 5467-80.

[81]   Bailly C. Contemporary challenges in the design of topoisomerase II inhibitors for cancer chemotherapy. Chemical reviews 2012 Jul 11; 112(7): 3611-40.

[82]   Petersen LN, Jensen PB, Sorensen BS, Engelholm SA, Spang-Thomsen M. Postincubation with aclarubicin reverses topoisomerase II mediated DNA cleavage, strand breaks, and cytotoxicity induced by VP-16. Invest New Drugs 1994; 12(4): 289-97.

[83]   Nitiss JL, Pourquier P, Pommier Y. Aclacinomycin A stabilizes topoisomerase I covalent complexes. Cancer Res 1997 Oct 15; 57(20): 4564-9.

[84]   Rubio GJ, Pinedo HM, Virizuela J, van Ark-Otte J, Giaccone G. Effects of suramin on human lung cancer cell lines. Eur J Cancer 1995; 31A(2): 244-51.

[85]   Lam ET, Au JL, Otterson GA, *et al.* Phase I trial of non-cytotoxic suramin as a modulator of docetaxel and gemcitabine therapy in previously treated patients with non-small cell lung cancer. Cancer Chemother Pharmacol 2010 Nov; 66(6): 1019-29.

[86]   Drake FH, Hofmann GA, Mong SM, *et al.* *In vitro* and intracellular inhibition of topoisomerase II by the antitumor agent merbarone. Cancer Res 1989 May 15; 49(10): 2578-83.

[87]   Pastor N, Dominguez I, Orta ML, *et al.* The DNA topoisomerase II catalytic inhibitor merbarone is genotoxic and induces endoreduplication. Mutat Res 2012 Oct-Nov; 738-739: 45-51.

[88]   Glover A, Chun HG, Kleinman LM, *et al.* Merbarone: an antitumor agent entering clinical trials. Invest New Drugs 1987; 5(2): 137-43.

[89]   Creighton AM, Hellmann K, Whitecross S. Antitumour activity in a series of bisdiketopiperazines. Nature 1969 Apr 26; 222(5191): 384-5.

[90]   Huang KC, Gao H, Yamasaki EF, *et al.* Topoisomerase II poisoning by ICRF-193. J Biol Chem 2001 Nov 30; 276(48): 44488-94.

[91]   Oestergaard VH, Knudsen BR, Andersen AH. Dissecting the cell-killing mechanism of the topoisomerase II-targeting drug ICRF-193. J Biol Chem 2004 Jul 2; 279(27): 28100-5.

[92]   Leopold WR, Shillis JL, Mertus AE, *et al.* Anticancer activity of the structurally novel antibiotic Cl-920 and its analogues. Cancer Res 1984 May; 44(5): 1928-32.

[93]   de Jong RS, Mulder NH, Uges DR, *et al.* Phase I and pharmacokinetic study of the topoisomerase II catalytic inhibitor fostriecin. Br J Cancer 1999 Feb; 79(5-6): 882-7.

[94]   Goodell JR, Ougolkov AV, Hiasa H, *et al.* Acridine-based agents with topoisomerase II activity inhibit pancreatic cancer cell proliferation and induce apoptosis. J Med Chem 2008 Jan 24; 51(2): 179-82.

[95]   Oppegard LM, Ougolkov AV, Luchini DN, *et al.* Novel acridine-based compounds that exhibit an anti-pancreatic cancer activity are catalytic inhibitors of human topoisomerase II. Eur J Pharmacol 2009 Jan 14; 602(2-3): 223-9.

[96]   Etchison RJ, B; Benoit, A; Ferguson, D; Kratzke, R. Efficacy of substituted 9-aminoacridine derivatives in small cell lung cancer. Invest New Drugs 2012.

[97]   Raza A, Jacobson BA, Benoit A, *et al.* Novel acridine-based agents with topoisomerase II inhibitor activity suppress mesothelioma cell proliferation and induce apoptosis. Invest New Drugs 2012 Aug; 30(4): 1443-8.

[98]   Teitelbaum AM, Gallardo JL, Bedi J, *et al.* 9-Amino acridine pharmacokinetics, brain distribution, and *in vitro/in vivo* efficacy against malignant glioma. Cancer Chemother Pharmacol 2012 Jun; 69(6): 1519-27.

[99]   Cornford EM, Young D, Paxton JW. Comparison of the blood-brain barrier and liver penetration of acridine antitumor drugs. Cancer Chemother Pharmacol 1992; 29(6): 439-44.

[100] Chene P, Rudloff J, Schoepfer J, *et al.* Catalytic inhibition of topoisomerase II by a novel rationally designed ATP-competitive purine analogue. BMC chemical biology 2009; 9: 1.

[101] Pentheroudakis G, Goussia A, Voulgaris E, *et al.* High levels of topoisomerase IIalpha protein expression in diffuse large B-cell lymphoma are associated with high proliferation, germinal center immunophenotype, and response to treatment. Leuk Lymphoma 2010 Jul; 51(7): 1260-8.

[102] Zhang S, Liu X, Bawa-Khalfe T, *et al.* Identification of the molecular basis of doxorubicin-induced cardiotoxicity. Nature medicine 2012 Nov; 18(11): 1639-42.

[103] Toyoda E, Kagaya S, Cowell IG, *et al.* NK314, a topoisomerase II inhibitor that specifically targets the alpha isoform. J Biol Chem 2008 Aug 29; 283(35): 23711-20.

[104] Pogorelcnik B, Perdih A, Solmajer T. Recent advances in the development of catalytic inhibitors of human DNA topoisomerase IIalpha as novel anticancer agents. Curr Med Chem 2013; 20(5): 694-709.

[105] Pogorelcnik B, Perdih A, Solmajer T. Recent developments of DNA poisons--human DNA topoisomerase IIalpha inhibitors--as anticancer agents. Curr Pharm Des 2013; 19(13): 2474-88.

[106] Fayad W, Fryknas M, Brnjic S, *et al.* Identification of a novel topoisomerase inhibitor effective in cells overexpressing drug efflux transporters. PLoS One 2009; 4(10): e7238.

[107] Salerno S, Da Settimo F, Taliani S, *et al.* Recent advances in the development of dual topoisomerase I and II inhibitors as anticancer drugs. Curr Med Chem 2010; 17(35): 4270-90.

CHAPTER 2

Janus Kinase 2 and Transforming Growth Factor Beta Signal Transduction Targeted Therapies in BCR/ABL-Negative Myeloproliferative Neoplasms

Vladan P. Čokić and Juan F. Santibáñez[*]

Laboratory for Experimental Hematology, Institute for Medical Research, University of Belgrade, Belgrade, Serbia

Abstract: The classic BCR/ABL-negative myeloproliferative neoplasms (MPNs), including polycythaemia vera (PV), essential thrombocythaemia (ET) and primary myelofibrosis (PMF), originate from a stem cell-derived clonal myeloproliferation represented with variable hematopoietic cell lineages and the possibility to convert to PMF and progress into acute myeloid leukemia. Their molecular pathogenesis has been associated with persistent and acquired gain-of-function mutations in the Janus kinase 2 (JAK2) and thrombopoietin receptor (MPL) genes. Furthermore, familial MPNs have an autosomal dominant inheritance with decreased penetrance. Additionally, mutations in TET2, IDH1/2, EZH2, and ASXL1 genes which appear to affect the epigenome of MPN patients have been described. The transforming growth factor-beta (TGF-β) signaling pathway has a defined role in regulating normal hematopoiesis and is frequently dysregulated in hematologic malignancies. During hematopoiesis, the TGF-β potently inhibits proliferation and stimulates cell differentiation and apoptosis. MPNs are resistant to normal homeostatic regulation by TGF-β mainly due to mutations or deletion of members of TGF-β signaling pathways or deregulation by oncoproteins. Despite the heterogeneity and genetic complexity of MPNs, the improvement in understanding of their pathogenetic mechanism of myeloid transformation, coupled with the increasing availability of agents acting as tyrosine kinase inhibitors, facilitated the development of therapeutics capable of suppressing the constitutive activation of the JAK/STAT pathway. In addition, advances in the TGF-β signaling area enable targeting it for the treatment of hematologic malignancies. In this chapter we will discuss new insights in the molecular pathomechanism of MPN, the new innovative JAK inhibitor drugs and potential therapeutic strategies by targeting TGF-β signaling as well as the potential combinatory use of JAK inhibitors and TGF-β signal transduction modulators for the treatment of BCR/ABL-negative MPNs.

Keywords: Angiogenesis, essential thrombocythemia, JAK2, JAK2 inhibitors, JAK-STAT pathway, myeloproliferative neoplasms, polycythemia vera, primary myelofibrosis, therapies, transforming growth factor-beta.

---

*Address correspondence to Juan F. Santibáñez: Laboratory for Experimental Hematology, Institute for Medical Research, University of Belgrade, Dr. Subotića 4, 11129 Belgrade, Serbia; Tel: +381 11 2685 788; Fax: +381 11 2643 691; E-mail: jfsantibanez@imi.bg.ac.rs

INTRODUCTION

Myeloproliferative neoplasms (MPNs) are a group of stem/progenitor cell-derived clonal disorders with defective regulation of myeloid cell proliferation because of hypersensitivity or independence from normal cytokine regulation, described by an overproduction of mature blood cells and an affinity to convert to acute myeloid leukemia (AML). This results in an overproduction of mature erythrocytes, granulocytes, and platelets. This myeloproliferation results from the absence of feedback regulation by mature cells, decreasing cytokine levels. Classical MPNs consist of chronic myelogenous leukemia (CML), polycythemia vera (PV), essential thrombocythemia (ET), and primary myelofibrosis (PMF). The cardinal features of the three main BCR-ABL negative MPNs are an increased red-cell mass in PV, a high megakaryocyte/platelet count in ET, and bone marrow fibrosis with the predominant megakaryocyte/granulocytic lineages in PMF. CML (not discussed here) is a MPN that is defined by its causative molecular lesion, the BCR-ABL fusion gene, which most commonly results from the Philadelphia translocation [1]. BCR-ABL-negative MPNs are associated with acquired mutations of tyrosine kinase. Janus kinase 2 (JAK2) is a non-receptor tyrosine kinase that acts as an important signal transducer in cytokine signalling and promoting growth, survival, and differentiation of various cell types. The *JAK2* mutation is valine-to-phenylalanine substitution at position 617 (V617F) that can be detected in approximately 95% of PV patients. Other *JAK2* mutations located in exon 12 can be found in 2-5% of PV patients, so virtually all PV patients carry hematopoietic cells affected by an activating mutation in the JAK2 protein [2]. In ET and PMF, the *JAK2* V617F mutation is found in approximately 50-60% of patients, while mutations in myeloproliferative leukemia virus oncogene (MPL), the receptor for thrombopoietin, have been reported in 5–10% of ET and PMF patients [3].

Transforming growth factor-beta (TGF-β) is pleiotropic factor, with different roles in health and disease, implicated in cell growth, proliferation, differentiation, inflammation, angiogenesis and cancer among others. In cancer TGF-β has been postulated as dual factor since it can inhibits early step of tumorigenesis, while it can promotes late stages of tumor progression. Cancer cells become refractory to TGF-β growth inhibitory effects by different mechanisms, including modifications in the components of TGF-β signaling, such as inactivating mutations or silencing in its type II TGF-β receptor (TBRII) and Smad4, and other not fully elucidated alterations [4, 5]. TGF-β is one of the most important players in the immune system regulation, posses' potent tumor immune-suppressive functions creating an immune-tolerant environment and allows cancer cells to escape from immune surveillance to finally support cancer progression [6, 7]. In MPNs, a downregulation of TBRII have been observed, meanwhile elevated levels of TGF-β in both blood and bone marrow may be implicated in myelofibrosis process. Here we will review clinical and molecular aspect of MNPs, the implication of TGF-β, and finally existing opportunities for TGF-β therapies, the targeting of JAK2 and some others therapies implicating epigenetic and immune-modulatory drugs in MPNs.

MYELOPROLIFERATIVE NEOPLASM

In the late 19th century a French physician Louis Henri Vaquez provided the first description of PV, as a condition of "persistent and excessive hypercellularity accompanied by cyanosis," while a German physician Gustav Hueck defined PMF [8, 9]. ET was last of the classic MPNs to be properly described (as hemorrhagic thrombocythemia) in 1934 by Emil Epstein and Alfred Goedel [10], both Austrian pathologists. In 1939, Vaughan and Harrison underscored the relationship between PMF, PV and ET, in terms of their origin from a common ancestral cell. William Dameshek, an American hematologist, presented that these disorders, along with CML, have many similar clinical and laboratory features, and grouped them as myeloproliferative disorders (MPDs) in 1951 [11]. In 2001, the World Health Organization (WHO) classification of myeloid neoplasms included the Dameshek-defined MPDs under the broader category of chronic myeloproliferative diseases (CMPDs), and also included chronic neutrophilic leukemia (CNL), chronic eosinophilic leukemia/hypereosinophilic syndrome (CEL/HES), and "CMPD, unclassifiable." At the time, the CMPDs were in turn considered to be 1 of 4 major categories of chronic myeloid neoplasms; the other 3 were myelodysplastic syndromes (MDS), "MDS/MPD overlap," and mast cell disease (MCD) [12]. In 2008, WHO revised the classification of MPD influenced by genetic abnormalities and better characterization of histological features. The MPD name has been changed in MPN. Diagnostic algorithms for PV, ET, and

PMF have considerably altered to contain information about *JAK2* V617F and related activating mutations. Other clinical, laboratory, and histological parameters have been integrated to permit diagnosis and categorization despite of *JAK2* V617F or similar mutations [13]. In establishing the MPNs as stem cell-derived clonal diseases (1976-81), an American physician Philip Fialkow and colleagues exploited previous observations by Ernest Beutler and Mary Frances Lyon regarding X chromosome mosaicism in female humans and mice [14]. Clinical investigation in MPNs entered the modern era with the creation of the Polycythemia Vera Study Group (PVSG) in 1967 by Louis Wasserman. Under his leadership, the PVSG performed a series of randomized trials in PV, first demonstrating that phlebotomy is superior to phlebotomy plus chlorambucil or P32, due to an increased incidence of leukemic transformation in patients treated with chlorambucil or P32. The PVSG subsequently reported that hydroxyurea is associated with a reduced risk of thrombosis compared with a historical series of patients managed with phlebotomy, and that high-dose antiplatelet therapy is associated with an increased risk of bleeding in PV [15]. Anthony Green and colleagues used candidate gene resequencing followed by allele-specific PCR to identify the *JAK2* V617F allele in PV, ET, and PMF [16]. Building on the key observation of Josef Prchal and colleagues that acquired uniparental disomy (UPD) of chromosome 9p24 is common in PV [17], Robert Kralovics, Radek Skoda, and their colleagues sequenced the gene in the minimal region of UPD to identify the *JAK2* V617F allele [18]. Levine and colleagues used an approach based on the previous identification of activating mutations in tyrosine kinases of other MPNs, and performed a systematic survey of the tyrosine kinases in PV using high throughput DNA resequencing that led to the identification of the recurrent mutation in *JAK2* in MPN [19]. James and colleagues also described a clonal and recurrent mutation in the auto-inhibitory JH2 pseudo-kinase domain of the *JAK2* gene in PV patients. The mutation is a guanine to thymidine substitution that results in a valine to phenylalanine substitution, at amino acid position - codon 617 of *JAK2*, induce constitutive tyrosine phosphorylation activity that supports cytokine hypersensitivity and erythrocytosis in a mouse model [20]. The mutation is not present in the germ line, consistent with the notion that *JAK2* V617F is acquired as a somatic disease allele in the hematopoietic compartment [21].

Polycythaemia Vera

PV is a chronic blood disorder marked by an abnormal increase in three types of phenotypically normal blood cells produced by bone marrow: red blood cells (RBCs), white blood cells (WBCs), and platelets. Although trilineage proliferation is observed, RBCs mass is most augmented. Most of the symptoms of PV are related to the increased volume of the patient's blood and its greater thickness (high viscosity). Eventually, PV may undergo hematologic evolution into PMF, AML and MDS. In addition to increased hemoglobin (>185 g/L in men, 165 g/L in women) is either panmyelosis in a bone marrow biopsy, a low serum erythropoietin (EPO) level, or EPO-independent *in vitro* erythroid colony formation [13].

Epidemiology

Median age at diagnosis is 61 years and gender distribution is close to 1:1. PV is a rare disease with an incidence rate estimated in Europe and in the United States to be approximately 1.9–2.3 new cases per 100,000 persons / year. The incidence of PV is highest for men aged 70–79 years (24 cases/100,000 persons per year) (Table **1**).

Pathogenesis

The discovery that 9pLOH is present in more than 30% of PV subjects, drew interest towards the 9p chromosomal region that encodes the *p16* and *JAK2* genes [17]. In 2005, diverse groups reported the first recurrent molecular abnormality of PV, represented by a point mutation in *JAK2* exon 14 [16, 18-20], that autonomously activates downstream signaling pathways, including JAK-STAT, PI3K/Akt and ERK1/2 MAPK. Characteristic features of PV are the presence of the *JAK2* V617F mutation (95%) or an equivalent mutation in exon 12 of *JAK* (4%). In most PV patients, unlike a minority of ET patients, only the mutated allele is found in hematopoietic cells (homozygosity) as a result of a process of mitotic recombination. However, patients with mutations in *JAK2* exon 12 mainly demonstrate an isolated erythrocytosis without associated increase of platelet number or white blood count [2]. The raise and clustering of enlarged mature and pleiomorphic megakaryocytes with multilobulated nuclei and proliferation of erythropoiesis, in a modest to obvious hypercellular bone marrow with hyperplasia of dilated sinuses, are the particular diagnostic features of untreated *JAK2* V617F positive PV. Because JAK2 exon 12–positive PV not have the classic myeloproliferative morphologic features, bone marrow samples may be hard to classify as MPN [22].

Clinical Presentation

The course of PV can be divided in 3 phases: (1) the pre-polycythemic phase characterized by a borderline or mild erythrocytosis often in combination with significant thrombocytosis (sometimes associated with thrombotic events), (2) the apparent polycythemic phase, and (3) the post-polycythemic phase defined by cytopenia (including anemia), bone marrow fibrosis, and extramedullary hematopoiesis (post-polycythemia myelofibrosis). Almost all patients are diagnosed when they are in the polycythemic phase and the first symptoms appear. Many patients are asymptomatic or present with nonspecific constitutional complaints. Palpable splenomegaly, pruritus and vasomotor symptoms are each expressed by about a third of the patients. Venous thrombosis and thrombocytosis are more frequent in women, while arterial thrombosis and palpable splenomegaly in men. Headache, dizziness, blurred vision, transient neurologic symptoms, and gastroduodenal lesions are mainly due to thrombotic events in the microvasculature. The greatest impact on morbidity and mortality is due to the thrombotic and hemorrhagic complications. Major arterial or venous thrombosis of the hepatic (Budd–Chiari syndrome), splanchnic, or portal veins can occur. Abnormal karyotype at diagnosis is documented in 12% of the studied patients and is more frequent in men. Increased serum lactate dehydrogenase level and leukoerythroblastosis are, respectively, documented in 50% and 6% of patients evaluated. There is no difference in survival between patients with *JAK2* V617F *vs* other *JAK2* mutations. Survival is negatively affected by older age, leukocytosis 15×10^9/L, venous thrombosis and abnormal karyotype. Cumulative hazard of leukemic transformation, with death as a competing risk, is 2.3% at 10 years and 5.5% at 15 years [23].

Differential Diagnosis

Absolute polycythemia can be due to an increase in the total red cell mass, secondary to fluid overload or liver dysfunction. On the contrary, relative polycythemia can occur with volume depletion. These cases are not reflective of absolute increase in cell counts; rather, they characterize volume status and occur briefly with resolution once patients become euvolemic. Autosomal-dominant primary familial PV and congenital erythrocytosis also have been described. These patients usually have a strong family history and present with low-serum EPO levels. Chronic tissue hypoxemia, impaired tissue oxygenation, endogenous production, or exogenous EPO administration can all cause secondary PV. These conditions are not associated with an absolute increase in cell counts. It is important to recognize that secondary causes of PV can occur as a normal physiological reaction to adjust to new surroundings (*i.e.*, high altitude) [24].

Diagnosis

Patients are diagnosed with PV if they present with both major criteria and 1 minor criterion or the first major criterion and 2 minor criteria. The 2008 World Health Organization diagnostic criteria are:

Major Criteria:

1)   Hgb >185 g/L (men) >165 g/L (women) or Hgb >170 g/L (men), or >150 g/L (women) if associated with a sustained increase of ≥ 20 g/L from baseline that is not associated with treatment of iron deficiency anemia;

2)   Presence of *JAK2* V617F or similar mutation.

Minor Criteria:

1)   Bone marrow trilineage myeloproliferation.

2)   Subnormal serum EPO level.

3)   Endogenous erythroid colony formation *in vitro*.

Treatment

The current recommendation for treatment is phlebotomy targeting a hematocrit (Hct) of <45 L/L and <42 L/L in men and women, respectively. All patients should receive low-dose aspirin. Interferon-α (IFN-α) or bulsulfan, another alkylating agent, is recommended in high-risk patients <65 years of age who cannot tolerate hydroxyurea or are refractory to standard therapy. Low risk patients are <60 years of age with no history of thrombosis, their therapy is low-dose aspirin plus phlebotomy. Low risk with extreme thrombocytosis patients are <60 years of age, no history of thrombosis but with platelet count $>1000\times10^9$/L, their therapy is low-dose aspirin if Ristocetin cofactor activity is <30% plus phlebotomy. Ristocetin Cofactor Activity evaluates the ability of von Willebrand factor to bind to platelets and stimulate primary hemostasis. Ristocetin is an antibiotic that augments von Willebrand factor binding to platelets, through a conformational change of platelet receptor glycoprotein Ib. Ristocetin Cofactor Activity <30% (normal range 50-160) confirms low levels of von Willebrand factors. High risk patients are ≥60 years of age, or with history of thrombosis and their therapy is low-dose aspirin, phlebotomy and hydroxyurea. It is no association between leukemic transformation and hydroxyurea use [23]. High-risk PV patients also receive pegylated IFN-α as first-line treatment. The current practice of targeting Hct <45 L/L for men and <42 L/L for women is founded on earlier studies estimating the cerebral blood flow (CBF) in patients with PV. Phlebotomy mediated a reduction in the Hct from a mean of 0.536 to 0.455 L/L, increased CBF by 73%, and decreased blood viscosity by 30%. Low-dose aspirin prophylaxis in PV patients reduced the cumulative rate of nonfatal myocardial infarction, cerebrovascular accident, pulmonary embolism, major venous thrombosis, and death from cardiovascular causes without significant risk of bleeding [24]. In addition to high rates of clinical and hematologic responses, IFN-α significantly reduced *JAK2* V617F allele burden involving complete molecular responses [25].

Prognosis

Patients are generally asymptomatic for many years. Median survival in untreated patients is estimated to be between 6 and 18 months, with CVA and CV thrombotic events presenting the highest mortality risk. PV is a chronic and incurable disease, and most patients develop post-PV PMF over time. The incidence of AML and MDS ranges is 5-10% after 10 years of observation in PV, with a time-dependent increase of risk. The risk seems higher (8-20%) in PMF and lower (2-5%) in ET. MPN patients with AML transformation have a median survival of 3 months from time of AML diagnosis. Outcome after AML transformation is not influenced by type of previous MPN treatment. In addition, hydroxyurea exposure, even at high doses, is not related with a significantly increased risk of transformation to AML/MDS [26]. Median overall survival was 20.3 years after a median follow-up of 16.3 years in patients with PV treated with hydroxyurea [27]. The cumulative incidence of AML/MDS in the hydroxyurea treatment is 6.6%, 16.5%, and 24.2% at 10, 15, and 20 years, respectively. The cumulative incidence of PMF at 10, 15, and 20 years for PV patients in the hydroxyurea treatment is 12.6%, 19.4%, and 26.9%, respectively. A major risk factor to progress to myelofibrosis seems to be the JAK2V617F allele load. It is currently unclear whether the observed incidence of AML/MDS should be attributed to the natural long-term evolution of PV, which is unaffected by palliative hydroxyurea therapy, or cumulative hydroxyurea therapy *per se* [27]. The life expectancy of well-treated PV patients is only moderately reduced, showing a 15-year survival of 65%. Vascular and non-vascular death rates are 1.7 and 1.8 deaths per 100 patients per year.

Essential Thrombocythaemia

ET is an acquired stem cell-derived clonal disease with expansion of the megakaryocytic/platelet line characterized by a continued increase in the platelet count, and a tendency for thrombosis or bleeding.

Epidemiology

The mean age at diagnosis of ET is approximately 60 years of age; however, up to 20% of patients are diagnosed at <40 years of age. ET has an annual incidence of 0.5–2.5 per 100 000 people. Female-to-male ratio is 1.8 [24] (Table 1).

Pathogenesis

Like PV, there are no specific cytogenetic abnormalities associated with ET; however, 7% of patients have deletion (20q), deletion (13q), +8, +9, and chromosome 1, 5, and 7 abnormalities. *JAK2* V617F and *MPL* may or may not be present [24]. Approximately half of the ET patients carry the *JAK2* V617F mutation; these patients mainly bear cells that are heterozygous for the mutation. About 5% of the ET patients are positive for a mutation in exon 10 of MPL and additional 5% bear a mutation in the adaptor protein LNK. The remaining ET patients (~1/3) do not display any known mutation affecting the JAK-STAT signaling pathway [28, 29].

Clinical Presentation

Up to 50% of patients are asymptomatic on presentation. In symptomatic patients, headaches and visual complaints are common. Erythromelalgia, paresthesias, seizures, bleeding diathesis when platelet counts >1000x10^9/L, and arterial or venous thrombosis can also be present. Compared to PV, pruritus, hypercatabolic conditions, and constitutional symptoms are less usually observed. In young women, recurrent first-trimester pregnancy loss can occur. Nearly 25% of patients have palpable mild to moderate splenomegaly; however, hepatomegaly is rare [24]. The clinical presentation of ET is dominated by a predisposition to vascular occlusive events and hemorrhages. Vascular occlusive events include thromboses in the cerebrovascular, coronary and peripheral arterial circulation. Thromboses of large arteries represent a major cause of mortality associated with the disease or can induce severe neurological, cardiac or peripheral arteries disabilities. Deep vein thrombosis also represents a potentially serious and life-threatening event due to the risk of pulmonary embolism, hepatic (Budd Chiari syndrome) or portal thrombosis. Aspirin-sensitive erythromelalgia, one of the most characteristic microvascular disturbances in ET, is described as burning painful and ulcerative toes. It is often accompanied by a warm, red or violet colored congested limb extremity. The ischemic attacks of digital arteries may subsequently progress towards small zones of limited necrosis or even peripheral gangrene with palpable arterial pulsations. Headaches are the most common neurological manifestations. Visual dysfunction manifests as attacks of diplopia and rapid reversible attacks of blurred vision. Bleeding in ET is often limited to frequent skin manifestations: bruising, subcutaneous hematomas, ecchymoses, and epistaxis or gum bleeding. There is an inverse relationship between von Willebrand Factor levels and platelet counts. Some patients with ET are asymptomatic [24].

Differential Diagnosis

Platelets are acute phase reactants; therefore, thrombocytosis can be related to a number of conditions, such as with malignancy, glucocorticoids and iron deficiency. Reactive thrombocytosis is transient and should resolve with treatment of the primary etiology. It is essential to know that extreme thrombocytosis with platelet counts $>1000x10^9$/L has been documented in inflammatory conditions, infections, functional or surgical postsplenectomy, trauma, blood loss, and rebound states, indicating that absolute platelet counts alone cannot distinguish between an autologous clonal process and secondary causes. Evaluation of iron stores can be helpful in distinguishing between ET and PV, as ET patients will be iron replete. It is important to note that ET has heterogeneous properties that overlap with PMF; in advanced cases, this can make diagnosis quite complex. Clinical and laboratory estimation is important to discriminate between them, and in the absence of extreme splenomegaly, anemia, teardrop anisopoikilocytosis, and leukoerythroblastosis, advanced ET, or "prefibrotic PMF," can safely be diagnosed [24].

Diagnosis

Isolated thrombocytosis of $450x10^9$/L or greater is generally seen with or without associated erythrocytosis or leukocytosis. Histologic evaluation is obligatory for diagnosis, and bone marrow biopsy usually exposes clusters of large, hyperlobulated, and mature megakaryocytes accompanied by granulocytic proliferation with a left shift in approximately 50% of cases [24]. Diagnosis of ET requires meeting all 4 major criteria. The 2008 World Health Organization diagnostic criteria are:

Major Criteria:

1)   Sustained platelet counts $\geq 450x10^9$/L;

2)   Bone marrow biopsy with predominant megakaryocyte proliferation with large and mature megakaryocytes. No or little granulocyte or erythroid proliferation.

3)   Not meeting WHO criteria for PV, PMF, CML, MDS, or other myeloid neoplasm.

4)   Demonstration of *JAK2* V617F or other clonal marker or no evidence of reactive thrombocytosis.

Treatment

Low risk ET patients are <60 years of age, with no history of thrombosis and platelet count $<1500 \times 10^9$/L without history of bleeding or acquired von Willebrand syndrome, no cardiovascular risk factors, such as smoking, hypercholesterolemia, or diabetes mellitus. Intermediate risk ET patients are neither low- nor high-risk category, while high risk patients are ≥ 60 years of age and with history of thrombosis. Current recommendations advise dual therapy with hydroxyurea plus low-dose aspirin in high-risk patients. All patients should receive low-dose aspirin [24]. High-risk patients with ET are also treated with pegylated IFN-α or anagrelide [28]. *JAK2* V617F-positive ET patients were more sensitive to therapy with hydroxyurea, but not anagrelide, than those without the *JAK2* mutation [30].

Prognosis

Around 10% of patients experience a thrombotic event and roughly 4% suffer a hemorrhagic episode. There is evidence that a high burden of *JAK2* V617F mutation also confers increased risk of thrombosis. Decreased survival is associated with age >60 years, leukocytosis $\geq 15 \times 10^9$/L, tobacco use, and diabetes mellitus. Transformation to other myeloid disorders and AML are relatively low in the first decade (1.4% and 9.1%, respectively) but increased by 8.1% and 28.3%, respectively, in the second decade and 24.0% and 58.5%, respectively, in the third decade. Age >60 years at diagnosis and leukocytosis are also found to be independent risk factors for decreased survival. Patients with none, one or both risk factors have median survival rates of 25.3, 16.9, and 10.3 years, respectively [31].

Primary Myelofibrosis

PMF is characterized by bone marrow fibrosis, splenomegaly, leukoerythroblastosis, extramedullary hematopoiesis, and a collection of debilitating symptoms. Myelofibrosis is defined as an increase in quantity and density of extracellular matrix (ECM) proteins, which normally provide a scaffold for the hematopoietic (stem and progenitor) cells in the bone marrow. In the revised classification, the diagnostic criteria of PMF are independent of disease stage and the presence of fibrosis at diagnosis. PMF can present as a primary disorder or evolve from PV or ET to post-PV PMF or post-ET PMF, respectively. A semi-quantitative grading of bone marrow fibrosis ranging from MF-0 (normal) to MF-3 (osteosclerosis) is adopted [32].

Epidemiology

Median age at diagnosis is approximately the mid-60s. It is the least common of the typical BCR-ABL-negative MPNs, with an annual ageand sex-adjusted rate of 1.46 per 100,000 persons per year, and carries a poor prognosis (Table **1**).

Pathogenesis

In PMF, clonal myeloproliferation is associated with reactive bone marrow fibrosis, osteosclerosis, angiogenesis, extramedullary hematopoiesis, and an abnormal cytokine expression. Ineffective erythropoiesis and extramedullary hematopoiesis are the main causes of anemia and organomegaly, respectively. It is currently assumed that aberrant cytokine production by clonal cells and host immune reaction contributes to PMF-associated bone marrow stromal changes, ineffective erythropoiesis, extramedullary hematopoiesis, cachexia, and constitutional symptoms. Bone marrow fibrosis in PMF is usually associated with *JAK2* V617F, trisomy 9, or del(13q). Approximately half of the patients with PMF carry the *JAK2* V617F mutation, whereas approximately 10% are positive for a mutation in exon 10 of MPL. Additionally, mutations in the adaptor proteins LNK or CBL can be found in PMF patients as well (each ~5%). The remaining PMF patients (~25%) do not display any known mutation affecting the JAK-STAT signaling pathway. PMF is characterized by enhanced proliferation mainly of the megakaryocytic lineage and the adjustment of the bone marrow structure including progressive myelofibrosis and hyperactive angiogenesis, which often go together with extramedullary hematopoiesis. The disease course can be divided in two phases: The prefibrotic or early phase is characterized by a hypercellular bone marrow (due to an increase of the megakaryocytic and the granulocytic lineages; erythropoiesis is often decreased) with no or slight reticulin fibrosis and an increased platelet count in the peripheral blood. The fibrotic phase displays a hypocellular bone marrow with marked reticulin and/or collagen fibrosis and also osteosclerosis. Megakaryocytes and platelets for illustration generate PDGF, TGF-β, or OSM, that stimulate fibroblast proliferation and activity. Inflammation and an aberrant activation of the JAK-STAT signaling pathway are also hallmarks of MPN irrespective of mutations influencing the JAK-STAT pathway [28].

Clinical Presentation

Many patients deny any symptoms or present with nonspecific complaints, such as fatigue. The majority of patients have moderate to severe splenomegaly because of extramedullary hematopoiesis, with associated complications such as early satiety, abdominal discomfort, and portal hypertension. Importantly, the clinical characteristics of post-polycythemic or post-ET myelofibrosis are the same as for PMF in the fibrotic phase and can only be distinguished when the initial disease is well diagnosed. Constitutional symptoms, hypermetabolic state, hepatomegaly and diarrhea may also be present. Anemia is the predominant laboratory feature with 36% of patients presenting with hemoglobin <100 g/L. It occurs secondary to decreased erythropoiesis, hemolysis, and, as thrombocytopenia and splenomegaly progress, hemorrhage and gastrointestinal bleeding. Leukocytosis or thrombocytopenia occurs in 10% and 16% of patients, respectively. Histologic evaluation is critical for diagnosis, and bone marrow biopsy typically reveals clusters of abnormal megakaryotes with hyperchromatic, intermittently folded, and bulky nuclei "dwarf megakaryocytes," excessively elevated number of hematopoietic progenitor cells staining positive for CD34[+] with or without significant reticulin and collagen fibrosis. In advanced stages, a bone marrow biopsy of an entirely fibrotic marrow will often yield a "dry tap" [24]. Moreover, the plasma levels of inflammatory cytokines (*e.g.*, IL1β, IL6, IL8, IFNγ, and TNFα) are highly increased. In the advanced stages, bone marrow failure results in replacement of the hematopoiesis to other organs. Most ordinary sites of extramedullary hematopoiesis are the spleen and the liver, but any other organ (*e.g.*, kidney, lung, or the gastrointestinal tract) can be affected. Bone marrow failure also leads to high levels of CD34$^+$ cells in the peripheral blood, which normally exist in the bone marrow [28].

Differential Diagnosis

PMF should be distinguished from other closely related myeloid neoplasms including CML, PV, ET, MDS, chronic myelomonocytic leukemia (CMML), and acute myelofibrosis. Myelofibrosis secondary to CML, AML, ET, or MDS can be difficult to distinguish from that of PMF. Polymerase chain reaction assay can be used to identify BCR-ABL, which is diagnostic of CML. AML presents with rapid disease development, pancytopenia, mild to no splenomegaly, and a high frequency of myeloblasts that contain Auer rods. As stated earlier, ET and PMF frequently have overlapping qualities; however, the presence of extreme splenomegaly, anemia, teardrop anisopoikilocytosis, and leukoerythroblastosis favors the diagnosis of PMF. MDS can be distinguished from PMF by the presence of dyserythropoiesis or dysgranulopoiesis on a peripheral smear [24]. Patients who otherwise fulfill the diagnostic criteria for PV should be labeled as "PV" even if they display extensive bone marrow fibrosis. Prefibrotic PMF can imitate ET in its presentation and careful morphologic assessment is required for distinguishing the two; megakaryocytes in ET are large and mature-appearing whereas those in prefibrotic PMF display abnormal maturation with hyperchromatic and irregularly folded nuclei [33].

Diagnosis

Diagnosis requires all 3 major criteria and 2 minor criteria according to 2008 WHO Diagnostic Criteria [24].

Major Criteria:

1)   Megakaryocyte proliferation and small to large megakaryocytes with an aberrant nuclear/cytoplasmic ratio and hyperchromatic and irregularly folded nuclei and dense clustering accompanied by either reticulin and/or

collagen fibrosis. Also, in the absence of reticulin fibrosis, megakaryocyte changes must be accompanied by increased bone marrow cellularity, granulocytic proliferation and decreased erythropoiesis;

2) Not meeting WHO criteria for CML, PV, MDS, or other myeloid neoplasm;

3) Demonstration of *JAK2* V617F or other associated mutations, or in the absence of above mutations no evidence of reactive bone marrow fibrosis;

Minor Criteria:

1) Leukoerythroblastosis.

2) Increased serum LDH.

3) Anemia.

4) Palpable splenomegaly.

Treatment

Current drug therapy for PMF is not curative and has not been shown to prolong survival. Therapeutic regimens are largely aimed at relieving symptoms and preserving quality of life. As for splenomegaly, cytoreductive therapy with hydroxyurea, radiation, or splenectomy may be considered. Splenectomy is associated with a high-morbidity and high-mortality rate and should only be performed on a select group of patients. Allogeneic stem cell transplant is the only curative therapy; however, the procedure is considered high risk with an estimated 1-year post stem cell transplant mortality rate approaching 30%, and an estimated survival of 50% within the same length of time [34]. Clinical trials involving inhibitors of the JAK tyrosine kinase have shown promising results as an alternative medical therapy for splenomegaly. Low or intermediate-1 risk asymptomatic patients with PMF can be observed without any therapeutic intervention. Particular therapy is considered only in the presence of symptoms. First-line drugs of choice for anemia include thalidomide and prednisone, an androgen preparation or danazol. PMF-associated anemia is usually treated with androgens (*e.g.*, testosterone enanthate 400–600 mg IM weekly, oral fluoxymesterone 10 mg three-times-a-day), prednisone (0.5 mg/kg/day), danazol (600 mg/day), thalidomide (50 mg/day), prednisone or lenalidomide (10 mg/day).

Response rates to each one of the mentioned drugs are in the vicinity of 15–25% and response durations average about one to two years [35]. First-line therapy for PMF-associated splenomegaly is hydroxyurea. Adverse reactions to hydroxyurea therapy are mostly bone pain, constitutional symptoms, pruritus, splenomegaly, and anemia. According to the International Working Group for Myelofibrosis Research and Treatment criteria, clinical improvement was achieved in 40% patients. Median duration of response is 13.2 months [36]. PMF patients with high or intermediate-2 risk disease should be considered for investigational drug therapy or allogeneic stem cell transplantation (ASCT). The estimated 5-year event-free and overall survival is 51% and 67%, respectively followed by ASCT from related or unrelated donors [37]. Overall survival is significantly reduced in multivariate analysis in PMF patients harboring *JAK2* wild-type compared with *JAK2* mutated patients. In this large study (139 patients), no significant influence on outcome is noted for the mutated allele burden. Moreover, achievement of *JAK2* V617F negativity after ASCT is significantly associated with a decreased incidence of relapse [38]. In a small study, which included 30 MPN patients, measurement of allele burden on day 28 after ASCT discriminates two prognostic groups: patients with a *JAK2* V617F allele burden >1% have a significantly higher risk of relapse of *JAK2* V617F positive neoplasia and a poorer overall survival [39].

Prognosis

In general, PMF is associated with a poor prognosis. Based on the International Working Group for Myelofibrosis Research and Treatment developed by a Dynamic International Prognostic Scoring System, 8 risk factors for decreased survival are: age >65 years, Hb <100 g/L, leukocyte count >25×10^9/L, circulating blasts >1%, presence of constitutional symptoms, presence of unfavorable karyotype, platelet count <100×10^9/L and presence of red cell transfusion need. Low risk patients do not have risk factors and their median survival is 15.4 years. Intermediate-1 patients have one risk factor and their median survival is 6.5 years. Intermediate-2 patients have two or three risk factors and their median survival is 2.9 years. High risk patients have four or more risk factors and their median survival is 1.3 years. Patients who are severely anemic with a platelet count <100×10^9/L and a high number of circulating immature cells have a high risk of developing AML. Patients diagnosed at >55 years of age have an average lifespan of 3-5 years, whereas patients diagnosed at <55 years of age have a median survival of 8-10 years [24]. Causes of death include leukemic progression that occurs in approximately 20% of patients but many patients also die of comorbid conditions including cardiovascular events and consequences of cytopenias including infection or bleeding secondary to bone marrow failure, portal hypertension or hepatic failure caused by hepatic vein thrombosis or extramedullary hematopoiesis [40].

Table 1:   Epidemiology of MPNs

	ET	PV	PMF
Incidence	0.59-2.53/100,000	1.9-2.3/100,000	0,4-1.46/100,000
The Median Age at Diagnosis	55 to 65 years	61 (18–95) F 62 (18–92) M 59 (19–95)	67
Female to Male Ratio	about 2:1	1:1,2	1:1
Median Survival (Years)	Low risk 25.3[23] Intermediate 16.9 High risk 10.3	14.1[16]	Low risk 15.4[25] Intermediate-1 6.5 Intermediate-2 2.9 High risk 1.3

Mutations in MPN

The mechanism by which *JAK2* V617F single mutation contributes to the pathogenesis of three clinically distinctive MPN remains undetermined. Several novel mutations have been described recently in chronic or blast-phase MPN.

The Gain of Function Founding Mutations

JAK2 V617F Mutation

JAK2 is essential in the signaling of cytokines with homodimeric receptors (Epo, Tpo, prolactin, leptin, and growth hormone). JAK2 also plays a central role in the signaling of cytokines employing the common β chain receptor (IL3, IL5, and GM-CSF), of certain members of the IL10 type cytokine family (IFNγ, IL19, IL20, and IL24), and of the IL12 type family members (IL12 and IL23). The *JAK2* V617F mutation results from a guanine to thymine change at nucleotide

1849 of the cDNA, in exon 14 of the gene. This valine is located at one of the predicted interfaces between JH1 and JH2 domains, and the change to a phenylalanine appears to relieve the inhibition of the JH2 domain on the kinase domain (Fig. **1**). The carboxyl JH1 domain contains the catalytic activity, whereas N-terminal JH7 domain is responsible for receptor binding. Normal activation of JAK2 is *via* cytokine-dependent phosphorylation of JH1 and JH2; the negative regulatory effect of JH2 on JH1 is essential for normal signaling. Binding of a ligand to its receptor results in receptor dimerization and stimulation of the JAK kinase activity that phosphorylate cytoplasmic domain of the receptor. There is evidence that constitutive signaling by *JAK2* V61F requires the homodimeric receptor, explaining why the *JAK2* V617F induced proliferation affects 3 myeloid lineages [28].

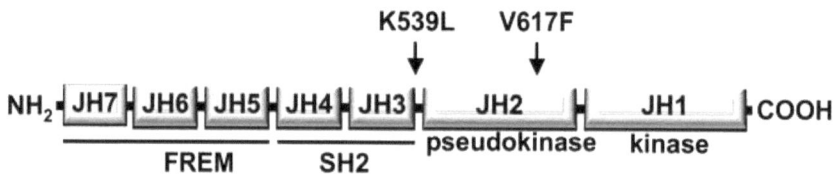

Fig. (1): Structure of JAK2 protein. JAK2 has seven distinct regions of homology, named JAK homology (JH) domains (JH1-7). The carboxyl terminus contains the kinase and pseudokinase domains labeled JH1 and JH2. The sequence of the JH2 pseudokinase domain is homologous to the kinase domain, but has not typical residues of active tyrosine kinases, making it catalytically inactive. The primary structure of JH3 and JH4 shares homology with Src-homology-2 (SH2) domains with a scaffold rather than a signaling role. Rounding off the N-terminus, the JH5-JH7 domains include a predicted FERM (Band-4.1, ezrin, radixin and moesin)-like motif which plays a role in appending JAKs to their cytokine receptors.

JAK2 Exon 12 Mutations

Scott and colleagues discovered several additional mutations in exon 12 of *JAK2* including K539L by sequencing *JAK2* in *JAK2* V617F-negative PV patients [2]. They include a point mutation (K539L), a double mutation (H538QK539L), a 2-amino acid deletion (N542-E543del) and a 2-amino acid deletion followed by an insertion (F537-K539delinsL). Several more point mutations, deletions, and insertions affecting *JAK2* exon 12 have been identified in PV patients since then. These mutations span the linker region between the SH2 and JH2 domains. Although not located in the pseudokinase domain, these mutations may modify the structure of the JH2 domain in a very similar fashion as V617F. However, in contrast to *JAK2* V617F, exon 12 mutations are not associated with ET and PMF, although *JAK2* exon 12 PV may progress to a secondary myelofibrosis. Compared with *JAK2* V617F-positive PV patients, those with exon 12 mutations have significantly higher hemoglobin level and lower platelet and leukocyte counts at diagnosis but similar incidences of thrombosis, myelofibrosis, leukemia, and death [41].

MPL Mutations

MPL encodes the thrombopoietin receptor which is a major regulator of megakaryocytopoiesis and platelet formation. Several gain-of-function mutations of *MPL* have been found in exon 10, resulting in the substitution of a tryptophan 515 to a leucine, lysine, asparagine, or alanine. The most commonly observed mutations of *MPL* are the W515L and W515K. Somatic gain of function mutations often affecting the amino acid residues W515 and S505 have been found in the *MPL* of patients with ET and PMF. Both *JAK2* exon 12 (K539L) and *MPL* (W515K/L) mutants have been shown to induce a MPN-like phenotype in murine bone marrow transplantation models. These *MPL* mutations have been found in up to 15% of *JAK2* V617F-negative ET or PMF [25].

Genes Implicated in Intracellular Signaling

LNK Mutations

LNK plays an important role in hematopoiesis by negatively regulating *JAK2* activation through its SH2 domain, thus inhibiting EPOR and MPL signaling. In addition, LNK negatively regulates c-KIT and FMS signaling [25]. The frequency of mutations in LNK is low. However, other mutations of LNK have been found in leukemic transformation of MPN at a greater frequency (~13%). Furthermore, mutations in adaptor proteins involved in the negative regulation of cytokine signaling, *i.e.*, LNK and CBL, have been described in ET and PMF patients [25].

CBL Mutations

The Casitas B-cell lymphoma (CBL) proteins are multifunctional adapter proteins with ubiquitin ligase activity. They are usually involved in negative regulation of receptor tyrosine kinase (RTK) by competitive blocking of signaling and they induce RTK proteosomal degradation by mediating ubiquitination in endosomes. However, CBL may have numerous targets other than RTK, including JAK2 and cytokine receptors such as MPL. Most mutated CBL forms behave as loss-of-function molecules having a dominant-negative effect not only on c-CBL but also on CBL-b, leading to an excessive sensitivity to a variety of growth factors. In the chronic phase of classic MPN, c-CBL mutations have been found in a low percentage of PMF patients (6%) but are not detected in a small series of PV and ET patients [42].

SOCS 1, 2, 3 Mutations

Suppressor of cytokine signaling (SOCS) proteins are significant negative regulators of JAK signaling through a classic feedback loop. Hypermethylation of CpG islands in SOCS1 and SOCS3 associated with a decrease in expression is found in *JAK2V617F* PV and ET as well as in *JAK2V617F* and *MPLW515-*mutation negative ET. SOCS2 may also inhibit JAK2V617F signaling, and its promoter is hypermethylated in some MPN. The association between SOCS3 promoter methylation and reduction of transcription is shown in *JAK2V617F-*negative patients with PMF [25].

Genes Implicated in Leukemic Transformation
IDH1/2

Leukemic transformation, or blast phase, occurs in approximately 15% of PMF patients and in < 10% of PV and ET patients. IDH1 and IDH2 encode isocitrate dehydrogenase 1 and 2, which are $NADP^+$ enzymes that catalyze the conversion of isocitrate to α-ketoglutarate (αKG). The analysis of 1473 patients with MPN reveal a low incidence of IDH1/2 mutations in chronic phase ET, PV, and MF (0.8%, 1.9%, and 4.2%, respectively), contrasting with a 21.6% frequency in blast phase [43].

RUNX1

The RUNX1/AML1 gene encodes a transcription factor with a major role in hematopoiesis. RUNX1 mutations are found in leukemic blasts of 30% examined post–MPN-AML patients, mostly localized in the RUNT domain [25].

TP53

TP53 gene encodes a main tumor suppressor protein p53 involved in different biologic activities, together with the control of cell-cycle checkpoints and apoptosis. TP53 mutations are not linked with the chronic phase of MPN, but mutated TP53 have been found in 20% of post–MPN-AML patients [25].

Genes Implicated in Epigenetic Regulation

ASXL1

Mutations in ASXL1 are frameshifts and stop mutations located within the 12th exon of the gene; they usually affect only one copy of the gene and result in the loss of the carboxyterminal PHD domain. The ASXL1 protein is a part of various DNA and histone regulatory complexes and participates in the deubiquitination of these complexes. The function of ASXL1 in hematopoiesis is still poorly understood [25]. It has been found a high incidence of ASXL1 mutation in PMF patients (20%), post-PV PMF (50%) and post-ET PMF (10%) and a low incidence in PV (7%) and ET (4%) patients, with the same incidence of ASXL1 mutations in *JAK2*wt and *JAK2* V617F patients [44].

TET2

The Ten-Eleven-Translocation2 (TET2) gene codes for a 2-oxoglutarate and Fe(II)-dependent hydroxylase that is able to hydroxylate methylated cytosine. TET2 mutations are found in approximately 14% of MPNs ranging from ET (11%) to PMF (19%). In roughly 20% of the patients, 2 mutations are observed, suggesting that the inactivation of a single copy of TET2 is sufficient for the transformation process [44].

EZH2

EZH1 and EZH2 proteins (enhancer of zeste homolog) belong to the polycomb repressive complex 2 (PRC2), a histone H3 lysine 27 (H3K27) methyltransferase that influences stem cell renewal by epigenetic repression of genes involved in cell fate decisions. PRC2 is involved in various cellular processes, including proliferation, differentiation, cell-identity maintenance, aging, and plasticity. EZH2 mutations are not observed in ET, but are seen in 3% of PV and 13% of PMF in small study [45].

miRNA

Additional mechanisms like epigenetic silencing, post-transcriptional regulation, or post-translational modifications could account for the development of different phenotypes. MicroRNAs (miRNA) are 18-24 nucleotides single-stranded non-protein-coding RNAs that function principally as gene repressors by binding to their target messenger RNAs. There is mounting data that miRNAs control hematopoiesis in hematopoietic stem cells and committed progenitor cells. Usually, miRNAs suppress their targets by either targeting RNA degradation or translation inhibition. Moreover, the evaluation of miRNA expression in MPN patients identified miRNA 10a and 150 to be differentially expressed [46]. In addition, it has not been observed any correlation between the miRNA expression levels and CD34$^+$ cell *JAK2* V617F allele burdens. This proposes that deregulated miRNAs may operate as an independent event from the abnormal JAK2 signaling in MPN pathogenesis and disease phenotype determination. Definitely, miRNAs may provide valuable targets as RNA-based inhibition can be designed based on sequence alone, while miRNAs are readily inhibited by antisense oligonucleotides whose effects can be enhanced by various adjustments. Perhaps the most attractive feature of miRNA-based therapy comes from the view that miRNA dysregulation generally is well-tolerated in normal tissues while can greatly influence pathological cells and tissues, making miRNA therapy a very strong in modulation of the disease process while avoiding unwanted toxicity in normal tissues [47].

Familial MPNs

Although most MPN cases appear to be sporadic, familial predisposition has been recognized for many years and epidemiological studies have indicated the presence of common susceptibility alleles. The general hypothesis is that a genetic predisposition exists, which secondarily leads to the development of the *JAK2V617F* mutation. Currently the *JAK2* 46/1 haplotype (also referred to as

'GGCC') is the strongest known predisposition factor for sporadic MPNs carrying a *JAK2* V617F mutation, explaining a large proportion of the heritability of this disorder. The same haplotype also predisposes to mutations in *JAK2* exon 12 as well as in the MPL. Females develop the disease earlier than men, while the general average age of onset is 46 years, notably younger than in sporadic cases of MPN which usually occur around the age of 60 years. In addition, one third of the families present various subtypes of MPN within a family, suggesting that a predisposing gene is not only limited to a single subtype but also contributing in other subtypes, further on supporting the hypothesis of a mutation in an early multipotent stem cell. 67% families present members with the same MPN subtype (homogeneous - majority being PV-PV pairs (36%)) and 33% families present members with different subtypes of MPN (heterogeneous - majority being PV-PMF pairs (17%)). Furthermore, a majority of familial MPNs follows an autosomal dominant (AD) inheritance with a reduced penetrance. The origin of MPNs may occur in at least three different settings: (a) sporadic, (b) familial associated with a genetic heterogeneity and environmental impact (c) AD inheritance with variable penetrance [48].

JAK-STAT Signaling Pathway

JAK-STAT (Janus associated kinase-signal transducer and activator of transcription) pathway is one of the critical intracellular signaling cascades in transduction of extracellular signals into the nucleus to control gene expression (Fig. **2**). A variety of cytokines and growth factors perform their physiological assignment through JAK-STAT pathway, including proliferation, differentiation, survival, and cell migration, playing a major role in hematopoiesis and immune system. JAK family has four cytoplasmic tyrosine kinases, JAK1-3 and Tyk2. Activated JAK-cytokine receptor complex recruits and phosphorylates STAT cytoplasmic transcription factors. Seven STAT proteins have been recognized in human cells, STAT1-6, as well as STAT5a and STAT5b. Phosphorylation of specific STAT proteins results in their dimerization and subsequent translocation into the nucleus to interact with different regulatory elements for gene expression [49]. Three major mechanisms have been implicated to negatively regulate the JAK-STAT pathway: tyrosine phosphatases, protein inhibitors of activated STATs (PIAS), and suppressors of cytokine signaling (SOCS) proteins. Src homology-2 (SH2) containing tyrosine phosphatase and CD45 transmembrane tyrosine phosphatase play a major role in modulating JAK-STAT pathway. SH2 containing tyrosine phosphatases include SHP1 and SHP2. Their SH2 domains allow attachment to the phospho-tyrosine residues present on activated receptors, JAKs or STAT proteins, leading to dephosphorylation of the substrates. PIAS family consists of $PIAS_1$, $PIAS_3$, PIASx and PIASy. $PIAS_3$ and PIASx interact with STAT3 and STAT4 respectively, while $PIAS_1$ and PIASy with STAT1. $PIAS_1$ and $PIAS_3$ exert negative regulation by blocking the DNA binding of STAT1 and STAT3, respectively. On the other hand, PIASx and PIASy repress the transcriptional activity of STAT1 and STAT4 by recruiting co-repressor molecules such as histone deacetylases [49]. The SOCS family is composed of SOCS-1 to SOCS-7 and cytokine-inducible SH2-containing protein (CIS). SOCS proteins are cytokine-induced negative feedback-loop regulators of JAK-STAT signaling. The central SH2 domain directs the target binding of each CIS/SOCS protein. By three mechanisms SOCS protein provides negative modulation: a) SOCS binds the phospho-tyrosine residues on the receptors and physically blocks the STATs from binding to its receptors; b) SOCS proteins can bind directly to its specific JAKs or to the receptors and inhibit the corresponding JAK kinase activity; c) SOCS associate with the elongin BC complex and cullin 2, accelerating the ubiquination of JAKs and presumably the receptors [50]. Regardless of JAK2V617F status, patients with PV exhibits high STAT3 and 5 activities, patients with ET have high STAT3 activity, whereas patients with PMF have low activities of both STAT3 and 5 [51].

Thrombosis

Multivariate study of PV patients revealed age >70 years, white blood cell count >13 × 10^9/L and thrombo-embolism at diagnosis as independent risk factors for survival [52]. The main prevalence of thrombosis in PMF is detected in combination of *JAK2* mutation and leukocytosis [53]. Some studies demonstrate that incidence of thrombotic complications in JAK2-positive ET patients is significantly higher than that in wild-type ET patients [54], while other could not identify *JAK2* V617F mutation as a risk factor for thrombosis in ET and PV [55].

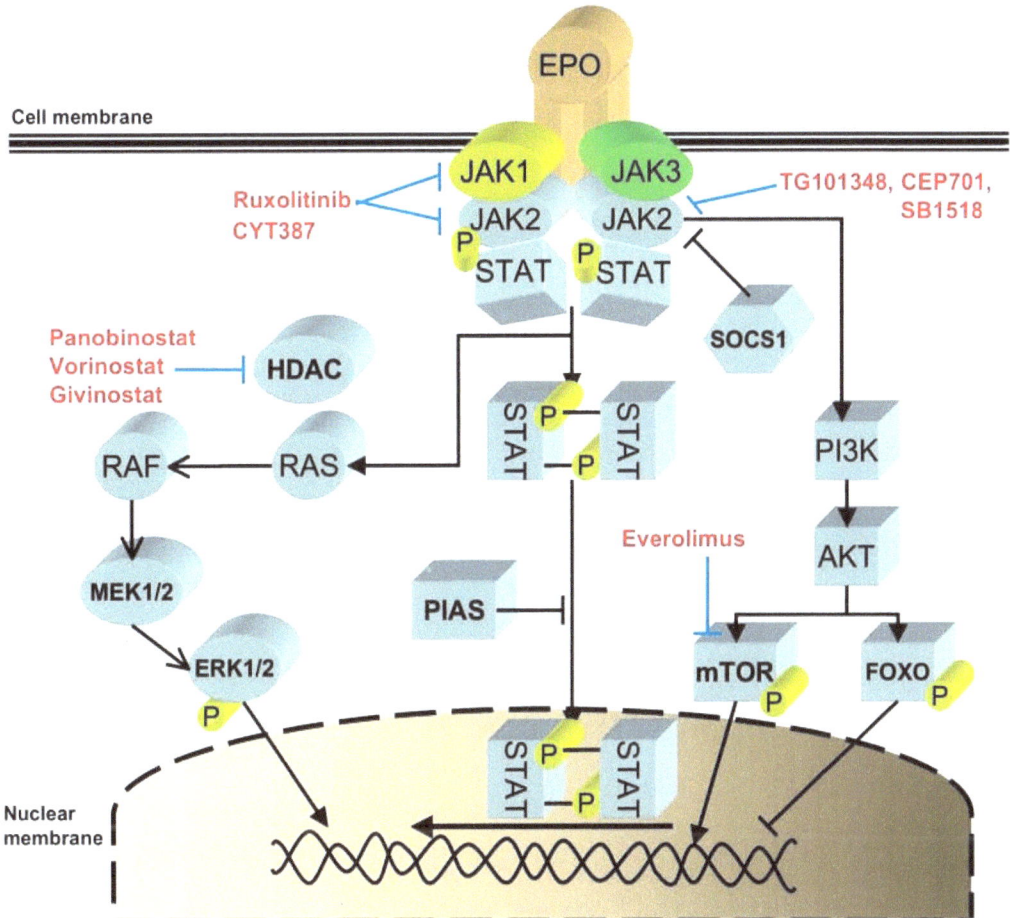

Fig. (2): JAK-dependent signaling with inhibitors. Activated JAK2 phosphorylate receptors on tyrosines, followed by STATs docking on phosphotysines and their JAK-dependent phosphorylation. STATs detach from the receptor and dimerize *via* SH2 domain. Protein inhibitors of activated STATs (PIAS) and suppressors of cytokine signaling (SOCS) act as negative regulators of JAK/STAT pathways. JAK intracellular non-receptor tyrosine kinase-triggered pathways include STAT, Ras GTPases/mitogen-activated protein kinases (MAPKs)/extracellular signal-related kinases (ERKs), phosphatidylinositol 3-kinase (PI3K)/Akt/mammalian target of rapamycin (mTOR). Ras/Raf/MEK/ERK and PI3K/PTEN/AKT signaling cascades play critical roles in the transmission of signals from growth factor receptors to regulate gene expression and prevent apoptosis.

Adenosine diphosphate (ADP)-induced platelet aggregation and thrombin generation are significantly increased in ET and PV, more prominent in *JAK2* V617F positive patients [56]. Recently, it has been found that platelets from *JAK2* V617F positive ET patients have significantly reduced phosphorylation of the PI3 kinase substrate Akt, and reduced activation of Rap1 in response to thrombopoietin, ADP, and thrombin [57]. In addition, it has been shown a novel EpoR-independent Rap1/Akt signaling pathway, activated by *JAK2* V617F in circulating PV red blood cells, responsible for Lutheran blood group/basal cell adhesion molecule activation [58]. Inhibition of PI3K/AKT signaling by allosteric AKT inhibitor MK-2206 reduced the growth of both *JAK2* V617F- or *MPL* W515L-expressing cells. In addition, MK-2206 mutually with ruxolitinib inhibit the growth of *JAK2* V617F-mutant megakaryoblastic cell line. Also, MK-2206 suppresses colony formation from hematopoietic progenitor cells of PMF patients, improve hepatosplenomegaly and reduce megakaryocyte burden in the bone marrow, liver and spleen of mice with MPLW515L-induced MPN [59]. ET patients with thrombotic events displayed higher monocyte CD25 levels, as well as *JAK2* V617F-positive patients [60]. Plasma P- and E-selectin levels are significantly elevated in ET and PV patients [61]. Cytoreductive treatment halves the occurrence of re-thrombosis in patients with PV and ET, particularly with first arterial thrombosis, while the *JAK2* V617F-positive ET patients are more sensitive to therapy with hydroxyurea than those without the *JAK2* mutation [30].

Involvement of the NO Pathway in MPN and Hydroxyurea Mechanism of Action

It has been hypothesized that chronic inflammation *via* oxidative stress, with increased levels of reactive oxygen species (ROS) in the bone marrow, may produce a high-risk microenvironment for induction of mutations caused by oxidative damage to DNA in hematopoietic cells of MPN [62]. Oxidative stress has carcinogen effect in MPN and promotes the development of thrombotic risk [63]. Increased ROS concentrations reduce the amount of bioactive NO by chemical inactivation to form toxic peroxynitrite [64]. The nitric oxide (NO) derivatives are significantly increased in ET patients treated with hydroxyurea compared to non-hydroxyurea treated ET and controls [61]. The endogenous NO and exogenously applied NO donors exert an antithrombotic effect *in vivo* through a direct suppression of platelet aggregation. Furthermore, eNOS exerts a powerful antithrombotic effect upon the vascular components of thrombosis but has a more subtle effect on the duration of thrombotic responses that are platelet-mediated [65]. We demonstrated that during erythroid differentiation endothelial NO synthase (eNOS) mRNA and protein levels diminishing progressively, as does the production of NO derivatives and cyclic adenosine monophosphate (cAMP) levels, but guanosine 3',5'-cyclic monophosphate (cGMP) levels are constant [66]. Hydroxyurea, a cytostatic used in therapy of MPN, increases intracellular cGMP and cAMP levels in erythroid progenitors and endothelial cells, as well as intracellular calcium [67, 68]. We verified that hydroxyurea can directly interact with the deoxy-heme of soluble guanylyl cyclase and activate cGMP production. These data add to an expanding appreciation of the role of hydroxyurea as an inducer of the NO/cGMP pathway in erythroid progenitors [69]. Although sickle-cell anemia is not an MPN, fact that AML/MDS development is an unusual incident, following many years of hydroxyurea treatment in patients with sickle-cell anemia, provides additional support for no connection between hydroxyurea treatment and AML transformation [26]. Moreover, we found that NO production and eNOS protein levels are increased by hydroxyurea and proteasome inhibitors in endothelial cells [70, 71]. This hydroxyurea stimulation is mediated by posttranscriptional augmentation in eNOS levels *via* inhibition of the proteasome activity [70]. Hydroxyurea induces rapid and transient phosphorylation of eNOS at Ser1177 *via* cAMP-dependent protein kinase (PKA). In addition, hydroxyurea NOS-dependent increase in endothelial-cell production of NO is reliant on PKA and AKT activity. These studies create a mechanism, by which hydroxyurea may induce cellular NO levels and enhance the angiogenic influence of NO in MPN [67]. Further on, we have used microarray analysis to examine JAK-STAT and AKT pathway-coupled genes in erythroid progenitors through ontogeny. Some JAK-STAT signaling pathway-linked genes are steadily upregulated (PIM1, SOCS2, MYC), while others are downregulated (PTPN6, PIAS, SPRED2) during EPO-stimulated erythroid differentiation [72]. Moreover, hypoxia increases endothelial cell capacity to produce NO in response to EPO by induction of both EPO receptor and eNOS [73, 74]. During treatment of erythroid progenitors, we demonstrated that hydroxyurea augmented SOCS1 gene expression, participating in inhibition of JAK-STAT signaling [75].

Hydroxyurea is now considered as the therapy for PV and ET patients older than 60 years and with severe thrombohemorrhagic complications, controlling increased blood cell counts and splenomegaly, as well as reducing the incidence of major vascular events in randomised clinical trials and in retrospective and non-controlled historical cohorts of patients with MPN [76]. The ability of hydroxyurea to reduce the *JAK2* V617F allelic load in PV and ET patients has been reported with contradictory results. In first small studies, it has been shown that hydroxyurea therapy (median duration: 15 months) reduces the percentage of *JAK2* V617F by >30% in 13/25 patients (4/8 PV, 9/17 ET) [77], and by 55% in 72% of the 18 PV and ET patients after 4 months and prolongs up to 12 months [78]. In the following larger study of 104 PV and 68 ET patients, the median follow-up time is 3.1 years and no evolution to PMF or AML occurred. A small (less than 10%), still statistically significant, reduction in V617F allele burden was observed only in newly hydroxyurea treated ET patients. Interestingly, in both PV and ET, changes in V617F allele burden under hydroxyurea are more prominent in women than in males [79]. Next, the *JAK2* V617F allele burden dynamics is prospectively analysed in 26 PV and 21 ET patients treated with hydroxyurea. PV patients receiving hydroxyurea have a significantly higher percentage of initial *JAK2* V617F alleles than those managed only with phlebotomies, whereas no significant difference is between treated and control ET patients. Hydroxyurea significantly reduces the *JAK2* V617F allelic ratio in PV and ET patients (50% with molecular response), as well as in comparison to non treated PV and ET patients (57%). A progressive decrease of the *JAK2* V617F allele load in PV *versus* ET patients over time is observed, with the difference from baseline levels being statistically significant at 36 months (PV - 22.9% and ET - 9.55%) [80]. The effect of hydroxyurea on the *JAK2* V617F allele burden is also evaluated in 8 PV and 13 ET patients with a median period of follow up of 20/21 months, where the percentage of *JAK2*-V617F allele burden tend to stay steady during hydroxyurea therapy [81].

Transforming Growth Factor Beta

TGF-β belongs to a large family of structurally related cell regulatory proteins of about more than 40 mammalian members, including activins-inhibins, bone morphogenetic proteins and growth and differentiation factors. TGF-βs has been involved in different biological processes, which include cell growth, differentiation, development and tumorigenesis [82]. In mammals three structurally isoforms are expressed (TGF-β 1, 2 and 3), and encoded by three distinct genes located on chromosomes 19q13, 1q41 and 14q24, respectively [83]. TGF-β1 is synthesized as homodimeric 75 kd precursor protein consisting of three domains, the signal peptide, latency associated peptide (LAP) and the mature TGF-β. This precursor is intra-cellulary cleaved by furin-type convertase to form an inactive complex, in which 25 kDa dimeric TGF-β remains noncovalently bound to LAP forming the small latent complex (SCL) [84]. Also, the SCL can be associated to the latent TGF-β binding protein (LTBP) rising to the large latent complex (LCC). Secreted complex is unable to associate with its cognate receptor and remain covalently associated to the ECM. Activation of TGF-β signaling pathways is primarily regulated by release of bioactive TGF-β, from the latent complex, which is stored in significant amounts in the ECM of many different tissues. Interestingly, the activation of a small fraction of latent TGF-β is capable of generating maximal cellular responses [83]. TGF-β is activated by releasing the dimer from LAP. Many mechanisms have been proposed for TGF-β activation, those including proteolytic cleavage by plasmin and metalloproteinases, acidic microenvironments, reactive oxygen species, or *via* interactions with proteins such as thrombospodin and integrins [84-86].

TGF-βs initiates signaling by binding cell-surface serine/threonine kinase receptors types I and II (TBRI/ALK5 and TBRII), respectively (Fig. **3**), which form heteromeric complexes in the presence of dimerized ligands [82]. TGF-β/TBRII complex recruits and transphosphorylates TBRI, in addition this complex may activates a second type I receptor, named activin receptor-like kinase-1 (ALK1) and mainly expressed in endothelial cells. Activated TBRI initiates intracellular signaling by phosphorylation of the cytoplasmic mediators, Smad2 and Smad3 by ALK5, Smad1,-5 and -8 by ALK1 [86-88]. Also, ALK1 can be activated by bone morphogenetic proteins (BMPs) such BMP9 and BMP10 [89]. Inactivation of the kinase domain of TβRI abrogates signaling, emphasizing the importance of the type 1 receptor for cell responsiveness to TGF-β1 [86, 90]. The phosphorylation of Smad2,3 by TBRI induces the release from the inner face of plasma membrane, where they are retained by endonfin or the anchor for receptor activation (SARA). Then a hetetromeric complex is formed with the common Smad4, translocated to the nucleus, where in collaboration with other transcription factors, coactivators or corepressors proteins, form a transcriptional regulatory complex that activates or repress different target genes transcription [82, 87, 90].

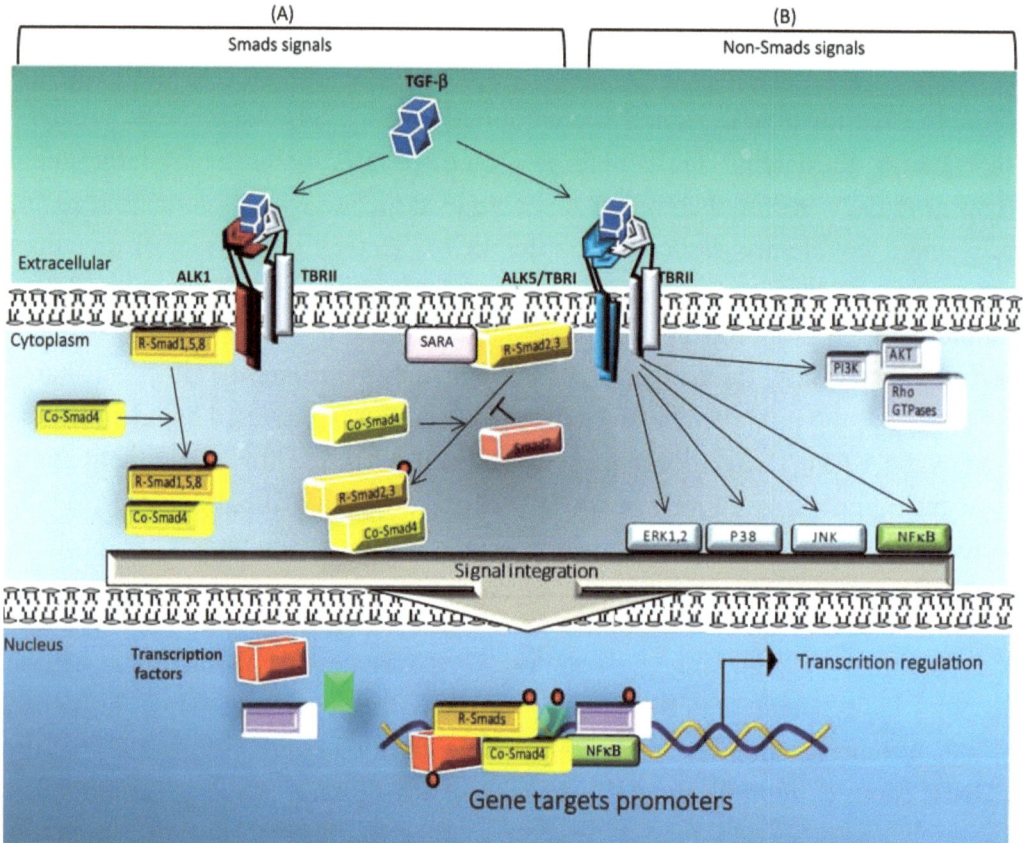

Fig. (3): TGF-β signaling. TGF-β signaling comprises two groups of a set of intracellular transduction pathway: Smads signals and Non-Smads signals. When TGF-β1 is active bind to its cell surface type II receptor (TβRII) inducing the activation of TGF-β type I receptor (ALK1 or ALK5) forming a heterotetrameric complex. **A)** Smads signals: TGF-β can activates ALK1 and triggered the activation of Smad1,5 and 8, which interact with co-Smad4 and translocated to the nucleus. Similarly, active ALK5 in the complex activates Smad2,3 which in turn promotes the Smads releasing from complexes with SARA from the inner face of plasmatic membrane. Then, Smad2,3 interact with co-Smad4 forming a heteromeric complex to be translocated into the cell nucleus. In the nucleus Smads complexes may interact with other transcription factor and co-repressors and co-activators to modulate gene expression. **B)** Non-Smad signals: Active TGF-β-receptors complex in turn active ERK1/2, p38, JNK and NF-κB pathways. Additionally, receptor activated complexes can activate PI3K provoking the activation of AKT and the Small Rho GTPases. The activation of Non-Smad signals pathways in turn initiate transcriptional or non-transcriptional activities to regulate cellular responses. Adapted from [84].

TGF-β1 signaling is regulated by the expression of other components of Smads, the inhibitory Smads proteins (Smad6 and Smad7 or I-Smads). Mainly, Smad7 antagonize TGF-β by interacting with TBRI, leading to its degradation. Smad6 in turn preferentially inhibits BMP signaling by disrupting the Smad1–Co-Smad interaction, and forming an inactive Smad1–Smad6 complex [91]. Smads1 and 5 induce Smad6 expression, whereas Smad3 induces Smad7 expression triggering an inhibitory feedback loop that suppresses TGF-β-mediated effects [83]. The TGF-β /receptor/Smads cascade is subjected to post-translational modification which finely regulates TGF-β signaling, process such as phosphorylation/ dephosphorylation, sumoylation and ubiquitination that reversible regulate their stability and availability. Another level of regulation is the internalization and recycling of the ligand–receptor complexes *via* either lipid rafts/caveolae or clathrin-coated vesicles, which can modulate signaling as well as protein degradation in the proteasome [92].

Besides to the canonical Smad2,3 pathway, TGF-β1 activates several non-canonical intracellular signal pathways (Fig. **3**), normally called as non-Smads pathway, including: mitogen-activated protein kinases (MAPK), ERK1/2, JNK and p38; PI3K (phosphoinositide 3-kinase)/AKT1,2 and mTOR which have a role as cells survival mediators; NF-κB (nuclear factor κB), Ciclooxygenase-2 and prostaglandins; the small GTPase proteins Ras, Rho family (Rho, Rac1 and Cdc42) among others [93-97]. The plethoric capability of TGF-β1 to activate different signal transduction pathways, partially can explain the pleiotropic competence of TGF-β to regulate many functions at molecular, biochemical and biological levels.

TGF-β and Immune System

The immune system is a complex, developed and organized body structure whose firm equilibrium is required for an accurate homeostasis during the life. Disorders of the immune system can result in autoimmune, inflammatory diseases and cancer [98]. The immune system is potent and precisely regulated to guarantee reaction against disorders; this regulation requires a complex crosstalk between the innate and adaptive system by secretion of cytokines and cell-cell interaction.

One of the most important players in the immune system regulation is the pleiotropic cytokine TGF-β [99].

In cancer, TGF-β is the most potent immune-suppressive cytokine; it can act on cancer cells, "non-transformed cells" in the tumor microenvironment and distal cells in the host. TGF-β suppresses antitumor immune responses creating an immune-tolerant environment and allows cancer cells to escape from immune surveillance to finally support cancer progression [6, 7]. TGF-β1 is the most highly expressed isoform in the immune system; however the importance of TGF-β as master regulator of mammalian immune system function and homeostasis was not highlighted until the observations that *tgf-b1*-knockout mice exhibited lethal multi-organ inflammatory disease, primarily as consequence of deregulation in T cells compartments [99-101]. Meanwhile, *Smad3*-deficient mice died due to a primary defect in immune function, the mice exhibits inflammatory lesions in several organs, defects in the responsiveness and chemotaxis of neutrophils, T and B cells [102]. *Smad3*-deficient T cells are defective in Treg cell differentiation with altered induction of Treg cell-specific genes. Conversely to defective Treg cell induction, *smad3*-deficient T cells have an enhanced propensity to develop into Th17 cells in the presence of TGF-β and IL-6 [103, 104].

Smad2 Mouse knockouts are embryonic lethal (before E8.5) due to failure to create an anterior-posterior axis, gastrulation and mesoderm formation [105, 106]. However, on the contrary to the Smad3 T-cell deletion, T-cell specific *Smad2* deficient cells reveal significant defects in their differentiation to the Th17 linage, supporting the notion that Smad2 and Smad3 plays a non-redundant role to the generation of Th17 cells [103, 107]. In turn, double *Smad2,3* knockout mice develop a fatal lymphoproliferative disorder phenocoping *tgf-b* deficient mice [108]. In addition, the transgenic targeting of T cells with a truncated TBRII expression resulted in a severe autoimmune reaction characterized by multifocal inflammation, similar to that seen in *tgf-b1* deficient mice, and autoantibody production [99, 109].

Although some tumors express tumor specific antigens, which can be recognized by immune system, tumor specific immune responses often fail to eradicate them because tumors evade immune surveillance by a variety of strategies [6]. TGF-β downregulates the MHC Class I molecules in malignant cells making them invisible to the immune system, acts on T cells, natural killer cells, monocytes/macrophages, neutrophils, and dendritic cells. TGF-β can affect the initiation and stimulation of both primary and secondary immune responses as well as to suppress antitumor effector cells [110, 111]. TGF-β negatively regulates the immune response of lymphoid compartment by activating the conversion of naive T-cells toward regulatory T-cells (Tregs), by inhibition of B and T cells, by effector cytokines production (including IL-2, IL-4 and IFN-γ), and by inducing Th17 differentiation enhancing the secretion of pro-inflammatory cytokine IL-17 [112-114]. TGF-β1 also has profound effects in innate immune cells compartment; TGF-β promotes the recruitment of monocytes to the tumor and may induce monocyte to macrophage differentiation [4]. TGF-β has been shown to suppress the macrophage expression of MIP-1α, MIP-2, CXCL1, IL-1β, IL-8, GM-CSF and IL-10 [114], moreover in tumor-associated macrophages TGF-β1 provokes its polarization from M1 toward a protumorigenic M2 phenotype. Furthermore, macrophages by producing TGF-β may participate to the enhancement of tumor growth and angiogenesis, while increase of TGF-β levels within the tumor can help cancer cells to escape from immune surveillance [115-117]. In neutrophils, TGF-β may inhibits the ability of these cells to eliminate cancer cells-expressing Fas-Ligand, and like in macrophages TGF-β promotes tumor-associated neutrophils from N1 toward protumorigenic N2 phenotype, thus creating a tolerant tumor microenvironment [118, 119]. In tumor linked dendritic cells, TGF-β represses the expression of MHC class II, CD40, CD80, CD86, TNF-α, IL-12, and CCL5/Rantes. As a consequence, these dendritic cells become functionally defective because of its immature phenotype, and promote the expansion of Treg associated with TGF-β-dependent tumor progression [120-124].

TGF-β, secreted by cells in the tumor microenvironment, contributes to the progression and malignancy of cancer cells. Commonly in cancer, elevated TGF-β plasma levels have been associated with the advanced stage and poorer clinical outcome. In breast, prostate, pancreatic and renal cell cancers elevated levels of plasma TGF-β have been associated with advanced stage, metastases, and poorer clinical outcome [125-128]. It is believed that the active TGF-β produced by the tumor and local stroma cells contributes to the cancer progression and metastatic potential through autocrine and paracrine effects. Elevated serum levels of TGF-β have been observed in patients with myeloma, where both malignant and bone marrow stromal cells are the source of TGF-β. TGF-β levels are also elevated in non–Hodgkin's lymphoma and high-grade lymphomas, cutaneous T cell lymphomas with a T-regulatory phenotype, and in splenic marginal zone lymphomas as myelofibrosis [7].

TGF-β in Myeloproliferative Neoplasms

As it is mentioned above, the three types of Philadelphia-negative MPNs (PV, ET, PMF) are clonal hematological neoplasms in which an increased risk of arterial thrombosis occurs [129]. The rise in proliferative capacity, benefit for the clonal expansion, in MPN clones can originate either from a hypersensitivity to mitogenic cytokines, loss of the proliferative inhibitory cytokines, and changes in the expression or homeostasis of cytokine balance. TGF-β is believed to be one of the most potent regulators of proliferation in human and murine hematopoietic systems [130-133].

Aberrant expression of TGF-β resulted in profound changes in the genetic stability of cells leading to alteration of cell differentiation, cell interaction with the host environment, and the generation of therapy resistant disease. Malignant cell resistance to TGF-β is frequently due to loss, silencing, or mutational inactivation of genes in the TGF-β signaling pathway including the type I and type II receptors and receptor-associated and common-mediators Smads [7]. In MPNs, lack of the inhibitory TGF-β effects may explain the expansion of the cell clone.

Histomorphological findings in the bone marrow of ET patients are loose clusters of predominantly large to giant megakaryocytes. The megakaryocytes display a normal maturation with hyperlobulated and staghorn-like nuclei [134]. In normal cell megakaryocytes proliferation is generally inhibited by TGF-β1, but in ET a decrease in Smad4 expression in megakaryocytes have been associated with refractory megakaryocyte colony-forming units in response to TGF-β1. Notably, the ectopic expression of Smad4 restored the megakaryocyte sensitivity to TGF-β1, while a decrease in TBRII expression have been observed in ET cells [135, 136] suggesting a critical role of the loss of sensitivity to TGF-β in the pathogenesis of ET [137].

PV is characterized by a trilineage proliferation of the erythroid, myeloid and megakaryocytic cell lines, resulting in mainly increased erythrocytes. Although 95% of the PV patients carry *JAK2* V617F mutation, a decrease in TBRII expression has been observed, potentially collaborating to the clonal expansion [136, 137].

The constitutional symptoms are mediated by the abnormal release of cytokines from clonal megakaryocytes as a result of emperipolesis in PMF. In the bone marrow of prefibrotic PMF an overall hypercellularity is evident, including prominent growth of abnormally differentiated and giant megakaryocytes [134]. In PMF, the expression of TBRI seems to be normal in CD34$^+$ cells; while a decrease in both TBRII mRNA and protein expression is reported [138].

Abnormal TGF-β regulation and function are implicated in a rising quantity of fibrotic pathologies [82], so it is no surprise that TGF-β is one of the main and most important candidates to study in the promotion of myelofibrosis. TGF-β induces fibroblasts to proliferate, produce and secrete ECM proteins, prevent ECM degradation by enhancing the expression of proteases inhibitors [139]. Although, very few ET patients (<10%), and about 30% of the PV patients develop myelofibrosis during progress of disease [134, 140].

One of the PMF clinical features is a diffuse bone marrow fibrosis with a prominent megakaryocyte hyperproliferation and abnormal morphology. The current pathogenetic hypothesis is that clonal proliferation of megakaryocytes and/or monocytes leads to abnormal cytokine release, responsible for the detrimental stromal reaction characterized by collagen fibrosis and new bone formation (osteogenesis or osteosclerosis) [139].

The level of both bioactive and total TGF-β in peripheral blood and bone marrow plasma have been found higher in patients with PMF, PV or ET than healthy controls, and intriguingly TGF-β is found mostly in a latent form [141]. When the expression of TGF-β is analyzed in megakaryocytes of bone marrow in patients with PMF and ET, megakaryocyte latent TGF-β1 immunoexpression is higher in both pre-fibrotic and fibrotic stages of PMF compared to ET and controls [142]. It is possible that a high level of latent form ensures a sustainable and chronic delivery of active TGF-β, increasing fibroblast activation and tissue fibrosis, while blocking of TGF-β activation can control pathological bone marrow fibrosis.

Mouse model for the pathogenesis of myelofibrosis supported the fundamental role of TGF-β1 in this disorder. In MPL/thrombopoietin overexpression-induced mouse myeloproliferative disorder, lethally irradiated wild-type recipients were transplanted with bone marrow cells, previously *ex vivo* infected with TPO-encoding retroviruses, from either *tgf-b* -/- or *tgf-b* +/+ mice. Although in both cases animals developed myeloproliferative syndrome, in mice receiving bone marrow from *tgf-b1* null mice no sign of myelofibrosis is detected [139, 143]. Interestingly, in myelofibrosis-developing mice, a four- to eight-fold increase in level of TGF-β1 has been found in plasma and spleen fluids. While, no increase in TGF-β1 plasma level is detected in *tgf-b1* null-cell-engrafted mice [139, 143]. Similar results are observed in another model of myelofibrosis by decreasing GATA-1 expression, where the development of myelofibrosis is associated with high levels of TGF-β1 in bone marrow and spleen fluids. Moreover, TPO treatment of GATA-1(low) mice restored the GATA-1 content in megakaryocytes and stopped the progress of both defective thrombocytopoiesis and fibrosis. These data indicate that the TPO (high) and GATA-1(low) alterations are linked in an upstream-downstream relationship along a pathobiologic pathway leading to development of myelofibrosis in mice and possibly analogous mechanism may function during the development of human PMF [137, 144]. Furthermore, the adenoviral inhibition of TGF-β1, by TBRII-Fc transduction, in TPO-induced myelofibrosis greatly reduced the bone marrow fibrosis development [145]. In addition, these animal models propose the opportunity to clarify the primary mechanism for the abnormal bone growth or osteosclerosis in PMF [143]. In spite of the host/graft combination, all animals that developed the myeloproliferative syndrome with severe myelofibrosis are coupled with an elevated TGF-β1 plasma level. Intriguingly, osteosclerosis is correlated with marked increase in osteoprotegerin (OPG) plasma level. By contrast, no such phenomenon could be seen in hosts with an OPG-impaired background and no OPG is detectable in the circulation [143]. OPG is a decoy secreted receptor that prevents RANK-L binding to its receptor RANK, thus inhibiting osteoclastogenesis [146]. OPG expression is regulated by TGF-β in bone marrow stroma cells contributing to the inhibition of osteoclatogenesis [147]. Also, TGF-β can contribute in the induction of osteoblast proliferation, while the increased plasma OPG levels do not correlate with TGF-β1 expression [148]. The growth of both OPG and TGF-β have profound effects in bone marrow, either by inhibiting osteoclastogenesis or by increasing osteoblast proliferation, that converge in the development of osteosclerosis.

It is believed that TGF-β1 is the most important cytokine involved in the promotion of myelofibrosis, but the mechanisms leading to its local activation in the bone marrow environment are not well elucidated. One of the main source of TGF-β in PMF are the platelets, that contain alpha-granules releasing thrombospondin-1 (TSP-1), and TSP-1 has been shown to activate latent TGF-β1 [149]. But conversely to expected, recently have been demonstrated the TSP-1 is not the major activator of TGF-β1 in TPO-induced myelofibrosis [150], and because platelet releases from *tsp-1* null mice contain active TGF-β1, it is suggested that other important mechanisms of physiological activation of TGF-β1 probably exist [151]. Interestingly, megakaryocytes from PMF patients express and secrete high amount of TGF-β1 and the matrix- metalloproteinase-9 (MMP-9), while MMP-9 is one of the potent activator of latent-TGF-β [152, 153]. It is possible that the increase in MMP-9, and also in other matrix proteinases, may enlighten the activation of TGF-β1 in PMF.

In PMF both megakaryocytes and monocytes seems to be the highly TGF-β's producers [154, 155], but the mechanism involved in the regulation of TGF-β expression remain to be clarified. Although it is presumable that, *JAK2* V617F-driven, megakaryocyte-derived TGF-β is responsible for myelofibrosis in the human MPNs [156], the implication of this mutation in the regulation of TGF-β1 expression is not clear. Interestingly, it is demonstrated that JAK2 mediates TGF-β-induced fibrosis in systemic sclerosis [157]. Therefore, does wild-type JAK2 participates in TGF-β1-induced myelofibrosis is worthy to be addressed in further studies.

Lately, the constitutive activation of NF-κB in megakaryocytes and monocytes from PMF patients has been associated with the increased TGF-β1 production [158, 159], predisposing the NF-κB as potential therapeutic target to reduce the high TGF-β production by PMF's megakaryocytes and monocytes. TGF-β could be one of the main targets either directly or indirectly in PMF and other disease with fibrosis based to its effects in angiogenesis and induction of ECM proteins [160].

Tumor Angiogenesis

Tumor-associated angiogenesis is originally defined as the formation and developing of new blood vessel by the proliferation of endothelial cells from pre-existing vessels [161, 162]. Tumor growth, primary or metastatic tumor, over a certain size, ~2-4 mm^3, requires influx of oxygen and nutrients, and efflux of waste and toxin products [161, 163]. A development of a new blood vasculature is obligatory to supply components for tumor cells metabolism simultaneously with a rapid tumor growth. One of the first evidences of angiogenic activity in tumors is vessel dilation, following by heterogeneity in vessel diameter and distribution [162]. During angiogenesis, a well-orchestrated serial of events and stages take place: in activation phase endothelial cells suffer shape changes encompassed with their proliferation, a degradation of basement membrane and directional migration toward tumor angiogenic stimuli; in the second resolution phase, endothelial cells decrease/stop proliferative or migration behaviors, smooth muscle cells and pericytes are recruited to enable stabilization of new vessels and functional lumen formation to permit a suitable blood flow [161, 164].

Induction of tumor angiogenesis is regulated at several levels, including stimulatory and inhibitory growth factors and cellular programs whose balanced equilibrium is kept firmly under homeostasis conditions [161, 165]. Interestingly, tumor associated vasculature is distinct to normal vasculature, in late stages of tumor development it loses all hierarchical features and becomes chaotic in organization and tortuous, unstable and porous [161, 166, 167].

TGF-β1 and Tumor Angiogenesis

TGF-β has an important role in the regulation of physiological and tumor angiogenesis, supported by numerous *in vitro* and *in vivo* studies [163, 164]. TGF-β is rich in the tumor microenvironment and regulates endothelial cells as well as surrounding vascular components such as smooth muscle cells and pericytes. In tumor stroma, TGF-β1 may trigger transformation of fibroblast into myofibroblast and consequently into smooth muscle cells or pericytes supporting angiogenesis [161, 168, 169].

In endothelial cells, TGF-β may signalize through two kind of type I receptors, ALK1 and ALK5, with evident opposing effects on angiogenesis [164, 170]. The activation of ALK1 by TGF-β induces Smad1,5 phosphorylation to stimulate endothelial cells proliferation, migration and tubulogenesis [171], associated with activation phase of angiogenesis. The activation of ALK5 induces Smad2,3 phosphorylation and inhibits endothelial cells proliferation, while induces fibronectin and plasminogen activator inhibitor PAI-1, and then negatively regulates endothelial cell migration, events related to resolution phase of angiogenesis [172].

The TGF-β type III receptor endoglin also play important role in angiogenesis. The equilibrium of both ALK1 and ALK5 activation in endothelial cells by TGF-β is finely regulated by endoglin. Endoglin binds TGF-β1 and can form heteromeric complex with ALK5-TBRII, inhibiting Smad3 signaling, and with ALK1-TBRII is vital for Smad1 signaling [170, 173, 174]. Intriguingly, endoglin, equally to Smad3 inhibition, induces an increase of Smad2 half life and activity [175], suggesting that endoglin may differentially and finely regulate Smad2 and Smad3 in endothelial cells. In addition, it is shown that caveolin-1 positively modulate ALK1, while inhibits ALK5 signaling [176, 177]. Furthermore, ALK1 can directly antagonize ALK5 signaling, whereas kinase activity of ALK5 is essential for maximal ALK1 activation, suggesting the ALK1-ALK5 cross-talk may present a fine tune regulation of TGF-β signaling in endothelial cells [171, 178].

In vivo, the role of TGF-β in the development of vascular system have been supported by knockout mice; *alk1* deficient mice die at midgestation with severe vascular abnormalities, both yolk sac and the embryo fail to develop and produce mature vascular tree, finally fusion of major arteries and veins is observed [179, 180]. *Alk5* knockout mice exhibit defects of the yolk sac and placenta, lack of circulating erythrocytes, defective vascular development, and they die at midgestation [181]. *TbRII* knockout mice die in midgestation, around E10.5, with impaired yolk sac hematopoiesis and vasculogenesis [182]. *Endoglin* knockout mice are embryonic lethal at E11.5 with defective vascular development, both in the yolk sac and in the embryo, with affected vascular smooth muscle cells [183]. Meanwhile, *Smad5* deficient mice are embryonic lethal between E7.5 and 8.5 due to multiple embryonic and extra-embryonic defects, involved in angiogenesis since embryos do not develop functional blood vessels [184, 185]. Finally, the endothelial specific *Smad4* deletion produces embryos with severe cardiovascular defects and died at E10.5 [186]. TGF-β1 also regulates vascular smooth muscle cell differentiation, as well as endothelial cell and vascular smooth muscle cell interactions [172]. In smooth muscle cells, TGF-β1 stimulates SM22α actin transcription, and inhibits cell proliferation and migration [187-189].

Endothelial cells produce latent TGF-β that upon endothelial cells - smooth muscle cells interaction can be activated to induce smooth muscle cell differentiation and function. Additionally, TGF-β stimulates smooth muscle cells to produce VEGF, which in turn can influence the growth and differentiation of both endothelial and smooth muscle cells [172, 190, 191]. Furthermore, TGF-β can induce endothelial-mesenchymal transdifferentiation converting endothelial cells into stromal cells, as an important source of cancer-associated fibroblast (CAFs) which are known to facilitate tumor development [192, 193].

Tumors or cancer cells can produce and secrete elevated levels of TGF-β, produced by the tumor and local stroma, which contributes to the progression and metastatic potential of cancer through autocrine and paracrine effects [7]. In breast cancer, high levels of TGF-β1 correlate with increased angiogenesis as well as bad patient prognosis. Neutralizing anti-TGF-β1 antibodies reduce angiogenesis and tumor development of renal carcinoma cells *in vivo*. Prostate carcinoma cells overexpressing TGF-β produces an enhancement of angiogenesis in tumor xenografts, reverted by blocking TGF-β antibodies [194, 195].

TGF-β1 not only directly affects tumor vasculature and angiogenesis, it induces production of angiogenic factors, such as VEGF, FGF, CTGF and PDGF from different cell types in the tumor microenvironment [163, 196, 197]. In addition, hypoxia and TGF-β1 have a similar effect on VEGF expression in human endothelial cells [198]. Finally, TGF-β regulates tumor angiogenesis by induction of proangiogenic proteases such as MMPs, which contributes not only by activating latent TGF-β, but also during ECM degradation activates angiogenic growth factors [199].

Angiogenesis in Myeloproliferative Neoplasms

The role of angiogenesis both in pathogenesis of solid tumors and hematological malignances has been well recognized. In the neoplastic bone marrow a disbalance occur in cells, cytokines and growth factors, and in the architecture of bone marrow ECM, finely regulated during physiological angiogenesis. The bone marrow cancer cells and local stroma cells may produce several factors, which in an autocrine and paracrine fashion lead to an augmentation in tumor-associated vascularity [161, 165, 200]. In MPN, significantly increased microvessel density (MVD) and VEGF expression have been described [201].

In PMF, the angiogenesis is more prominent than in PV or ET, since a 70% of PMF patients have a high grade of angiogenesis, in comparison to 33% of the patients with PV, and 12% of the ET cases [202]. Interestingly, in PMF the increase in MVD correlates with cellullarity and megakaryocyte clumping, which also correlates with the increase of spleen size and the overall survival [128, 203, 204]. The clonal proliferation of megakaryocytes in PMF has been demonstrated with amplified production of several cytokines, such as TGF-β, bFGF, PDGF and VEGF, with crucial roles in development of myelofibrosis and induction of bone marrow angiogenesis [205-207].

The constitutive expression and secretion of VEGF in human megakaryocytes can be increased by either a paracrine or an autocrine mechanism, and expression of both VEGF and its receptor VEGFR in MPNs suggest an increased MVD [200, 208, 209]. VEGF protein is detected principally in erythroid cells of the bone marrow, whereas the percentage of bone marrow VEGF positive cells completely correlate with serum levels of VEGF in MPN patients [210]. The angiogenic factor VEGF levels are particularly elevated in ET patients with high leuko-cytosis, but after hydroxyurea therapy they become markedly lower [211]. Intriguingly, in 90% of the patients with PV there are increased serum VEGF levels and splenomegaly [212]. Meanwhile, Alonci *et al.* [213] have been demonstrated that circulating VEGF is increased, whereas the VEGFR2 levels did not change in PMF, PV and ET.

In addition, an increase in circulating endothelial progenitors cells (EPC) are found in PMF and PV patients, and in circulating endothelial cells in all three MPNs subsets, suggesting endothelial cell proliferation and active angiogenesis which can be secondary to the augmentation of angiogenic cytokines [213].

VEGF expression is regulated by others cytokines, for example tumor necrosis factor-alpha and TGF-β that induce VEGF expression in cancer cells [200]. TGF-β stimulates VEGF expression in the recruited hematopoietic cells, resulting in activated angiogenesis and vascular remodeling. This VEGF induction is p38 and ERK1/2 MAPK dependent [214]. TGF-β1 induction of angiogenesis involves a rapid and transient apoptotic effect mediated by VEGF/VEGFR2 activation of p38 MAPK [215]. The promoter response of VEGF to TGF-β1 is upregulated by the transfection of hypoxia-inducible factor (HIF)-2α but downregulated by HIF-1α. Both HIF-1α and HIF-2α are induced by TGF-β1, although Smad3 cooperates with HIF-2α in TGF-β1 activation of VEGF transcription [216]. Although in MPNs both VEGF and TGF-β1 are highly expressed, the mutual interaction between VEGF and TGF-β1 and its impact in MNPs angiogenesis remains to be elucidated.

Mendiger *et al.* have found that MPNs cases with high *JAK2* V617F mutant allele burden show significantly increments in MVD and VEGF expression, suggesting JAK mutations may influence MNPs angiogenesis [201]. The mutational activation of *JAK2* results in constitutive phosphorylation of STAT proteins, and the activation of STAT3 induces an upregulation of VEGF expression and increases of tumor angiogenesis [217]. Bone marrow of PMF patients and all *JAK2* V617F positive patients shows a significantly higher pSTAT3 expression compared to control. pSTAT3 is observed in immature and mature myeloid cells as well as in endothelial cells, and the percentage of pSTAT3 is higher in *JAK2* V617F patients compared with normal *JAK2*. In addition the increase of pSTAT3 significantly correlates with the increase in MVD [218]. Interestingly, phosphorylated STAT5 is also increased and has been correlated with MVD in MPNs patients [218], and the importance of STAT5-VEGF in angiogenesis is supported by the study of Yang *et al.*, where the constitutive activation of STAT5 induces the expression of VEGF in endothelial cells [219]. In addition, recently it is shown that *JAK2* V617F-STAT5 axis promotes expression of oncostatin M (OSM) in neoplastic myeloid cells, and OSM induces the expression of VEGF and the growth of fibroblast and microvascular endothelial cells, indicating that MNPs cells carrying *JAK2* mutations may contribute to bone marrow angiogenesis by expressing OSM [220]. Another role of *JAK2* V617F mutation in angiogenesis came from the study identifying *JAK2* V617F mutation in the EPC [221]. An appropriate number of circulating EPC is a fundamental element for the maintenance of vascular homeostasis, and dysfunction in endothelial compartment may induce the progress of MNPs. *JAK2* V617F mutation has been detected in part of EPC isolated from a patient with idiopathic splanchnic thrombosis who subsequently developed a *JAK2* V617F PV [221, 222]. Several data confirm the common clonal origin for both hematopoietic and endothelial cell lineage in MPNs and other hematological disease, since the presence of the molecular markers trisomy 8 and *JAK2* V617F mutation are found in the liver endothelial cells of patients with Budd-Chiari syndrome [213, 223]. Moreover, CD34$^+$ cells isolated from PV and PMF patients harboring *JAK2* V617F mutation are capable of generating both wild type and *JAK2* mutated endothelial like cells when transplanted into NOD/SCID mice [221, 224]. Recently, positive *JAK2* V617F spleen endothelial cells from myelofibrosis patients have been reported, suggesting the participation of these endothelial cells in the increasing of MVD in spleen microenvironment during the development of splenomegaly [225].

Actually, during the embryonic development, hematopoietic and endothelial cells derived from a common precursor called hemangioblast, which arises from mesoderm [226]. *JAK2* V617F mutation or specific chromosome alterations have been identified in endothelial progenitors derived from the hematopoietic lineage (the so-called colony forming unit-endothelial cells CFU-ECs) [222] supporting the existence of a common hematopoietic and endothelial bilineage progenitor in MPNs [227]. The exact role of this *JAK2* V617F mutated endothelial cells, to the increase of MVD in MPNs, need further studies to be elucidated, as well as responses of these cells to the angiogenic stimuli by cytokines such as VEGF and TGF-β.

THERAPIES IN MYELOPROLIFERATIVE NEOPLASMS AND TGF-β SIGNALING

JAK2 Inhibitors

Although *JAK2* V617F is not found in all patients with ET and PMF, an aberrant activation of the JAK-STAT signaling pathway plays a central role in the pathogenesis of most PV, ET, and PMF patients. The JAK-STAT pathway not only drives myeloproliferation but also mediates the activity of inflammatory cytokines, whose levels are commonly increased in PMF patients. Following the identification of *JAK2* mutation, several inhibitors have been developed and are in various stages of clinical trials [228]. Similar to other tyrosine kinase inhibitors in current use, JAK2 inhibitors target the adenosine triphosphate (ATP) binding site at the tyrosine kinase domain and not the pseudokinase domain, thus affecting both mutated and wild-type kinases. In fact, clinical trials of these compounds have demonstrated improvements in constitutional symptoms and splenomegaly in patients with both mutated and wild-type *JAK2* PMF. It is believed that these drugs may act not only through inhibition of neoplastic cell proliferation, but also by downregulating signaling through proinflammatory cytokine receptors. Cotreatment with the hsp90 inhibitor AUY922 and JAK2- tyrosine kinase inhibitor TG101209 induces significantly more apoptosis of human $CD34^+$ MPN than normal hematopoietic progenitor cells [229]. These inhibitors include (Fig. **2**), but are not limited to:

Ruxolitinib (INCB018424)

To date, only ruxolitinib has received approval by the FDA (in November 2011) and the European Commission (in August 2012) for the treatment of intermediate- and high-risk PMF (primary and post-PV/ET). Ruxolitinib is a JAK1 and JAK2 inhibitor. The basis of its approval are two phase III clinical studies for PMF

(COMFORT I (*vs.* placebo) and II (*vs.* best available therapy)) which provide evidence that application of ruxolitinib leads to the reduction of spleen size and an improvement of myelofibrosis-related constitutional symptoms. Patients treated with ruxolitinib experienced relief of abdominal discomfort, early satiety, night sweats, itching and musculoskeletal pain. In addition, ruxolitinib decreases leukocytosis and thrombocytosis as well as inflammatory cytokine levels and thereby enhances the patients' quality of life. Long-term results from the phase 3 COMFORT-I study have shown that ruxolitinib-treated patients have a survival advantage over the control groups [230]. The responses are not specific for *JAK2* mutation. Interestingly, also the requirement of blood transfusions (due to the side effects of anemia and thrombocytopenia), observed in the early phases for patients receiving ruxolitinib, decrease to rates similar to the control groups [29]. Other investigators reported that in ruxolitinib-treated patients survival is not different from that of standard therapy in PMF patients [231]. Phase II results of ruxolitinib in PV patients, resistant to hydroxyurea therapy, are successful, with 97% reaching the target hematocrit (≤0.45) without phlebotomy and 61% of accessible patients showing about 50% reduction in palpable spleen length. Importantly, most patients experience a reduction or complete resolution in PV-associated symptoms including pruritis, night sweats and bone pain. Similar to the situation with PMF, changes in *JAK2* V617F load are modest. Two Phase III studies are currently evaluating the use of ruxolitinib in PV (RESPONSE and RELIEF; NCT01243944 and NCT01632904) [232].

TG101348 (SAR302503)

TG101348, an inhibitor described to be specific for JAK2 with activity on both wild type and mutant JAK2, is also evaluated in a phase II clinical trial in patients with high- or intermediate-risk primary or post-PV/ET PMF. In addition to the effect on splenomegaly, the majority of patients with constitutional symptoms, fatigue and pruritus have a durable resolution without a measurable effect on proinflammatory cytokines. A spleen response of 47% is seen after one year of treatment. Very interestingly, a significant decrease in *JAK2* V617F allele burden is observed at 12 months of therapy. Adverse events included nausea, vomiting, diarrhea, anemia, and thrombocytopenia. When tested in a phase I clinical trial in PMF patients, it leads to the normalization of leukocytosis and thrombocytosis. A multinational, randomized, placebo controlled phase III trial has been launched recently for patients with high risk PMF [233]. Similar to ruxolitinib, testing of TG101348 in PV and ET has begun (NCT01420783).

CYT387

A phase I/II trial of CYT387, a potent ATP-competitive small molecule JAK1/2 inhibitor, has been performed in patients with high- or intermediate-risk primary or post-PV/ET PMF. Anemia and spleen responses are 59% and 48%, respectively. The median duration of anemia response is 20 weeks, irrespective of the dose. Most patients experience constitutional symptoms improvement including pruritus, night sweats and bone pain. Adverse reactions include thrombocytopenia and mild peripheral neuropathy. Plasma cytokine and gene expression studies suggest a broad anticytokine drug effect [234]. It is worth to mention that responses are also seen in patients who had previously failed ruxolitinib or SAR302503. Surprisingly, 58% of transfusion-dependent patients become transfusion independent. Transient light headedness and hypotension are the common adverse events [49].

Lestaurtinib (CEP701)

Lestaurtinib is an orally available indolocarbazole derivative. As a tyrosine kinase inhibitor, lestaurtinib inhibits fms-like tyrosine kinase-3 (FLT3), JAK2 and JAK3. A phase II clinical study of CEP701 is performed in 22 *JAK2* V617F-positive PMF patients. Therapy with CEP701 has modest efficacy, with most responses consisting of reduction of spleen size. There is no improvement in the bone marrow fibrosis or *JAK2* V617F allelic burden. Main side effects are myelosuppression and mild but frequent gastrointestinal disturbances in PMF patients [235]. In another phase 2 study, lestaurtinib is given to 39 high-risk patients with *JAK2* V617F-positive PV (n=27) or ET (n=12). After 18 weeks of therapy, a significant decrease in spleen size is reported in 83% of the patients, while 6 patients develop thrombosis [236].

Pacritinib (SB1518)

Pacritinib is an innovative pyrimidine-based macrocycle that shows a unique kinase profile with selective inhibition of JAK2, both wild-type and mutated

JAK2 V617F, and FLT3. It inhibits JAK-STAT signaling pathway through caspase-dependent apoptosis. Pacritinib shows potent effects on cellular JAK/STAT pathways, inhibiting tyrosine phosphorylation on JAK2 (Y221) and downstream STATs. As a consequence pacritinib has potent anti-proliferative effects on myeloid cell lines driven by mutant or wild-type JAK2 or FLT3, resulting from cell cycle arrest and induction of apoptosis. Pacritinib given orally has been evaluated in a phase II study on 34 previously treated primary or post PV/ET PMF patients. Significant reductions in spleen size are observed and a trend for reduction in myelofibrosis-associated symptoms is also seen. Gastrointestinal-related adverse events are the most common toxicities reported [237].

Histone Deacetylase Inhibitors

Panobinostat (LBH589)

Deacetylase inhibitors are a class of novel agents that lead to increased acetylation of intracellular proteins implicated in oncogenic pathways. Panobinostat is a pan-histone deacetylase (HDAC) inhibitor with nanomolar inhibitor activity against class I, II, and IV deacetylase inhibitors. *In vitro* studies with MPN cells demonstrated that panobinostat depletes the mutant *JAK2* V617F protein and inhibits JAK-mediated intracellular signaling. The down-regulation of the *JAK2* V617F protein is shown to occur through inhibition of the association with HSP90, leading to proteasomal degradation of the *JAK2* V617F protein [238]. The phase II study evaluated the efficacy and safety of panobinostat in patients with higher-risk PMF. The results of this study also demonstrate that panobinostat inhibits JAK/STAT signaling, decreases inflammatory cytokine levels, and decreases *JAK2* V617F allele burden in patients with PMF, suggesting that panobinostat is biologically active. However, clinical efficacy is lower than expected, with only one patient demonstrating a clinical response according to International Working Group for Myelofibrosis Research and Treatment (IWG-MRT) criteria. Panobinostat is poorly tolerated at the dose and schedule evaluated, and only 16 of 35 patients completed ≥2 cycles of treatment. Common adverse events are thrombocytopenia and diarrhea [239]. Currently, two studies (NCT01693601 and NCT01433445) are testing the combination of ruxolitinib and panobinostat. The combination of ruxolitinib and panobinostat is found to have a more profound effect on splenomegaly, as well as on bone marrow and spleen histology, compared with either agent alone in mouse models of *JAK2* V617F-driven disease [240]. Treatment with panobinostat dose-dependently deplete JAK2, p-STAT5, p-STAT3, p-ERK1/2, and p-AKT levels, without significantly affecting STAT5, STAT3, AKT, and ERK1/2 levels in CD34$^+$ primary PMF cells. In the same cells, cotreatment with panobinostat and TG101348 results in greater inhibition of STAT5 and STAT3 phosphorylation than either agent alone [238]. Phosphorylation of STAT3 and STAT5 in granulocytes from patients with PMF is significantly less inhibited with CEP701 in comparison to PV and ET, while sensitivity to inhibition does not correlate with *JAK2* V617F clonal burden [241].

Vorinostat (MK0683)

Vorinostat as an inhibitor of histone deacetylases is analyzed in phase II multi-centre study that included 63 patients (19 ET, 44 PV). Vorinostat shows effectiveness by normalizing elevated leukocyte and platelet counts, resolving pruritus and significantly reducing splenomegaly. 65% of the patients experienced a decrease in *JAK2* V617F allele burden. However, vorinostat is associated with significant side effects resulting in a high discontinuation rate. A lower dose of vorinostat in combination with conventional and/or novel targeted therapies may be acceptable in future studies [242].

Givinostat (ITF2357)

A phase II study with givinostat (a novel histone-deacetylases inhibitor) is conducted in 29 *JAK2* V617F-positive MPN patients (12 PV, 1 ET, 16 PMF) as second line. Among 13 PV/ET patients, 1 complete and 6 partial responses are documented at study. Three major responses are registered among 16 PMF patients. Pruritus disappeared in most patients and reduction of splenomegaly is observed in 75% of PV/ET and 38% of PMF patients. Reverse transcription PCR identified a trend to reduction of the *JAK2* V617F allele burden. Givinostat is well tolerated and could induce hematological response in most PV and some PMF patients [243]. In following phase II study givinostat in combination with hydroxyurea are examined in 44 *JAK2* V617F-positive PV patients unresponsive to the maximum tolerated dose of hydroxyurea. The median weekly dose of hydroxyurea at baseline is per 1000 mg in the 50 and 100 mg givinostat groups. The combination of givinostat and hydroxyurea is generally well tolerated. Complete/partial response and control of pruritus is observed in 50-55% and 64-67% of patients receiving givinostat, respectively after 12 weeks of treatment. The 42% phlebotomy-dependent patients at baseline become phlebotomy-independent on treatment. In this study givinostat exhibits only modest effects on spleen size [244].

mTOR Inhibitor

Everolimus

It has been accomplished a phase 1/2 study with everolimus, an mTOR inhibitor, in 39 high- or intermediate-risk primary or post PV/post ET PMF subjects. Responses are evaluated in 30 patients of phase 2. No dose-limiting toxicity is observed in phase 1 up to 10 mg/d. Rapid and sustained splenomegaly reduction of > 50% and > 30% occurred in 20% and 44% of subjects, respectively. Most frequent extrahematologic toxicities include grade 1–2 stomatitis and transient grade 1–2 hypertriglyceridemia and hypercholesterolemia. A total of 69% and 80% experienced complete resolution of systemic symptoms and pruritus. Response in leukocytosis, anemia, and thrombocytosis occurred in 15-25%. Clinical responses are not associated with reduced *JAK2* V617F burden, circulating CD34$^+$ cells, or cytokine levels. These results provide proof-of-concept that targeting mTOR pathway in myelofibrosis may be clinically relevant [245]. mTOR inhibitors also impaired the proliferation and prevented colony formation from MPN hematopoietic progenitors at doses significantly lower than healthy controls. Co-treatment of mTOR inhibitor with JAK2 inhibitor resulted in synergistic activity against the proliferation of *JAK2* V617F mutated cell lines and significantly reduced EPO-independent colony growth in patients with PV [246]. Although effective in reducing constitutional symptoms and splenomegaly, treatment with JAK-tyrosine kinase inhibitor does not ameliorate myelofibrosis or significantly improve survival of patients with advanced myelofibrosis. A treatment with the dual phosphoinositide-3-kinase (PI3K)/AKT and mTOR inhibitor BEZ235 attenuated PI3K/AKT and mTOR signaling, as well as induced cell-cycle growth arrest and apoptosis of the primary CD34$^+$ PMF cells. Cotreatment with BEZ235 and JAK2- tyrosine kinase inhibitors (TG101209 and SAR302503) synergistically induce lethal activity against the cultured and primary CD34$^+$ PMF cells while relatively sparing the normal CD34$^+$ hemopoietic progenitor cells [247].

Currently the benefits of therapy with JAK inhibitors in MPNs are palliative in nature. JAK2 inhibitors are aimed at a gene present in normal cells responsible in the development of normal hematopoiesis. Also, JAK-STAT pathway inhibition is likely to impact more differentiated cells in MPN, with minor effect on disease-initiating stem cells. Therefore, the adverse actions induced with JAK2 inhibitors, such as hematological toxicity and gastrointestinal symptoms seen in clinical trials, limit the efficiency of JAK2 inhibitors. The drug resistance to JAK2 inhibitors, by acquisition of mutations in the ATP-binding pocket of the tyrosine kinase domain of JAK2, can be expected as well as *via* the amplification of JAK2. However, JAK2 burden is slightly reduced in clinical trials, indicating that JAK2 inhibitors are capable to block the cytokine pathway responsible of the clinical symptoms, but are unable to target the main molecular mechanism and uncommitted hematopoietic progenitors that originates the MPN. Hence JAK2 inhibitors induce myelosuppression but cannot cure MPN, combinations with other compounds that may have therapeutic synergy with JAK2 inhibitors seem to be necessary [248].

Therapies beyond JAK2

It is supposed that *JAK2* mutation can contribute to the initiation and progression of MPNs, but it is important to point out that recent data has shown that none of the *JAK2* activating mutations in MPNs can be considered as a causal event [249]. Increasing evidences indicate that other genetic and/or epigenetic abnormalities can contribute to the initiation and progression of MPNs. DNA methylation, histone modification, and microRNA expression patterns, and epigenetic modification of genes critical for cell proliferation and survival (such us suppressors of cytokine signaling, polycythemia rubra vera-1, CXC chemokine receptor 4, and HDAC) can collectively influence gene expression and potentially contribute to MPN pathogenesis [250]. These epigenetic lesions serve as novel targets for experimental therapeutic interventions. There are numerous compounds with different mechanism of action undergoing clinical testing in MPNs, which alone or in combination with JAK2 inhibitors can improve the treatment for MPNs patients [251].

A phase III clinical trial of combination of ruxolitinib and azacitidine in patients with PMF and MDS/MPN is ongoing (NCT01787487). Azacitidine is hypomethylating agent which can relapse gene silencing and improve hematopoiesis in some patients with bone marrow failure [252]. In cancer, localized enhancement of methylation in CpG dinucleotides is observed, and often correlated with clinical features [253]. Azacitidine can reactivate tumor suppressor genes *via* demethylation of CpG islands in the promoter regions of the target genes to improve the effects of JAK2 inhibitor ruxolitinib.

A Phase I Study of 5-AZA-2'-Deoxycytidine and Depsipeptide/FR901228 in patients with relapsed/refractory leukemia, MDS, or MPN (NCT00114257) have been completed. FR901228 that predominantly inhibits selected class I HDAC is used for cancer treatment because of capacity to repair normal expression of genes involved in cell cycle arrest, cell differentiation and apoptosis induction [254]. In addition, HDACs inhibitors may induce JAK2 degradation and downregulate intracellular oncogenic signaling to overcome resistance to JAK2 inhibitors [251].

A multi-center study of pomalidomide, in adult patients with PMF and unclassifiable MPN, showed at least grade 1 bone marrow fibrosis and requiring therapy in ongoing phase II (NCT00949364). Pomalidomide is an immunomodulatory drug derived from thalidomide and was approved for patients with multiple myeloma [255]. Recently a study with pomalidomide, for myelofibrosis-associated anemia, showed that at low dose it is well tolerated but has modest clinical activity in myelofibrosis [256].

A phase I clinical trial is recruiting participants to determine side effects and best dose of veliparib when given together with topotecan hydrochloride with or without carboplatin in patients with relapsed or refractory acute leukemia, high-risk myelodysplasia, or aggressive myeloproliferative disorders. Veliparib is poly(ADP-ribose) polymerase (PARP) inhibitor, PARP catalyzes the polyADP-ribosylation of proteins involved in DNA repair and his inhibition may increases sensitivity to platinum derivates drugs [257]. Topotecan is a water-soluble semisynthetic camptothecin analogue that inhibits the intranuclear enzyme topoisomerase 1, blocking DNA replication. Topotecan has shown a synergistic interaction with cisplatin both *in vitro* and *in vivo*, suggesting a potential clinical interest [258].

A phase I and II clinical trials are active to characterize the safety and efficacy of STA-9090 (ganetespib) in subjects with hematologic malignancies, including MPNs (NCT00858572). Ganetespib (formerly known as STA-9090) is a unique resorcinolic triazolone inhibitor of Hsp90 that is currently in clinical trials for cancer treatment. Notably, evaluation of the microregional activity of ganetespib in tumor xenografts showed that ganetespib is efficiently distributed throughout tumor tissue, including hypoxic regions of the microvasculature, to inhibit proliferation and induce apoptosis [259].

Interferon-alpha (IFN-α) is a nonleukemogenic therapy of PV. Its use is limited by toxicity, leading to treatment discontinuation in approximately 20% of patients. In first phase II multicenter study of pegylated IFN-α-2a, in 40 PV patients, median follow-up was 31.4 months. At 12 months, 35 patients have hematologic complete responses. *JAK2* V617F decrease is observed in 89.6% of examined PV patients, being complete in 17% (undetectable *JAK2* V617F). Median %V 617F decreases from 45% before pegylated IFN-α-2a to 22.5%, 17.5%, 5%, and 3% after 12, 18, 24, and 36 months, respectively [260]. In second phase II study of pegylated IFN-α-2a in 83 patients (43 with PV and 40 with ET), after a median follow-up of 42 months, complete hematologic response is achieved in 76% of patients with PV and 77% of those with ET. This is accompanied by complete molecular response (undetectable *JAK2* V617F) in 18% of PV and 17% of ET patients. Serial sequencing of TET2, ASXL1, EZH2, DNMT3A, and IDH1/2 revealed that patients, failing to achieve complete molecular response, have a higher frequency of mutations outside the JAK-STAT pathway and are more likely to acquire new mutations during therapy. Patients with both *JAK2* V617F and TET2 mutations at the beginning of therapy have a higher *JAK2* V617F mutant allele burden and a less significant reduction in *JAK2*

V617F allele burden compared with JAK2 mutant/TET2 wild-type patients. It has been reported that with pegylated IFN-α-2a, the phlebotomy rate has been significantly reduced. A randomized trial of pegylated IFN-α-2a (PEGASYS) *vs* hydroxyurea in PV and ET in phase 3 is ongoing (NCT01259856). IFN-α-2a may affect early stem cell proliferation with immunomodulatory effects to stimulate latent stem cells to become targets for activated immune cells [261]. Pegylated IFN-α-2a inhibited burst-forming unit erythroid-derived colony formation by PV CD34^{+} cells, while increased the rate of apoptosis of PV CD34^{+} cells through the p38 mitogen-activated protein kinase pathway [262].

Finally, a trial to assess the safety and tolerability of GC-1008 in patients with PMF or post-PV/ET PMF has been completed (NCT01291784). GC-1008 (fresolimumab) is a human IgG4 kappa monoclonal antibody capable of neutralizing all mammalian isoforms of TGF-β (β1, β2, and β3) with high-affinity. Reversal of bone marrow fibrosis is still a therapeutic challenge in this disease, and mAbs targeting TGF-β, such as GC-1008, may inhibit TGF-β signaling in myelofibrosis and decrease fibrogenic stimuli with parallel interruption of myeloproliferation.

Therapies Targeting TGF-β Signaling

TGF-β signaling has been shown to control a range of cellular responses implicated in a number of diseases, including cancer, kidney disease and cardiovascular disease. The TGF-βs signaling pathway is an emerging and attractive target for therapy in these diseases [263]. Three major classes of TGF-β-based therapeutics are currently in study or human treatment of several diseases: (a) ligand traps, including monoclonal TGF-βs-neutralizing antibodies and soluble(s) TGF-β receptors; (b) antisense-molecule-mediated silencing of TGF-β ligands; and (c) small molecule inhibitor designed to block TGF-βs receptors kinase activity [82].

Ligands Trap

The pan-TGF-β antibody GC-1008, as is mentioned above, has been tested in a phase I clinical trial in patients with myelofibrosis (NCT01291784), including PMF, post-

PV related myelofibrosis and post-ET related myelofibrosis, but the results have not been reported yet. This antibody also has been tested in cancer patients with renal cell carcinoma or malignant melanoma (NCT00356460, NCT00923169); in Phase II Trial for the treatment of pleural malignant mesothelioma, (NCT01112293), and GC-1008 is tested in phase I trials for idiopathic pulmonary fibrosis (NCT00125385). TGF-β1 is one of the main mediators in the fibrotic process, associated to both scarring and pathologies related to chronic inflammation. ISDIN has been develop as a peptide 144 (P144), a 14mer peptide from human TGF-β1 type III receptor (TβRIII/betaglycan) designed to block the interaction between TGF-β1 and TBR3, thus modulating TGF-β1 biological effects. Two clinical studies in phase II have been completed in 2013 for the treatment of skin fibrosis in systemic sclerosis (NCT00574613 and NCT00781053).

Antisense

Another promising approach which has entered clinical phase I and II trials is to inhibit TGF-β function by antisense oligonucleotides (AS-ODNs). A phase II trial with Lucanix (NovaRx Corporation), a TGF-β2 antisense gene-modified allogeneic tumor vaccine, is completed in patients with advanced non-small cell lung cancer (NCT01058785) and a phase III is ongoing (NCT00676507). The antitumorigenic effect of antisense oligonucleotides is supported by phase I/II trials with the TGF-β2 antisense compound AP12009 (Antisense Pharma). In comparison to standard chemotherapy, treatment with AP12009 resulted in prolonged survival of patients with anaplastic astrocytoma, and a phase III is ongoing (NCT00761280) [264]. Consistently, patients with high-grade glioma, in phase II trial, achieved a higher survival rate at 24 months and showed significantly more responders after 14 months when AP12009 treatment is compared to standard chemotherapy protocols (NCT00431561) [264]. Another phase I study (NCT00844064) investigating treatment of pancreatic neoplasms, melanoma and colorectal neoplasms is completed.

Receptors Inhibitors

Most of the strategies to inhibit TGF-β1 at the receptor kinase level use small molecule inhibitors, which typically bind to the ATP binding domain of the TGF-β receptors [265]. TβRI/ALK5 and TβRIII dual inhibitor LY2157299 is in clinical trial in patients with metastatic malignancies, including malignant glioma, hepatocellular carcinoma and pancreatic cancer. A number of companies have developed ATP-mimetic drugs that target the kinase catalytic site of TBRI. Although these small molecule inhibitors are not completely specific like most other kinase inhibitors, they are very effective at inhibiting Smad2/3 phosphorylation (Fig. **3**). Preclinical *in vitro* and *in vivo* studies have shown the usefulness of these compounds in prevention and treatment of several experimental diseases.

Tumors require new blood vessels to support their metastasis and growth. New treatments are aimed at preventing these blood vessels [82]. Since its expression is mostly restricted to endothelial cells, ALK1 and endoglin may represent promising target to antiangiogenic therapies in cancer [266]. A clinical phase II study testing a human anti-ALK1 antibody PF-03446962 (Pfizer) in patients with Transitional Cell Carcinoma of Bladder is ongoing (NCT01620970). Dalantercept/ACE-041 as a soluble fusion protein containing the extracellular domain of ALK1 fused to a human Fc domain (ALK1-Fc fusion protein), with potential antiangiogenic and antineoplastic activities, is being tested in clinical trials of patients with squamous cell carcinoma of the head and neck, endometrial cancer, ovarian, fallopian tube, or primary peritoneal cancer (NCT01458392, NCT01642082 and NCT01720173). The type III receptor endoglin also appears as a promissory target for anti-angiogenic therapies: a phase I trial using a human/murine chimeric anti-endoglin monoclonal antibody TRC105 (Tracon Pharmaceuticals Inc.) in patients with solid cancer has been completed (NCT00582985). Now several approaches have been tested in clinical trials, a combination of TRC105 with bevacizumab (a recombinant humanized monoclonal antibody directed against the VEGF) is being tested for glioblastoma multiforme and metastatic kidney cancer (NCT01648348 and NCT01727089).

Other Opportunities to the Control of TGF-β signaling in Human Diseases

Strategies to disrupt intracellular Smad signaling appear to be promising approach in the control of TGF-β signaling [82]. Several preclinical approaches confirmed efficacy of endogenous / synthetic Smad inhibitors, Smad sequestration or targeting degradation in several diseases *in vitro* and *in vivo* [265]. Gene transfer of inhibitory Smad7, Smad7 induction by hepatocyte growth factor or by BB3 (a HGF synthetic analog) showed antifibrotic properties in animal models [266, 267]. SiS3 specifically inhibited Smad3, showing antitumor activities in vitro [268]. Paclitaxel/Taxol, an anticancer drug that stabilizes the microtubules, attenuated hepatic fibrosis by inhibiting TGF-β signaling [269]. A thioredoxin-A SARA aptamers in mammalian cells blocked epithelial-mesenchymal transformation and related TGF-β responses without generally inhibiting Smad-dependent signaling [270].

The plethoric signal transduction pathways downstream of TGF-β (Fig. **4**) provide multiple opportunities for TGF-β-targeting therapies. In recent studies, the protein tyrosine kinase c-Abelson (c-Abl) is shown to be activated by TGF-β in fibroblasts, and to mediate some of the profibrotic effects independent of Smad signaling. Moreover, c-Abl is found to be constitutively phosphorylated in the lesional skin of patients with systemic sclerosis. It has been shown that Imatinib blocks the induction of c-Abl activity and fibrotic gene responses elicited by TGF-β, while normalizes collagen overproduction in explanted systemic sclerosis fibroblasts [265].

Recently, a substantial interest is aimed to the commonly used drugs as an anti-TGF-β therapy. For example, Tranilast an antagonist of angiotensin II, that prevents mast cell degranulation and which is currently used for the treatment of asthma, allergic rhinitis and atopic dermatitis, have been shown potent anti-fibrotic effects in sclerotic fibroblast, as well in animal models of fibrosis. Tranilast may inhibit TGF-β1 secretion, Smads and ERK1 activation [271, 272].

In cancer, the loss of TGF-β signaling occurs early in cancer development and contributes to tumor progression. The loss of TGF-β responsiveness frequently occurs at the level of the TGF-β type II receptor which has been identified as a tumor suppressor gene. Because the most frequent cause of TβRII silencing is through epigenetic mechanisms, growing efforts are in the line to the re-expression of TβRII by using HDAC inhibitors as epigenetic therapies to exploit the suppressive tumor role of TGF-β signaling pathway [273]. The

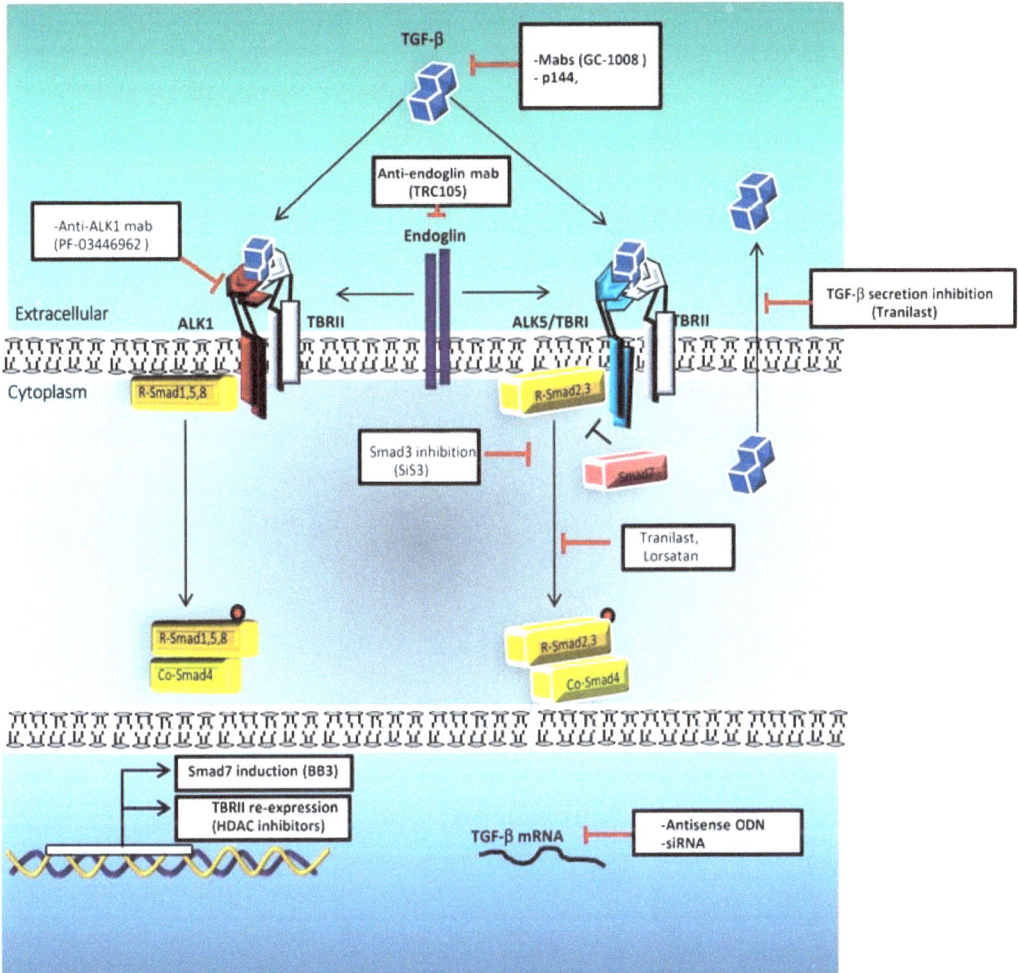

Fig. (4): Therapeutic opportunities to target TGF-β signaling pathways. TGF-β signaling pathways can be targeting at different levels, by targeting: TGF-β binding to cellular receptors; signaling receptors such ALK1 by monoclonal antibodies (Mabs) or ALK5 by small chemical inhibitors, and Endoglin by specific Mabs; inhibiting Smad2,3 signaling; inducing the expression of the inhibitory Smad7 or re-expression of TBRII; blocking TGF-β expression; and finally by inhibiting TGF-β secretion. For further details see the text. Adapted from [82].

treatment of *in vitro* cell lines, resistant to TGF-β induced growth inhibition, with HDAC inhibitors 5 aza-2′ deoxycytidine, MS275, TSA and sodium butyrate restored the expression of TβRII [273-275]. Although the use is limited to epigenetic silencing of TβRII, reactivation of the TβRII may lead to therapeutic benefit related to growth inhibition and apoptotic effects of the TGF-β signaling pathway.

CONCLUDING REMARKS

A significant number of new drugs with JAK2 target are currently at varying stages of clinical evaluation, and very recently Ruxolitinib (JAK1/2 inhibitor) became the first-in-class JAK inhibitor to obtain approval by the Food and Drug Administration for use in intermediate-2 and high-risk myelofibrosis. JAK2 inhibitors are currently tested also in patients with PV/ET refractory or intolerant to conventional therapy. Clinical trials using various pharmacologic inhibitors that target the JAK-STAT pathway in PMF have resulted in meaningful and significant advance in splenomegaly, coupled clinical manifestations, and disease linked constitutional symptoms. MPNs are a heterogeneous group of disorders and unlike BCR-ABL1-positive CML, are unlikely to be determined by a single mutation. Further survey to estimate new types of JAK2 inhibitors whether alone or in combination with other therapies such as immunomodulatory agents, histone deacetylase inhibitors, DNA methyltransferase inhibitors and other targeted agents may help to expand results in myelofibrosis and may help resolve some of the presently observed limitations in single JAK2 inhibitor therapy.

The pathophysiology of PMF and ET without mutation of *JAK2* or *MPL* (approximately 40% of patients) remained unknown until now. At the last meeting of the American Society of Hematology (ASH) held in New Orleans from December 7 to 10, 2013, two European teams [276, 277] reported in two abstracts similar results in cohorts of patients with PMF or ET. Both teams have shown that almost all patients, having no abnormality of JAK2 or MPL, have acquired abnormality of the gene encoding calreticulin (CALR). CALR is a protein essential to the function of endoplasmic reticulum by controlling both the folding of newly synthesized proteins and by maintaining calcium balance by fixing the free calcium in endoplasmic reticulum [278]. A role for CALR has already been mentioned in the pathophysiology of some cancers [279]. The abnormalities found by both teams are insertions or deletions in the last exon (exon 9) of *CALR* gene, resulting in a shift in the reading frame, and therefore to the formation of an abnormal protein. The two most commonly detected variants correspond either to a deletion of 52 base pairs (variant L367fs*46) or an insertion of 5 base pairs (variant K385fs*47). Interestingly, the different variants generate a shift in the reading frame of base pair, resulting in the loss of most of the C-terminal domain of the protein, and the portion of CALR responsible for the migration of protein of the Golgi to the endoplasmic reticulum, which could lead to a compromised fixation of the molecule to the endoplasmic reticulum. Moreover, the authors of the first study [276] show that overexpression of the most common mutation in *CALR* (variant L367fs*46) in Ba/F3 cells, dependent on IL-3 for proliferation, resulted in a loss of the cell dependence towards IL-3 together with a constitutive phosphorylation of STAT5 in mutant *CALR* cells. Also, the same authors have shown that these Ba/F3 cells with mutant *CALR* are sensitive to inhibitors of JAK family kinases. This indicates that the JAK-STAT signaling is involved in IL-3 - independent growth of Ba/F3 cells with the mutant *CALR*. This discovery supports previous observation that the responses to JAK2 inhibitor (Ruxolitinib) are not specific for *JAK2* mutation [29].

The remarkable efforts made by researches, using a combination of cellular and molecular systems, have contributed to our current knowledge of the modulatory mechanisms that provide the diversity of TGF-β signaling system. Although extraordinary advances in the understanding of TGF-β signaling have been done, it is still necessary to specify the individual role of many members of the family, as well as the transcriptional activities triggered by Smad and non-Smad pathways supporting tumor development. High-throughput drug screening has been used to find chemical compounds that selectively regulate TGF-β family system and some of them are currently being used in clinical trials to treat TGF-β-implicated human diseases. A crucial discovery of new compounds with high specificity has made it possible to finely target TGF-βs expression, receptor binding and kinase activities, intracellular signal transduction and gene transcription to modulate TGF-β effects on tumor progression.

In MPNs, TGF-β may have a dual role in the regulation and development of disease. MPNs proliferation seem to be refractory to inhibition induced by TGF-β, where cells have decreased expression of type II TGF-β receptors, while the re-expression of this receptors may recover the response of MPNs cells to TGF-β. Conversely, TGF-β has been implicated in the development of myelofibrosis with potential role in the increase of MVD often observed in bone marrow, and an anti-TGF-β targeting appears as a choice for the treatment. Several ongoing clinical trials are performed to target components of TGF-β signaling, these protocols in combination with the traditional or anti-JAK2 therapies, may increase the therapeutic efficiency in MPNs. Elucidating the complex interplay and roles of TGF-β, JAK2 and others actors in MPNs scenario, is critical challenge for understanding of their participation in the initiation and progression of MPN, to eventually uncover the combinatory therapeutic targets for future treatment of MPNs.

ACKNOWLEDGEMENTS

We apologize to those colleagues whose work, although relevant to the issues within this review, has not been included due to space limitations. This work was supported by Ministry of education, science and technological development of the Republic of Serbia (grants 175024, 175053 and 175062).

CONFLICT OF INTEREST

The authors confirm that this chapter content have no conflict of interest.

REFERENCES

[1]　Swerdlow SH, Campo E, Harris NL, *et al*. WHO Classification of Tumours of Haematopoietic and Lymphoid Tissues. Lyon, France: IARC Press; 2008.

[2]　Scott LM, Tong W, Levine RL, *et al*. JAK2 exon 12 mutations in polycythemia vera and idiopathic erythrocytosis. N Engl J Med 2007; 356; 459-68.

[3]　Beer PA, Campbell P, Scott LM, *et al*. MPL mutations in myeloproliferative disorders: analysis of the PT-1 cohort. Blood 2008; 112; 141-9.

[4]　Bierie B, Moses HL. TGF-beta and cancer. Cytokine Growth Factor Rev 2006; 17(1-2); 29-40.

[5]　Padua D, Massagué J. Roles of TGFbeta in metastasis. Cell Res 2009; 19(1); 89-102.

[6]　Park HY, Wakefield LM, Mamura M. Regulation of Tumor Immune Surveillance and Tumor Immune Subversion by TGF-β. Immune Network 2009; 9(4); 122-6.

[7]　Teicher BA. Transforming growth factor-beta and the immune response to malignant disease. Clin Cancer Res 2007; 13(21); 6247-51.

[8]　Heuck G. Zwei Falle von Leukemie mit eigenthumlichen Blutresp. Knockenmarksbefund (Two cases of leukemia with peculiar blood and bone marrow findings, respectively). Arch Pathol Anat Physiol Virchows. 1879; 78; 475-96.

[9]   Vaquez H. Sur une forme speciale de cyanose s'accompagnant d'hyperglobulie excessive et persistante (On a special form of cyanosis accompanied by excessive and persistent erythrocytosis). Cornpt. Rend. Soc. de Biol. 1892; 44; 384–8.

[10]   Epstein E, Goedel A. Hamorrhagische thrombozythamie bei vascularer schrumpfmilz (Hemorrhagic thrombocythemia with a vascular, sclerotic spleen). Virchows Archiv A Pathol Anat Histopathol 1934; 293; 233–48.

[11]   Dameshek W. Some speculations on the mycloproliferative syndromes. Blood. 1951; 6(4); 372-5.

[12]   Vardiman JW, Brunning RD, Harris NL. WHO histological classification of chronic myeloproliferative diseases. In: JaffeES, HarrisNL, SteinH, VardimanJW, eds. World Health Organization Classification of Tumors: Tumours of the Haematopoietic and Lymphoid Tissues. Lyon, France: International Agency for Research on Cancer (IARC) Press; 2001; 17-44.

[13]   Vardiman JW, Thiele J, Arber DA, *et al*. The 2008 revision of the World Health Organization (WHO) classification of myeloid neoplasms and acute leukemia: rationale and important changes. Blood 2009; 114; 937-51.

[14]   Tefferi A. The history of myeloproliferative disorders: before and after Dameshek. Leukemia 2008; 22; 3–13.

[15]   Levine RL, Gilliland DG. Myeloproliferative disorders. Blood. 2008; 112; 2190-8.

[16]   Baxter EJ, Scott LM, Campbell PJ, *et al*. Acquired mutation of the tyrosine kinase JAK2 in human myeloproliferative disorders. Lancet 2005; 365; 1054-61.

[17]   Kralovics R, Guan Y, Prchal JT. Acquired uniparental disomy of chromosome 9p is a frequent stem cell defect in polycythemia vera. Exp Hematol 2002; 30; 229-36.

[18]   Kralovics R, Passamonti F, Buser AS, *et al*. A gain-of-function mutation of JAK2 in myeloproliferative disorders. N Engl J Med 2005; 352; 1779-90.

[19]   Levine RL, Wadleigh M, Cools J, *et al*. Activating mutation in the tyrosine kinase JAK2 in polycythemia vera, essential thrombocythemia, and myeloid metaplasia with myelofibrosis. Cancer Cell 2005; 7; 387-97.

[20]   James C, Ugo V, Le Coue´dic JP *et al*. A unique clonal JAK2 mutation leading to constitutive signalling causes polycythaemia vera. Nature 2005; 434; 1144-8.

[21]   Delhommeau F, Jeziorowska D, Marzac C, Casadevall N. Molecular aspects of myeloproliferative neoplasms. Int J Hematol 2010; 91; 165-73.

[22]   Michiels JJ. Bone marrow histopathology and biological markers as specific clues to the differential diagnosis of essential thrombocythemia, polycythemia vera and prefibrotic or fibrotic agnogenic myeloid metaplasia. Hematol J. 2004; 5(2); 93-102.

[23]   Tefferi A, Rumi E, Finazzi G, *et al*. Survival and prognosis among 1545 patients with contemporary polycythemia vera: an international study. Leukemia 2013; 27(9); 1874-81.

[24]   Kim J, Haddad RY, Atallah E. Myeloproliferative neoplasms. Dis Mon 2012; 58(4); 177-94.

[25]   Vainchenker W, Delhommeau F, Constantinescu SN, Bernard OA. New mutations and pathogenesis of myeloproliferative neoplasms. Blood 2011; 118(7); 1723-35.

[26]   Björkholm M, Derolf AR, Hultcrantz M, *et al*. Treatment-Related Risk Factors for Transformation to Acute Myeloid Leukemia and Myelodysplastic Syndromes in Myeloproliferative Neoplasms. J Clin Oncol 2011; 29(17); 2410-5.

[27]   Kiladjian JJ, Chevret S, Dosquet C, Chomienne C, Rain JD. Treatment of polycythemia vera with hydroxyurea and pipobroman: final results of a randomized trial initiated in 1980. J Clin Oncol 2011; 29(29); 3907-13.

[28]   Gäbler K, Behrmann I, Haan C. JAK2 mutants (*e.g.*, JAK2V617F) and their importance as drug targets in myeloproliferative neoplasms. JAKSTAT 2013; 2(3); e25025.

[29]   Verstovsek S, Kantarjian H, Mesa RA, *et al*. Safety and efficacy of INCB018424, a JAK1 and JAK2 inhibitor, in myelofibrosis. N Engl J Med. 2010; 363(12); 1117-27.

[30]   Campbell PJ, Scott LM, Buck G, *et al*. Definition of subtypes of essential thrombocythaemia and relation to polycythaemia vera based on JAK2 V617F mutation status: a prospective study. Lancet 2005; 366(9501); 1945-53.

[31]   Wolanskyj AP, Schwager SM, McClure RF, *et al*. Essential thrombocythemia beyond the first decade: life expectancy, long-term complication rates, and prognostic factors. Mayo Clin Proc 2006; 81(2); 159-66.

[32]   Thiele J, Kvasnicka HM, Facchetti F, Franco V, Walt J, Orazi A. European consensus on grading bone marrow fibrosis and assessment of cellularity. Haematologica 2005; 90; 1128-32.

[33]   Kvasnicka HM, Thiele J. Prodromal myeloproliferative neoplasms: The 2008 WHO classification. Am J Hematol 2010; 85; 62-9.

[34]   Ballen KK, Shrestha S, Sobocinski KA, *et al*. Outcome of transplantation for myelofibrosis. Biol Blood Marrow Transplant 2010; 16; 358-67.

[35]   Tefferi A. Primary myelofibrosis: 2013 update on diagnosis, risk-stratification, and management. Am J Hematol 2013; 88(2); 141-50.

[36]   Martínez-Trillos A, Gaya A, Maffioli M, *et al*. Efficacy and tolerability of hydroxyurea in the treatment of the hyperproliferative manifestations of myelofibrosis: results in 40 patients. Ann Hematol 2010; 89(12); 1233-7.

[37]   Kröger N, Holler E, Kobbe G, *et al*. Allogeneic stem cell transplantation after reduced-intensity conditioning in patients with myelofibrosis: a prospective, multicenter study of the Chronic Leukemia Working Party of the European Group for Blood and Marrow Transplantation. Blood 2009; 114(26); 5264-70.

[38]   Alchalby H, Badbaran A, Zabelina T, *et al*. Impact of JAK2V617F mutation status, allele burden, and clearance after allogeneic stem cell transplantation for myelofibrosis. Blood 2010; 116(18); 3572-81.

[39]   Lange T, Edelmann A, Siebolts U, *et al*. JAK2 p.V617F allele burden in myeloproliferative neoplasms one month after allogeneic stem cell transplantation significantly predicts outcome and risk of relapse. Haematologica 2013; 98(5); 722-8.

[40]   Mesa RA, Li CY, Ketterling RP, *et al*. Leukemic transformation in myelofibrosis with myeloid metaplasia: A single-institution experience with 91 cases. Blood 2005; 105; 973-7.

[41]   Passamonti F, Elena C, Schnittger S, *et al*. Molecular and clinical features of the myeloproliferative neoplasm associated with JAK2 exon 12 mutations. Blood 2011; 117(10); 2813-6.

[42]   Grand FH, Hidalgo-Curtis CE, Ernst T, *et al*. Frequent CBL mutations associated with 11q acquired uniparental disomy in myeloproliferative neoplasms. Blood 2009; 113(24); 6182-92.

[43]   Pardanani A, Lasho TL, Finke CM, Mai M, McClure RF, Tefferi A. IDH1 and IDH2 mutation analysis in chronic- and blast-phase myeloproliferative neoplasms. Leukemia 2010; 24(6); 1146-51.

[44] Brecqueville M, Rey J, Bertucci F, *et al*. Mutation analysis of ASXL1, CBL, DNMT3A, IDH1, IDH2, JAK2, MPL, NF1, SF3B1, SUZ12, and TET2 in myeloproliferative neoplasms. Genes Chromosomes Cancer 2012; 51(8); 743-55.

[45] Ernst T, Chase AJ, Score J, *et al*. Inactivating mutations of the histone methyltransferase gene EZH2 in myeloid disorders. Nat Genet 2010; 42(8); 722-6.

[46] Gebauer N, Bernard V, Gebauer W, Feller AC, Merz H. MicroRNA expression and JAK2 allele burden in bone marrow trephine biopsies of polycythemia vera, essential thrombocythemia and early primary myelofibrosis. Acta Haematol 2013; 129(4); 251-6.

[47] Zhan H, Cardozo C, Raza A. MicroRNAs in myeloproliferative neoplasms. Br J Haematol 2013; 161(4); 471-83.

[48] Ranjan A, Penninga E, Jelsig AM, Hasselbalch HC, Bjerrum OW. Inheritance of the chronic myeloproliferative neoplasms. A systematic review. Clin Genet 2013; 83(2); 99-107.

[49] Furqan M, Mukhi N, Lee B, Liu D. Dysregulation of JAK-STAT pathway in hematological malignancies and JAK inhibitors for clinical application. Biomark Res. 2013;1(1); 5.

[50] Tamiya T, Kashiwagi I, Takahashi R, Yasukawa H, Yoshimura A. Suppressors of cytokine signaling (SOCS) proteins and JAK/STAT pathways: regulation of T-cell inflammation by SOCS1 and SOCS3. Arterioscler Thromb Vasc Biol. 2011; 1(5); 980-5.

[51] Teofili L, Martini M, Cenci T, *et al*. Different STAT-3 and STAT-5 phosphorylation discriminates among Ph-negative chronic myeloproliferative diseases and is independent of the V617F JAK-2 mutation. Blood. 2007; 1(1); 354–359.

[52] Bonicelli G, Abdulkarim K, Mounier M, *et al*. Leucocytosis and thrombosis at diagnosis are associated with poor survival in polycythaemia vera: a population-based study of 327 patients. Br J Haematol 2013; 160; 251-4.

[53] Barbui T, Carobbio A, Cervantes F, *et al*. Thrombosis in primary myelofibrosis: incidence and risk factors. Blood 2010; 115; 778-82.

[54] Finazzi G, Rambaldi A, Guerini V, Carobbo A, Barbui T. Risk of thrombosis in patients with essential thrombocythemia and polycythemia vera according to JAK2 V617F mutation status. Haematologica. 2007; 92; 135-6.

[55] Caramazza D, Caracciolo C, Barone R, *et al*. Correlation between leukocytosis and thrombosis in Philadelphia-negative chronic myeloproliferative neoplasms. Ann Hematol 2009; 88; 967-71.

[56] Panova-Noeva M, Marchetti M, Russo L, *et al*. ADP-induced platelet aggregation and thrombin generation are increased in Essential Thrombocythemia and Polycythemia Vera. Thromb Res 2013; 132; 88-93

[57] Moore SF, Hunter RW, Harper MT, *et al*. Dysfunction of the PI3 kinase/Rap1/integrin α(IIb)β(3) pathway underlies *ex vivo* platelet hypoactivity in essential thrombocythemia. Blood 2013; 121; 1209-19.

[58] De Grandis M, Cambot M, Wautier MP, *et al*. JAK2V617F activates Lu/BCAM-mediated red cell adhesion in polycythemia vera through an EpoR-independent Rap1/Akt pathway. Blood 2013; 121; 658-65.

[59] Khan I, Huang Z, Wen Q, *et al*. AKT is a therapeutic target in myeloproliferative neoplasms. Leukemia. 2013 Sep;27(9):1882-90.

[60] Goette NP, Lev PR, Heller PG, *et al*. Monocyte IL-2Ralpha expression is associated with thrombosis and the JAK2V617F mutation in myeloproliferative neoplasms. Cytokine 2010; 51; 67-72.

[61]   Cella G, Marchetti M, Vianello F, *et al*. Nitric oxide derivatives and soluble plasma selectins in patients with myeloproliferative neoplasms. Thromb Haemost 2010; 104; 151-6.

[62]   Hasselbalch HC. Perspectives on chronic inflammation in essential thrombocythemia, polycythemia vera, and myelofibrosis: is chronic inflammation a trigger and driver of clonal evolution and development of accelerated atherosclerosis and second cancer? Blood 2012; 119(14); 3219-25

[63]   Musolino C, Allegra A, Saija A, *et al*. Changes in advanced oxidation protein products, advanced glycation end products, and s-nitrosylated proteins, in patients affected by polycythemia vera and essential thrombocythemia. Clin Biochem 2012; 45; 1439-43.

[64]   Förstermann U. Nitric oxide and oxidative stress in vascular disease. Pflugers Arch 2010; 459; 923-39.

[65]   Moore C, Tymvios C, Emerson M. Functional regulation of vascular and platelet activity during thrombosis by nitric oxide and endothelial nitric oxide synthase. Thromb Haemost 2010; 104; 342-9.

[66]   Cokic VP, Schechter AN. The Effects of Nitric Oxide on Red Cell Development and Phenotype. Curr Top Dev Biol 2008; 82; 169-215.

[67]   Cokic VP, Beleslin-Cokic BB, Tomic M, Stojilkovic SS, Noguchi CT, Schechter AN. Hydroxyurea induces the eNOS-cGMP pathway in endothelial cells. Blood 2006; 108(1); 184-91.

[68]   Cokic VP, Smith RD, Beleslin-Cokic BB, *et al*. Hydroxyurea induces fetal hemoglobin by the nitric oxide-dependent activation of soluble guanylyl cyclase. J Clin Invest 2003; 111; 231-39.

[69]   Cokic VP, Andric SA, Stojilkovic SS, Noguchi CT, Schechter AN. Hydroxyurea nitrosylates and activates soluble guanylyl cyclase in human erythroid cells. Blood 2008; 111(3); 1117-23.

[70]   Cokic VP, Beleslin-Cokic BB, Noguchi CT, Schechter AN. Hydroxyurea increases eNOS protein levels through inhibition of proteasome activity. Nitric Oxide 2007; 16(3); 371-8.

[71]   Cokic VP, Beleslin-Cokic BB, Smith RD, *et al*. Stimulated stromal cells induce gamma-globin gene expression in erythroid cells *via* nitric oxide production. Exp Hematol 2009; 37; 1230-7.

[72]   Cokic VP, Bhattacharya B, Beleslin-Cokic BB, Noguchi CT, Puri RK, Schechter AN. JAK-STAT and AKT pathway-coupled genes in erythroid progenitor cells through ontogeny. J Transl Med 2012; 10; 116.

[73]   Beleslin-Cokic BB, Cokic VP, Yu X, Weksler BB, Schechter AN, Noguchi CT. Erythropoietin and hypoxia stimulate erythropoietin receptor and nitric oxide production by endothelial cells. Blood 2004; 104; 2073-80.

[74]   Beleslin-Cokic BB, Cokic VP, Wang L, *et al*. Erythropoietin and hypoxia increase erythropoietin receptor and nitric oxide levels in lung microvascular endothelial cells. Cytokine 2011; 54(2); 129-35.

[75]   Cokic VP, Smith RD, Biancotto A, Noguchi CT, Puri RK, Schechter AN. Globin gene expression in correlation with G protein-related genes during erythroid differentiation. BMC Genomics 2013; 14; 116.

[76]   Finazzi G, Barbui T. Evidence and expertise in the management of polycythemia vera and essential thrombocythemia. Leukemia 2008; 22(8); 1494-502.

[77]   Girodon F, Schaeffer C, Cleyrat C, *et al.* Frequent reduction or absence of detection of the JAK2-mutated clone in JAK2V617F-positive patients within the first years of hydroxyurea therapy. Haematologica 2008; 93(11); 1723-7.

[78]   Ricksten A, Palmqvist L, Johansson P, Andreasson B. Rapid decline of JAK2V617F levels during hydroxyurea treatment in patients with polycythemia vera and essential thrombocythemia. Haematologica 2008; 93(8); 1260-1.

[79]   Antonioli E, Carobbio A, Pieri L, *et al.* Hydroxyurea does not appreciably reduce JAK2 V617F allele burden in patients with polycythemia vera or essential thrombocythemia. Haematologica 2010; 95(8); 1435-8.

[80]   Besses C, Alvarez-Larrán A, Martínez-Avilés L, *et al.* Modulation of JAK2 V617F allele burden dynamics by hydroxycarbamide in polycythaemia vera and essential thrombocythaemia patients. Br J Haematol 2011; 152(4); 413-9.

[81]   Zalcberg IR, Ayres-Silva J, de Azevedo AM, Solza C, Daumas A, Bonamino M. Hydroxyurea dose impacts hematologic parameters in polycythemia vera and essential thrombocythemia but does not appreciably affect JAK2-V617F allele burden. Haematologica 2011; 96(3); e18-20.

[82]   Santibanez JF, Quintanilla M, Bernabeu C. TGF-β/TGF-β receptor system and its role in physiological and pathological conditions. Clin Sci (Lond) 2011; 121(6); 233-51.

[83]   Dobaczewski M, Chen W, Frangogiannis NG. Transforming growth factor (TGF)-β signaling in cardiac remodeling. J Mol Cell Cardiol 2011; 51(4); 600-6.

[84]   Santibanez JF. Transforming growth factor-Beta and urokinase-type plasminogen activator: dangerous partners in tumorigenesis-implications in skin cancer. ISRN Dermatol 2013; 597927.

[85]   Yu Q, Stamenkovic I. Cell surface-localized matrix metalloproteinase-9 proteolytically activates TGF-beta and promotes tumor invasion and angiogenesis. Genes Dev 2000; 14(2); 163-76.

[86]   Perera M, Tsang CS, Distel RJ, *et al.* TGF-beta1 interactome: metastasis and beyond. Cancer Genomics Proteomics 2010; 7(4); 217-29.

[87]   Shi Y, Massagué J. Mechanisms of TGF-beta signaling from cell membrane to the nucleus. Cell 2003; 113(6); 685-700.

[88]   ten Dijke P, Hill CS. New insights into TGF-beta-Smad signalling. Trends Biochem Sci 2004; 29(5); 265-73.

[89]   David L, Feige JJ, Bailly S. Emerging role of bone morphogenetic proteins in angiogenesis. Cytokine Growth Factor Rev 2009; 20(3); 203-12.

[90]   Feng XH, Derynck R. Specificity and versatility in tgf-beta signaling through Smads. Annu Rev Cell Dev Biol 2005; 21; 659-93.

[91]   Itoh S, ten Dijke P. Negative regulation of TGF-beta receptor/Smad signal transduction. Curr Opin Cell Biol 2007; 19(2); 176-84.

[92]   Kang JS, Liu C, Derynck R. New regulatory mechanisms of TGF-beta receptor function. Trends Cell Biol 2009; 19(8); 385-94.

[93]   Santibanez JF, Kocic J. Transforming growth factor-beta superfamily, implications in development and differentiation of stem cells. BioMolecular Concepts 2012; 3(5); 429-45.

[94]   Santibáñez JF, Kocić J, Fabra A, Cano A, Quintanilla M. Rac1 modulates TGF-beta1-mediated epithelial cell plasticity and MMP9 production in transformed keratinocytes. FEBS Lett 2010; 584(11); 2305-10.

[95]   Santibañez JF. JNK mediates TGF-beta1-induced epithelial mesenchymal transdifferentiation of mouse transformed keratinocytes. FEBS Lett 2006; 580(22); 5385-91.

[96]   Santibáñez JF, Iglesias M, Frontelo P, Martínez J, Quintanilla M. Involvement of the Ras/MAPK signaling pathway in the modulation of urokinase production and cellular invasiveness by transforming growth factor-beta(1) in transformed keratinocytes. Biochem Biophys Res Commun 2000; 273(2); 521-7.

[97]   Tobar N, Villar V, Santibanez JF. ROS-NFkappaB mediates TGF-beta1-induced expression of urokinase-type plasminogen activator, matrix metalloproteinase-9 and cell invasion. Mol Cell Biochem 2010; 340(1-2); 195-202.

[98]   Franks AL, Slansky JE. Multiple associations between a broad spectrum of autoimmune diseases, chronic inflammatory diseases and cancer. Anticancer Res 2012; 32(4); 1119-36.

[99]   Worthington JJ, Fenton TM, Czajkowska BI, Klementowicz JE, Travis MA. Regulation of TGFβ in the immune system: an emerging role for integrins and dendritic cells. Immunobiology 2012; 217(12); 1259-65

[100]   Shull MM, Ormsby I, Kier AB et al. Targeted disruption of the mouse transforming growth factor-β1 gene results in multifocal inflammatory disease. Nature 1992; 359; 693-9.

[101]   Kulkarni AB, Huh CG, Becker D, et al. TGF-β1 null mutation in mice causes excessive inflammatory response and early death. Proc Natl Acad Sci USA 1993; 90; 770-4.

[102]   Yang X, Letterio JJ, Lechleider RJ, et al. Targeted disruption of SMAD3 results in impaired mucosal immunity and diminished T cell responsiveness to TGF-β. EMBO J 1999; 18; 1280-91.

[103]   Malhotra N, Kang J. SMAD regulatory networks construct a balanced immune system. Immunology. 2013; 139(1); 1-10.

[104]   Martinez GJ, Zhang Z, Chung Y, et al. Smad3 differentially regulates the induction of regulatory and inflammatory T cell differentiation. J Biol Chem 2009; 284; 35283–6.

[105]   Nomura M, Li E. Smad2 role in mesoderm formation, left-right patterning and craniofacial development. Nature 1998; 393; 786-90.

[106]   Weinstein M, Yang X, Li C, Xu X, Gotay J, Deng CX. Failure of egg cylinder elongation and mesoderm induction in mouse embryos lacking the tumor suppressor smad2. Proc Natl Acad Sci USA 1998; 95; 9378-83.

[107]   Malhotra N, Robertson E, Kang J. SMAD2 is essential for TGF beta-mediated Th17 cell generation. J Biol Chem 2010; 285(38); 29044-8.

[108]   Takimoto T, Wakabayashi Y, Sekiya T et al. Smad2 and Smad3 are redundantly essential for the TGF-β-mediated regulation of regulatory T plasticity and Th1 development. J Immunol 2010; 185; 842-55.

[109]   Gorelik L, Flavell RA. Abrogation of TGF-β signaling in T cells leads to spontaneous T cell differentiation and autoimmune disease. Immunity 2000; 12; 171-81.

[110]   Kao JY, Gong Y, Chen CM, Zheng QD, Chen JJ. Tumor-derived TGF-beta reduces the efficacy of dendritic cell/tumor fusion vaccine. J Immunol 2003; 170(7); 3806-11.

[111]   Geiser AG, Letterio JJ, Kulkarni AB, Karlsson S, Roberts AB, Sporn MB. Transforming growth factor beta 1 (TGF-beta 1) controls expression of major histocompatibility genes in the postnatal mouse: aberrant histocompatibility antigen expression in the pathogenesis of the TGF-beta 1 null mouse phenotype. Proc Natl Acad Sci U S A 1993; 90(21); 9944-8.

[112]   Han G, Li F, Singh TP, et al. The pro-inflammatory role of TGFβ1: a paradox? Int J Biol Sci 2012; 8(2); 228-35.

[113] Yoshimura A, Wakabayashi Y, Mori T. Cellular and molecular basis for the regulation of inflammation by TGF-beta. J Biochem 2010; 147(6); 781-92.

[114] McDonald PP, Fadok VA, Bratton D, Henson PM. Transcriptional and translational regulation of inflammatory mediator production by endogenous TGF-beta in macrophages that have ingested apoptotic cells. J Immunol 1999; 163(11); 6164-72.

[115] Mantovani A, Sozzani S, Locati M, Allavena P, Sica A. Macrophage polarization: tumor-associated macrophages as a paradigm for polarized M2 mononuclear phagocytes. Trends Immunol 2002; 23(11); 549-55.

[116] Mantovani A, Locati M. Tumor-associated macrophages as a paradigm of macrophage plasticity, diversity, and polarization: lessons and open questions. Arterioscler Thromb Vasc Biol 2013; 33(7); 1478-83.

[117] Park CC, Bissell MJ, Barcellos-Hoff MH. The influence of the microenvironment on the malignant phenotype. Mol Med Today 2000; 6(8); 324-9.

[118] Chen JJ, Sun Y, Nabel GJ. Regulation of the proinflammatory effects of Fas ligand (CD95L). Science 1998; 282(5394); 1714-7.

[119] Fridlender ZG, Albelda SM. Tumor-associated neutrophils: friend or foe? Carcinogenesis 2012; 33(5); 949-55.

[120] Ghiringhelli F, Puig PE, Roux S, *et al*. Tumor cells convert immature myeloid dendritic cells into TGF-beta-secreting cells inducing CD4+CD25+ regulatory T cell proliferation. J Exp Med 2005; 202(7); 919-29.

[121] Wrzesinski SH, Wan YY, Flavell RA. Transforming growth factor-beta and the immune response: implications for anticancer therapy. Clin Cancer Res 2007; 13(18 Pt 1); 5262-70.

[122] Geissmann F, Revy P, Regnault A, *et al*. TGF-beta 1 prevents the noncognate maturation of human dendritic Langerhans cells. J Immunol 1999; 162(8); 4567-75.

[123] Chaux P, Favre N, Bonnotte B, Moutet M, Martin M, Martin F. Tumor-infiltrating dendritic cells are defective in their antigen-presenting function and inducible B7 expression. A role in the immune tolerance to antigenic tumors. Adv Exp Med Biol 1997; 417; 525-8.

[124] Tian M and Schiemann WP. The TGF-β Paradox in Human Cancer: An Update. Future Oncol 2009; 5(2); 259–271.

[125] Ivanovic V, Todorovic-Rakovic N, Demajo M, *et al*. Elevated plasma levels of transforming growth factorB1 (TGF-B1) in patients with advanced breast cancer: association with disease progression. Eur J Cancer 2003; 39; 454-61.

[126] Wikstrom P, Stattin P, Franck-Lissbrant I, Damber JE, Bergh A. Transforming growth factor B1 is associated with angiogenesis, me tastasis, and poor clinical outcome in prostate cancer. Prostate 1998; 37; 19-29.

[127] Friess H, Yamanaka Y, Buchler M, *et al*. Enhanced expression of transforming growth factor b isoforms in pancreatic cancer correlates with decreased survival. Gastroenterology 1993; 105; 1846-5.

[128] Wunderlich H, Steiner T, Kosmehl H, *et al*. Increased transforming growth factor B1 plasma level in patients with renal cell carcinoma: a tumor-specific marker? Urol Int 1998; 60; 205-7.

[129] Redondo S, Navarro-Dorado J, Ramajo M, Medina Ú, Tejerina T. The complex regulation of TGF-β in cardiovascular disease. Vasc Health Risk Manag 2012; 8; 533-9.

[130] Keller JR, McNiece IK, Sill KT, *et al*. Transforming growth factor beta directly regulates primitive murine hematopoietic cell proliferation. Blood 1990; 75; 596-602.

[131] Ohta M, Greenberger JS, Anklesaria P, Bassols A, Massague J. Two forms of transforming growth factor-beta distinguished by multipotential haematopoietic progenitor cells. Nature 1987; 329; 539-41.

[132] Li MO, Wan YY, Sanjabi S, *et al.* Transforming growth factor-beta regulation of immune responses. Annu Rev Immunol 2006; 24; 99–146.

[133] Wahl SM. Transforming growth factor-beta: innately bipolar. Curr Opin Immunol 2007; 19;55-62.

[134] Koopmans SM, van Marion AM, Schouten HC. Myeloproliferative neoplasia: a review of clinical criteria and treatment. Neth J Med 2012; 70(4); 159-67.

[135] Kuroda H, Matsunaga T, Terui T, *et al.* Decrease of Smad4 gene expression in patients with essential thrombocythaemia may cause an escape from suppression of megakaryopoiesis by transforming growth factor-beta1. Br J Haematol 2004; 124; 211-20.

[136] Rooke HM, Vitas MR, Crosier PS, Crosier KE. The TGF-beta type II receptor in chronic myeloid leukemia: analysis of microsatellite regions and gene expression. Leukemia 1999; 13; 535-41.

[137] Dong M, Blobe GC. Role of transforming growth factor-beta in hematologic malignancies. Blood 2006; 107(12); 4589-96.

[138] Le Bousse-Kerdiles MC, Chevillard S, Charpentier A, *et al.* Differential expression of transforming growth factor-beta, basic fibroblast growth factor, and their receptors in CD34 hematopoietic progenitor cells from patients with myelofibrosis and myeloid metaplasia. Blood. 1996; 88; 4534-46

[139] Chagraoui H, Wendling F, Vainchenker W. Pathogenesis of myelofibrosis with myeloid metaplasia: Insight from mouse models. Best Pract Res Clin Haematol 2006; 19(3); 399-412.

[140] Vannucchi AM. Management of myelofibrosis. Hematology Am Soc Hematol Educ Program 2011; 2011; 222–30.

[141] Campanelli R, Rosti V, Villani L, *et al.* Evaluation of the bioactive and total transforming growth factor β1 levels in primary myelofibrosis. Cytokine 2011; 53(1); 100-6.

[142] Ponce CC, de Lourdes F Chauffaille M, Ihara SS, Silva MR. The relationship of the active and latent forms of TGF-β1 with marrow fibrosis in essential thrombocythemia and primary myelofibrosis. Med Oncol 2012; 29(4); 2337-44.

[143] Chagraoui H, Komura H, Tulliez E, *et al.* Prominent role of TGF-beta 1 in thrombopoietin-induced myelofibrosis in mice. Blood 2002; 100; 3495–503.

[144] Vannucchi AM, Bianchi L, Paoletti F, *et al.* A pathobiologic pathway linking thrombopoietin, GATA-1, and TGF-beta1 in the development of myelofibrosis. Blood 2005; 105; 3493-501.

[145] Gastinne T, Vigant F, Lavenu-Bombled C, *et al.* Adenoviral-mediated TGF-beta1 inhibition in a mouse model of myelofibrosis inhibit bone marrow fibrosis development. Exp Hematol 2007; 35(1); 64-74.

[146] Simonet WS, Lacey DL, Dunstan CR, *et al.* Osteoprotegerin: a novel secreted protein involved in the regulation of bone density. Cell 1997; 89; 309–19.

[147] Takai H, Kanematsu M, Yano K, *et al.* Transforming growth factor-beta stimulates the production of osteoprotegerin/osteoclastogenesis inhibitory factor by bone marrow stromal cells. J Biol Chem 1998; 273(42); 27091-6.

[148] Chagraoui H, Tulliez M, Smayra T, *et al.* Stimulation of osteoprotegerin production is responsible for osteosclerosis in mice overexpressing TPO. Blood 2003; 101; 2983–89.

[149] Ahamed J, Janczak CA, Wittkowski KM, Coller BS. *In vitro* and *in vivo* evidence that thrombospondin-1 (TSP-1) contributes to stirring- and shear-dependent activation of platelet-derived TGF-beta1. PLoS One 2009; 4(8); e6608.

[150] Evrard S, Bluteau O, Tulliez M, *et al.* Thrombospondin-1 is not the major activator of TGF-β1 in thrombopoietin-induced myelofibrosis. Blood 2011; 117(1); 246-9.

[151] Abdelouahed M, Ludlow A, Brunner G, Lawler J. Activation of platelet-transforming growth factor beta-1 in the absence of thrombospondin-1. J Biol Chem 2000; 275(24); 17933-6.

[152] Ciurea SO, Merchant D, Mahmud N, *et al.* Pivotal contributions of megakaryocytes to the biology of idiopathic myelofibrosis. Blood 2007; 110(3); 986-93.

[153] Quintanilla M, del Castillo G, Kocic J, Santibanez JF. (2012) TGF-B and MMPs: A Complex Regulatory Loop Involved in Tumor Progression. In: Matrix Metalloproteinases: Biology, Functions and Clinical Implications. Editors: Namae Oshiro and Eiko Miyagi. Nova Science Publishers.

[154] Rameshwar P, Narayanan R, Qian J, Denny TN, Colon C, Gascon P. NF-kappa B as a central mediator in the induction of TGF-beta in monocytes from patients with idiopathic myelofibrosis: an inflammatory response beyond the realm of homeostasis. J Immunol 2000; 165(4); 2271-7.

[155] Cairo MS. Myelofibrosis with myeloid metaplasia: targeted therapy. Blood 2007; 110(1); 2-3.

[156] Kaushansky K. The chronic myeloproliferative disorders and mutation of JAK2: Dameshek's 54 year old speculation comes of age. Best Pract Res Clin Haematol 2007; 20(1); 5-12.

[157] Dees C, Tomcik M, Palumbo-Zerr K, *et al.* JAK-2 as a novel mediator of the profibrotic effects of transforming growth factor β in systemic sclerosis. Arthritis Rheum 2012; 64(9); 3006-15.

[158] Sato Y, Suda T, Suda J, *et al.* Multilineage expression of haemopoietic precursors with an abnormal clone in idiopathic myelofibrosis. Br J Haematol 1986; 64(4); 657-67.

[159] Komura E, Tonetti C, Penard-Lacronique V, *et al.* Role for the nuclear factor kappaB pathway in transforming growth factor-beta1 production in idiopathic myelofibrosis: possible relationship with FK506 binding protein 51 overexpression. Cancer Res 2005; 65; 3281-89.

[160] Barosi, B. Myelofibrosis with myeloid metaplasia: diagnostic definition and prognostic classification for clinical studies and treatment guidelines. J Clin Oncol 1999; 17(9); 2954-70.

[161] Tlsty TD, Coussens LM. Tumor stroma and regulation of cancer development. Annu Rev Pathol 2006; 1; 119-50.

[162] Ganss R. Tumor stroma fosters neovascularization by recruitment of progenitor cells into the tumor bed. J Cell Mol Med 2006; 10(4); 857-65.

[163] Naber HP, ten Dijke P, Pardali E. Role of TGF-beta in the tumor stroma. Curr Cancer Drug Targets 2008; 8(6); 466-72.

[164] Pardali E, Goumans MJ, ten Dijke P. Signaling by members of the TGF-beta family in vascular morphogenesis and disease. Trends Cell Biol 2010; 20(9); 556-67.

[165] Giordano FJ, Johnson RS. Angiogenesis: the role of the microenvironment in flipping the switch. Curr Opin Genet Dev 2001; 11(1); 35-40.

[166] Lafleur MA, Handsley MM, Edwards DR. Metalloproteinases and their inhibitors in angiogenesis. Expert Rev Mol Med 2003; 5(23); 1-39.

[167] McDonald DM, Baluk P. Significance of blood vessel leakiness in cancer. Cancer Res 2002; 62; 5381–85.

[168] Hirschi KK, Rohovsky SA, D'Amore PA. PDGF, TGFbeta, and heterotypic cell-cell interactions mediate endothelial cell-induced recruitment of 10T1/2 cells and their differentiation to a smooth muscle fate. J Cell Biol 1998; 141; 805–14.

[169] Chambers RC, Leoni P, Kaminski N, Laurent GJ, Heller RA. Global expression profiling of fibroblast responses to transforming growth factor-beta1 reveals the induction of inhibitor of differentiation-1 and provides evidence of smooth muscle cell phenotypic switching. Am J Pathol 2003; 162; 533–46.

[170] Blanco FJ, Santibanez JF, Guerrero-Esteo M, Langa C, Vary CP, Bernabeu C. Interaction and functional interplay between endoglin and ALK-1, two components of the endothelial transforming growth factor-beta receptor complex. J Cell Physiol 2005; 204(2); 574-84.

[171] Goumans MJ, Valdimarsdottir G, Itoh S, Rosendahl A, Sideras P, ten Dijke P. Balancing the activation state of the endothelium *via* two distinct TGF-beta type I receptors. EMBO J 2002; 21(7); 1743-53.

[172] Goumans MJ, Liu Z, ten Dijke P. TGF-beta signaling in vascular biology and dysfunction. Cell Res 2009; 19(1); 116-27.

[173] López-Novoa JM, Bernabeu C. The physiological role of endoglin in the cardiovascular system. Am J Physiol Heart Circ Physiol 2010; 299(4); H959-74.

[174] Lebrin F, Goumans MJ, Jonker L, *et al*. Endoglin promotes endothelial cell proliferation and TGF-beta/ALK1 signal transduction. EMBO J 2004; 23(20); 4018-28.

[175] Santibanez JF, Letamendia A, Perez-Barriocanal F, *et al*. Endoglin increases eNOS expression by modulating Smad2 protein levels and Smad2-dependent TGF-beta signaling. J Cell Physiol 2007; 210(2); 456-68.

[176] Santibanez JF, Blanco FJ, Garrido-Martin EM, Sanz-Rodriguez F, del Pozo MA, Bernabeu C. Caveolin-1 interacts and cooperates with the transforming growth factor-beta type I receptor ALK1 in endothelial caveolae. Cardiovasc Res 2008; 77(4); 791-9.

[177] Schwartz EA, Reaven E, Topper JN, Tsao PS. Transforming growth factor-beta receptors localize to caveolae and regulate endothelial nitric oxide synthase in normal human endothelial cells. Biochem J 2005; 390(Pt 1); 199-206.

[178] Goumans MJ, Valdimarsdottir G, Itoh S, *et al*. Activin receptor- like kinase (ALK)1 is an antagonistic mediator of lateral TGFβ/ALK5 signaling. Mol Cell 2003; 12; 817-28.

[179] Urness LD, Sorensen LK, Li DY. Arteriovenous malformations in mice lacking activin receptor-like kinase-1. Nat Genet 2000; 26(3); 328-31.

[180] Oh SP, Seki T, Goss KA, *et al*. Activin receptor-like kinase 1 modulates transforming growth factor- 1 signaling in the regulation of angiogenesis. Proc Natl Acad Sci USA 2000; 97; 2626–31.

[181] Larsson J, Goumans MJ, Sjostrand LJ, *et al*. Abnormal angiogenesis but intact hematopoietic potential in TGF- type I receptor-deficient mice. EMBO J 2001; 20; 1663–73.

[182] Oshima M, Oshima H, Taketo MM. TGF-beta receptor type II deficiency results in defects of yolk sac hematopoiesis and vasculogenesis. Dev Biol 1996; 179(1); 297-302

[183] Li DY, Sorensen LK, Brooke BS, *et al*. Defective angiogenesis in mice lacking endoglin. Science 1999; 284(5419); 1534-7.

[184] Yang X, Castilla LH, Xu X, *et al.* Angiogenesis defects and mesenchymal apoptosis in mice lacking SMAD5. Development 1999; 126(8); 1571-80.

[185] Weinstein M, Yang X, Deng C Functions of mammalian Smad genes as revealed by targeted gene disruption in mice. Cytokine Growth Factor Rev 2000; 11(1-2); 49-58.

[186] Lan Y, Liu B, Yao H, Li F, *et al.* Essential role of endothelial Smad4 in vascular remodeling and integrity. Mol Cell Biol 2007; 27(21); 7683-92.

[187] Qiu P, Ritchie RP, Fu Z, *et al.* Myocardin enhances Smad3-mediated transforming growth factor-beta1 signaling in a CArGbox-independent manner: Smad-binding element is an important cis element for SM22alpha transcription *in vivo*. Circ Res 2005; 97; 983-991.

[188] Feinberg MW, Watanabe M, Lebedeva MA, *et al.* Transforming growth factor-β1 inhibition of vascular smooth muscle cell activation is mediated *via* Smad3. J Biol Chem 2004; 279; 16388-93.

[189] Lin DW, Chang IC, Tseng A, *et al.* Transforming growth factor b up-regulates cysteine-rich protein 2 in vascular smooth muscle cells *via* activating transcription factor 2. J Biol Chem 2008; 283; 15003-14.

[190] Ding R, Darland DC, Parmacek MS, D'Amore PA. Endothelial- mesenchymal interactions *in vitro* reveal molecular mechanisms of smooth muscle/pericyte differentiation. Stem Cells Dev 2004; 13; 509-520.

[191] Yamamoto T, Kozawa O, Tanabe K, *et al.* Involvement of p38 MAP kinase in TGF-b-stimulated VEGF synthesis in aortic smooth muscle cells. J Cell Biochem 2001; 82; 591-598.

[192] Zeisberg EM, Potenta S, Xie L, Zeisberg M, Kalluri R. Discovery of endothelial to mesenchymal transition as a source for carcinoma associated fibroblasts. Zeisberg EM. Cancer Res 2007; 67(21); 10123-28.

[193] Potenta S, Zeisberg E, Kalluri R. The role of endothelial-to-mesenchymal transition in cancer progression. Br J Cancer 2008; 99(9); 1375-9.

[194] de Jong JS, van Diest PJ, van der Valk P, Baak JP. Expression of growth factors, growth inhibiting factors, and their receptors in invasive breast cancer. I: An inventory in search of autocrine and paracrine loops. J Pathol 1998; 184(1); 44-52.

[195] Ananth S, Knebelmann B, Grüning W, *et al.* Transforming growth factor beta1 is a target for the von Hippel-Lindau tumor suppressor and a critical growth factor for clear cell renal carcinoma. Cancer Res 1999; 59(9); 2210-6.

[196] Sunderkötter C, Goebeler M, Schulze-Osthoff K, Bhardwaj R, Sorg C. Macrophage-derived angiogenesis factors. Pharmacol Ther 1991; 51(2); 195-216.

[197] Pertovaara L, Kaipainen A, Mustonen T, *et al.* Vascular endothelial growth factor is induced in response to transforming growth factor-beta in fibroblastic and epithelial cells. J Biol Chem 1994; 269(9); 6271-4.

[198] Sánchez-Elsner T, Botella LM, Velasco B, Corbí A, Attisano L, Bernabéu C. Synergistic cooperation between hypoxia and transforming growth factor-beta pathways on human vascular endothelial growth factor gene expression. J Biol Chem 2001; 276(42); 38527-35.

[199] Benjamin MM, Khalil RA. Matrix metalloproteinase inhibitors as investigative tools in the pathogenesis and management of vascular disease. EXS 2012; 103; 209-79.

[200] Medinger M, Mross K. Clinical trials with anti-angiogenic agents in hematological malignancies. J Angiogenes Res 2010; 2; 10.

[201]   Medinger M, Skoda R, Gratwohl A, *et al.* Angiogenesis and vascular endothelial growth factor-/receptor expression in myeloproliferative neoplasms: correlation with clinical parameters and JAK2-V617F mutational status. Br J Haematol 2009; 146; 150–157

[202]   Kvasnicka HM, Thiele J. Bone marrow angiogenesis: methods of quantification and changes evolving in chronic myeloproliferative disorders. Histol Histopathol 2004; 19(4); 1245-60.

[203]   Mesa RA, Elliott MA, Tefferi A. Splenectomy in chronic myeloid leukemia and myelofibrosis with myeloid metaplasia. Blood Rev 2000; 14(3); 121-9.

[204]   Mesa RA, Hanson CA, Rajkumar SV, Schroeder G, Tefferi A. Evaluation and clinical correlations of bone marrow angiogenesis in myelofibrosis with myeloid metaplasia. Blood 2000; 96(10); 3374-80.

[205]   Le Bousse-Kerdilès MC, Martyré MC. Dual implication of fibrogenic cytokines in the pathogenesis of fibrosis and myeloproliferation in myeloid metaplasia with myelofibrosis. Ann Hematol 1999; 78(10); 437-44.

[206]   Le Bousse-Kerdilès MC, Martyré MC. Myelofibrosis: pathogenesis of myelofibrosis with myeloid metaplasia. French INSERM Research Network on Myelofibrosis with Myeloid Metaplasia. Springer Semin Immunopathol 1999; 21(4); 491-508.

[207]   Di Raimondo F, Palumbo GA, Molica S, Giustolisi R. Angiogenesis in chronic myeloproliferative diseases. Acta Haematol 2001; 106(4); 177-83.

[208]   Möhle R, Green D, Moore MA, Nachman RL, Rafii S. Constitutive production and thrombin-induced release of vascular endothelial growth factor by human megakaryocytes and platelets. Proc Natl Acad Sci U S A 1997; 94(2); 663-8.

[209]   Bellamy WT, Richter L, Frutiger Y, Grogan TM. Expression of vascular endothelial growth factor and its receptors in hematopoietic malignancies. Cancer Res 1999; 59(3); 728-33.

[210]   Berse B, Hunt JA, Diegel RJ, *et al.* Hypoxia augments cytokine (transforming growth factor-beta (TGF-beta) and IL-1)-induced vascular endothelial growth factor secretion by human synovial fibroblasts. Clin Exp Immunol 1999; 115; 176-82.

[211]   Treliński J, Wierzbowska A, Krawczyńska A, *et al.* Plasma levels of angiogenic factors and circulating endothelial cells in essential thrombocythemia: correlation with cytoreductive therapy and JAK2-V617F mutational status. Leuk Lymphoma 2010; 51; 1727-33.

[212]   Murphy P, Ahmed N, Hassan HT. Increased serum levels of vascular endothelial growth factor correlate with splenomegaly in polycythemia vera. Leuk Res 2002; 26(11); 1007-10.

[213]   Alonci A, Allegra A, Bellomo G, *et al.* Evaluation of circulating endothelial cells, VEGF and VEGFR2 serum levels in patients with chronic myeloproliferative diseases. Hematol Oncol 2008; 26; 235–9.

[214]   Fang S, Pentinmikko N, Ilmonen M, Salven P. Dual action of TGF-β induces vascular growth *in vivo* through recruitment of angiogenic VEGF-producing hematopoietic effector cells. Angiogenesis 2012; 15; 511-9.

[215]   Ferrari G, Cook BD, Terushkin V, Pintucci G, Mignatti P. Transforming growth factor-beta 1 (TGF-beta1) induces angiogenesis through vascular endothelial growth factor (VEGF)-mediated apoptosis. J Cell Physiol 2009; 219; 449-58.

[216]   Chae KS, Kang MJ, Lee JH, *et al.* Opposite functions of HIF-α isoforms in VEGF induction by TGF-β1 under non-hypoxic conditions. Oncogene 2011; 30; 1213-28.

[217]   Niu G, Wright KL, Huang M, *et al.* Constitutive Stat3 activity up-regulates VEGF expression and tumor angiogenesis. Oncogene 2002; 21; 2000–8.

[218] Koopmans SM, Bot FJ, Schouten HC, Janssen J, van Marion AM. The involvement of Galectins in the modulation of the JAK/STAT pathway in myeloproliferative neoplasia. Am J Blood Res 2012; 2(2); 119-27.

[219] Yang X, Meyer K, Friedl A. STAT5 and prolactin participate in a positive autocrine feedback loop that promotes angiogenesis. J Biol Chem 2013; 288(29); 21184-96.

[220] Hoermann G, Cerny-Reiterer S, Herrmann H, *et al*. Identification of oncostatin M as a JAK2 V617F-dependent amplifier of cytokine production and bone marrow remodeling in myeloproliferative neoplasms. FASEB J 2012; 26(2); 894-906.

[221] Nuzzolo ER, Iachininoto MG, Teofili L. Endothelial progenitor cells and thrombosis. Thromb Res. 2012; 129(3); 309-13.

[222] Yoder MC, Mead LE, Prater D, *et al*. Redefining endothelial progenitor cells *via* clonal analysis and hematopoietic stem/progenitor cell principals. Blood 2007; 109(5); 1801-1809.

[223] Sozer S, Fiel MI, Schiano T, Xu M, Mascarenhas J, Hoffman R. The presence of JAK2V617F mutation in the liver endothelial cells of patients with Budd-Chiari syndrome. Blood 2009; 113(21); 5246-9.

[224] Sozer S, Ishii T, Fiel MI, Wang J, *et al*. Human CD34+ cells are capable of generating normal and JAK2V617F positive endothelial like cells *in vivo*. Blood Cells Mol Dis 2009; 43(3); 304-12.

[225] Rosti V, Villani L, Riboni R, *et al*. Spleen endothelial cells from patients with myelofibrosis harbor the JAK2V617F mutation. Blood 2013; 121(2); 360-8.

[226] Yoshimoto M, Yoder MC. Developmental biology: Birth of the blood cell. Nature 2009; 457(7231); 801-3.

[227] Sun T, Zhang L. Thrombosis in myeloproliferative neoplasms with JAK2V617F mutation. Clin Appl Thromb Hemost 2013; 19(4); 374-81.

[228] Sonbol MB, Firwana B, Zarzour A, Morad M, Rana V, Tiu RV. Comprehensive review of JAK inhibitors in myeloproliferative neoplasms. Ther Adv Hematol 2013; 4(1); 15-35.

[229] Fiskus W, Verstovsek S, Manshouri T, *et al*. Heat shock protein 90 inhibitor is synergistic with JAK2 inhibitor and overcomes resistance to JAK2-TKI in human myeloproliferative neoplasm cells. Clin Cancer Res 2011; 17(23); 7347-58.

[230] Verstovsek S, Kantarjian HM, Estrov Z, *et al*. Long-term outcomes of 107 patients with myelofibrosis receiving JAK1/JAK2 inhibitor ruxolitinib: survival advantage in comparison to matched historical controls. Blood 2012; 120(6); 1202-9.

[231] Tefferi A, Litzow MR, Pardanani A. Long-term outcome of treatment with ruxolitinib in myelofibrosis. N Engl J Med 2011; 365; 1455–1457.

[232] Verstovsek S, Passamonti F, Rambaldi A, *et al*. Long-Term Efficacy and Safety Results From a Phase II Study of Ruxolitinib in Patients with Polycythemia Vera. Blood 2012; 120; A804.

[233] Pardanani A, Gotlib JR, Jamieson C, *et al*. Safety and efficacy of TG101348, a selective JAK2 inhibitor, in myelofibrosis. Journal of Clinical Oncology 2011; 29; 789–796.

[234] Pardanani A, Laborde RR, Lasho TL, *et al*. Safety and efficacy of CYT387, a JAK1 and JAK2 inhibitor, in myelofibrosis. Leukemia 2013; 27(6); 1322-7.

[235] Santos FP, Kantarjian HM, Jain N, *et al*. Phase 2 study of CEP-701, an orally available JAK2 inhibitor, in patients with primary or post-polycythemia vera/essential thrombocythemia myelofibrosis. Blood 2010; 115(6); 1131-6.

[236] Moliterno AR, Hexner E, Roboz GJ, *et al.* An Open-Label Study of CEP-701 in Patients with JAK2 V617F-Positive PV and ET: Update of 39 Enrolled Patients. ASH Annual Meeting Abstracts. 2009; 1(22); 753.

[237] Verstovsek S, Deeg HJ, Odenike O, Zhu J, *et al.* Phase 1/2 study of SB1518, a novel JAK2/FLT3 inhibitor, in the treatment of primary myelofibrosis. Blood 2010; 116; 3082.

[238] Wang Y, Fiskus W, Chong DG, *et al.* Cotreatment with panobinostat and JAK2 inhibitor TG101209 attenuates JAK2V617F levels and signalling and exerts synergistic cytotoxic effects against human myeloproliferative neoplastic cells. Blood 2009; 114; 5024–5033.

[239] DeAngelo DJ, Mesa RA, Fiskus W, *et al.* Phase II trial of panobinostat, an oral pan-deacetylase inhibitor in patients with primary myelofibrosis, post-essential thrombocythaemia, and post-polycythaemia vera myelofibrosis. Br J Haematol. 2013; 162(3); 326-35.

[240] Evrot E, Ebel N, Romanet V, *et al.* JAK1/2 and Pan-Deacetylase Inhibitor Combination Therapy Yields Improved Efficacy in Preclinical Mouse Models of JAK2V617F-Driven Disease. Clin Cancer Res. 2013; 19(22); 6230-41.

[241] Kalota A, Jeschke GR, Carroll M, Hexner EO. Intrinsic resistance to JAK2 inhibition in myelofibrosis. Clin Cancer Res. 2013; 19(7); 1729-39.

[242] Andersen CL, McMullin MF, Ejerblad E, *et al.* A phase II study of vorinostat (MK-0683) in patients with polycythaemia vera and essential thrombocythaemia. Br J Haematol 2013 ; 162(4); 498-508.

[243] Rambaldi A, Dellacasa CM, Finazzi G, *et al.* A pilot study of the Histone-Deacetylase inhibitor Givinostat in patients with JAK2V617F positive chronic myeloproliferative neoplasms. Br J Haematol. 2010 Aug; 150(4); 446-55.

[244] Finazzi G, Vannucchi AM, Martinelli V, *et al.* A phase II study of Givinostat in combination with hydroxycarbamide in patients with polycythaemia vera unresponsive to hydroxycarbamide monotherapy. Br J Haematol. 2013; 161(5); 688-94.

[245] Guglielmelli P, Barosi G, Rambaldi A, *et al.* Safety and efficacy of everolimus, a mTOR inhibitor, as single agent in a phase 1/2 study in patients with myelofibrosis. Blood 2011; 118(8); 2069-76.

[246] Bogani C, Bartalucci N, Martinelli S, *et al.* mTOR inhibitors alone and in combination with JAK2 inhibitors effectively inhibit cells of myeloproliferative neoplasms. PLoS One. 2013; 8(1); e54826.

[247] Fiskus W, Verstovsek S, Manshouri, *et al.* Dual PI3K/AKT/mTOR inhibitor BEZ235 synergistically enhances the activity of JAK2 inhibitor against cultured and primary human myeloproliferative neoplasm cells. Mol Cancer Ther. 2013 May; 12(5); 577-88.

[248] Bellido M, Te Boekhorst PA. JAK2 Inhibition: Reviewing a New Therapeutical Option in Myeloproliferative Neoplasms. Adv Hematol. 2012; 2012; 535709.

[249] Tefferi, A. Novel mutations and their functional and clinical relevance in myeloproliferative neoplasms: JAK2, MPL, TET2, ASXL1, CBL, IDH and IKZF1. Leukemia 2010; 24; 1128–1138.

[250] Mascarenhas J, Roper N, Chaurasia P, Hoffman R. Epigenetic abnormalities in myeloproliferative neoplasms: a target for novel therapeutic strategies. Clin Epigenetics 2011; 2(2); 197-212.

[251] Santos FP, Verstovsek S. What is next beyond janus kinase 2 inhibitors for primary myelofibrosis? : Curr Opin Hematol 2013; 20(2); 123-9.

[252] Steensma DP. Can hypomethylating agents provide a platform for curative therapy in myelodysplastic syndromes? Best Pract Res Clin Haematol 2012; 25(4); 443-51.

[253] Mikeska T, Bock C, Do H, Dobrovic A. DNA methylation biomarkers in cancer: progress towards clinical implementation. Expert Rev Mol Diagn 2012; 12(5); 473-87.

[254] Ververis K, Hiong A, Karagiannis TC, Licciardi PV. Histone deacetylase inhibitors (HDACIs): multitargeted anticancer agents. Biologics 2013; 7; 47-60.

[255] Lacy MQ, McCurdy AR. Pomalidomide. Blood 2013; 122(14):2305-2309.

[256] Daver N, Shastri A, Kadia T, *et al*. Modest activity of pomalidomide in patients with myelofibrosis and significant anemia. Leuk Res 2013; pii; S0145-2126(13)00234-8.

[257] Cheng H, Zhang Z, Borczuk A, *et al*. PARP inhibition selectively increases sensitivity to cisplatin in ERCC1-low non-small cell lung cancer cells. Carcinogenesis 2013; 34(4); 739-49.

[258] Zanaboni F, Grijuela B, Giudici S, *et al*. Weekly topotecan and cisplatin (TOPOCIS) as neo-adjuvant chemotherapy for locally-advanced squamous cervical carcinoma: Results of a phase II multicentric study. Eur J Cancer 2013; 49(5); 1065-72.

[259] Ying W, Du Z, Sun L, *et al*. Ganetespib, a unique triazolone-containing Hsp90 inhibitor, exhibits potent antitumor activity and a superior safety profile for cancer therapy. Mol Cancer Ther 2012; 11(2); 475-84.

[260] Kiladjian JJ, Cassinat B, Chevret S, *et al*. Pegylated interferon-alfa-2a induces complete hematologic and molecular responses with low toxicity in polycythemia vera. Blood 2008; 112(8); 3065-72.

[261] Quintás-Cardama A, Abdel-Wahab O, Manshouri T, *et al*. Molecular analysis of patients with polycythemia vera or essential thrombocythemia receiving pegylated interferon α-2a. Blood 2013; 122(6); 893-901.

[262] Lu M, Zhang W, Li Y, Berenzon D, *et al*. Interferon-alpha targets JAK2V617F-positive hematopoietic progenitor cells and acts through the p38 MAPK pathway. Exp Hematol 2010; 38; 472-80.

[263] Otten J, Bokemeyer C, Fiedler W. Tgf-Beta superfamily receptors-targets for antiangiogenic therapy? J Oncol 2010; 2010; 317068.

[264] Bogdahn U, Schneider T, Oliushine V, *et al*. Randomized, active-controlled phase IIb study with trabedersen (AP 12009) in recurrent or refractory high-grade glioma patients: basis for phase III endpoints. Journal of Clinical Oncology 2007; 27(15s); abstract 2037.

[265] Pennison M, Pasche B. Targeting transforming growth factor-beta signaling. Curr Opin Oncol 2007; 19(6); 579-85.

[266] Mitchell D, Pobre EG, Mulivor AW, *et al*. ALK1-Fc inhibits multiple mediators of angiogenesis and suppresses tumor growth. Mol Cancer Ther 2010; 9(2); 379-88.

[267] Shukla MN, Rose JL, Ray R, Lathrop KL, Ray A, Ray P. Hepatocyte growth factor inhibits epithelial to myofibroblast transition in lung cells *via* Smad7. Am J Respir Cell Mol Biol 2009; 40(6); 643-53.

[268] Jinnin M, Ihn H, Tamaki K. Characterization of SIS3, a novel specific inhibitor of Smad3, and its effect on transforming growth factor-beta1-induced extracellular matrix expression. Mol Pharmacol 2006; 69(2); 597-607.

[269] Zhou J, Zhong DW, Wang QW, Miao XY, Xu XD. Paclitaxel ameliorates fibrosis in hepatic stellate cells *via* inhibition of TGF-beta/Smad activity. World J Gastroenterol 2010; 16(26); 3330-4.

[270] Zhao BM, Hoffmann FM. Inhibition of transforming growth factor-beta1-induced signaling and epithelial-to-mesenchymal transition by the Smad-binding peptide aptamer Trx-SARA. Mol Biol Cell 2006; 17(9); 3819-31.

[271] Yamada H, Tajima S, Nishikawa T. Tranilast inhibits collagen synthesis in normal, scleroderma and keloid fibroblasts at a late passage culture but not at an early passage culture. J Dermatol Sci 1995; 9; 45–47.

[272] Xu Q, Norman JT, Shrivastav S, *et al*. *In vitro* models of TGF-beta-induced fibrosis suitable for high-throughput screening of antifibrotic agents. Am J Physiol Renal Physiol 2007; 293; F631–F640.

[273] Chowdhury S, Ammanamanchi S, Howell GM. Epigenetic Targeting of Transforming Growth Factor beta Receptor II and Implications for Cancer Therapy. Mol Cell Pharmacol 2009; 1(1); 57-70.

[274] Venkatasubbarao K, Ammanamanchi S, Brattain MG, Mimari D, Freeman JW. Reversion of transcriptional repression of Sp1 by 5 aza-2′ deoxycytidine restores TGF-beta type II receptor expression in the pancreatic cancer cell line MIA PaCa-2. Cancer Res 2001; 61; 6239–47.

[275] Huang W, Zhao S, Ammanamanchi S, Brattain M, Venkatasubbarao K, Freeman JW. Trichostatin A induces transforming growth factor beta type II receptor promoter activity and acetylation of Sp1 by recruitment of PCAF/p300 to a Sp1. NF-Y complex. J Biol Chem 2005; 280; 10047–54.

[276] Gisslinger H, Harutyunyan AS, Nivarthi H, *et al*. Frequent Mutations in the Calreticulin Gene CALR in Myeloproliferative Neoplasms. Blood 2013; 122(21); LBA-1.

[277] Massie C, Baxter EJ, Nice FL, *et al*. The Genomic Landscape of Myeloproliferative Neoplasms: Somatic Calr Mutations in the Majority of JAK2-Wildtype Patients. Blood 2013; 122(21); LBA-2.

[278] Wang WA, Groenendyk J, Michalak M. Calreticulin signaling in health and disease. Int J Biochem Cell Biol 2012; 44(6); 842-6.

[279] Zamanian M, Veerakumarasivam A, Abdullah S, Rosli R. Calreticulin and cancer. Pathol Oncol Res. 2013; 19(2); 149-54.

Frontiers in Anti-Cancer Drug Discovery, 2014, 3, 109-150   109

CHAPTER 3

Targeted Anti-Cancer Therapy, Acquiring and Overcoming Multi-Drug Resistance

Milica Pesic, Jasna Bankovic and Nikola Tanic[*]

Institute for Biological Research "Sinisa Stankovic", University of Belgrade, Belgrade, Serbia

Abstract: Although advances have been made in reducing mortality rates and improving survival, cancer is still the second world cause of death among men and women. Such an unfavorable prognosis is a consequence of its complex genetic nature that makes it difficult to diagnose and treat. Moreover, due to inherent ability of cancer cells to acquire resistance to cytotoxic agents, most therapies eventually fail, resulting in resumption of disease progression. Therefore, the call for the discovery of less toxic, more selective, and more effective agents to treat cancer has become most urgent. At this moment, molecular targeted therapy looks most promising. Small-molecule and antibody therapeutics against targets implicated in PI3K-Akt pathway such as EGFR (*e.g.,* cetuximab, gefitinib), erbB2 (trastuzumab, lapatinib), mTOR (sirolimus, temsirolimus), in tumor angiogenesis such as VEGFR (bevacizumab, sunitinib) and αvβ3 integrin receptors (cilengitide) as well as against other tyrosine kinases such as Abl (imatinib, nilotinib), have delivered clinical efficacy in certain disease settings. The emergence of these therapies has led to an era of treatments increasingly aimed at certain patient populations, and this has implications for the development of future novel treatments. However, cancer cells could develop the resistance to anti-cancer drugs in molecular targeted therapy, like in conventional chemotherapy, by several mechanisms. Resistance mechanisms include increased DNA damage repair, reduced apoptosis, altered drug metabolism and site of action, increased energy-dependent efflux of hydrophobic anticancer agents that enter cells. The latter refers to multi-drug resistance (MDR) which is one of the major and most common obstacles for the effective treatment of cancer. The most frequent mechanism underlying MDR is over-expression of P-glycoprotein (P-gp)/MDR1/ABCB1 which acts as an efflux pump for various hydrophobic anticancer drugs. Among them are anticancer drugs of previous generations (such as anthracyclines, Vinca alkaloids, taxanes, epipodophyllotoxins), of new generation (*e.g.,* imatinib, nilotinib, everolimus), as well as other tumor signal transduction inhibitors currently undergoing clinical investigation (aurora B kinase inhibitor AZD1152). The most striking feature of ABCB1 is its remarkable spectrum of substrates. Namely, ABCB1 recognizes and mediates the transport of thousands of substrates without specified structural determinants. Therefore, anti-ABCB1 therapy

*****Address correspondence to Nikola Tanic:** Institute for Biological Research "Sinisa Stankovic", University of Belgrade, Belgrade, Serbia; Tel: + 381 11 2078 410; Fax: +381 11 2761 433; E-mail: nikolata@sbb.rs

Atta-ur-Rahman & M. Iqbal Choudhary (Eds)

represents a significant step forward in cancer therapy. However, many things remain to be clarified, such as how to use anti ABCB1 therapeutics, what is the biological consequence of ABCB1-blockade, *etc*. We know that tumors are very diverse and plastic entities, able to adapt to various conditions. Lessons that we have learned in cancer research, taught us that the diversity of signal networks underlying tumor growth could eventually overcome our efforts in finding efficient therapeutic approaches. In this chapter, we present a reflection of new anti-cancer therapeutic strategies driven toward specific molecular targets, their benefits and limitations.

Keywords: ATP-binding cassette (ABC) transporters, multi-drug resistance (MDR), p53, P-glycoprotein (ABCB1), targeted anti-cancer therapy, tyrosine kinase inhibitor (TKI).

INTRODUCTION

The major clinical obstacle in cancer chemotherapy is the development of drug resistance. To overcome this problem, different combinatorial chemotherapy strategies with multiple agents exerting effects through different mechanisms have been designed. Unfortunately, cancer cells often develop multi-drug resistance (MDR), either intrinsic or acquired, to multiple classes of structurally unrelated drugs that do not have a common mechanism of action. Tumors with intrinsic drug resistance fail to respond to initial chemotherapy while the treatment with chemotherapeutic agents induces acquired resistance frequently observed in cancer patients [1, 2].

Several mechanisms are involved in the development of resistance to anti-cancer drugs:

1)   Decreased uptake of water-soluble drugs that enter cells *via* transporters;

2)   Increased DNA damage repair;

3)   Reduced apoptosis;

4)   Altered drug metabolism;

5)   Altered site of action;

6)   Increased energy-dependent efflux of hydrophobic anti-cancer agents [3].

This last point refers to the most relevant mechanisms underlying MDR - the cellular overproduction of P-glycoprotein (P-gp/MDR1/ABCB1), which is encoded by the *mdr1* gene and belongs to the large ATP-binding cassette (ABC) transporter family [4-6]. ABCB1 acts as an efflux pump for various hydrophobic anti-cancer drugs, such as anthracyclines, Vinca alkaloids, taxanes, epipodophyllotoxins, and some of the newer anti-cancer drugs (*e.g.,* imatinib, nilotinib, everolimus) [7], as well as other tumor signal transduction inhibitors currently undergoing clinical investigation (*e.g.,* the aurora B kinase inhibitor AZD1152) [8].

Generally, all hydrophobic small molecular mass compounds of foreign origin can be recognized and eliminated by ABC transporters, particularly ABCB1. Clinically used and FDA approved new targeted therapies interact with ABC transporters at the cellular and tissue barriers [9]. This so-called "chemo-immune" system recognizes new drugs as xenobiotics at the membrane level and protects intracellular targets from their action. Interestingly, induced expression of ABCB1 is probably a transient event that needs the presence of the cytotoxic drug to activate stress-activated molecular changes. Accordingly, clinical studies proved that chemotherapy-induced up-regulation of MDR transporter genes occurs rapidly (within 24 h) from the beginning of the treatment [10]. A similar trend was observed by comparing pre- and post-chemotherapy samples [10].

MDR transporters have been recognized as important determinants of the general ADME-Tox (absorption, distribution, metabolism, excretion, toxicity) properties of small molecules [9]. In the age of the individualized therapies, it is important to identify the molecular background of the concrete malignancy and xenobiotics-managing characteristics of each patient. Considering that MDR transporter expression shows great inter-individual variability, individual responses need to be followed as well as early changes in gene expression levels in patients, immediately after the treatment with chemotherapeutics. Therefore, new anti-cancer agents, including targeted drugs should be designed to evade the xenobiotic defense mechanisms.

MAIN MOLECULAR TARGETS IN CANCER

Cancer is usually associated with aberrant cell cycle progression and defective apoptosis induction due to the activation of proto-oncogenes and/or inactivation of tumor suppressor genes [11]. Proper strategies for combating cancer by inhibiting its deregulated proliferation, survival and anti-apoptotic signaling, are emerging in treatment of this metastatic and incurable disease.

One of the most promising targets is p53, a well-established and frequently mutated tumor suppressor in human cancer. p53 plays central role in cancer prevention and suppression. Consequently, its function has to be inactivated during carcinogenesis allowing most cancers to arise. Indeed, p53 is inactivated by point mutations in more than 50% of human cancers (http://www.iarc.fr/p53) with a majority of mutations occurring in the DNA binding domain, which either change wild-type (wt) p53 conformation or abolish its DNA contact [12].

Furthermore, in cancer carrying a wt p53, p53 is often degraded by over-expressed Mdm2 [13] or excluded from the nucleus where it acts as a transcriptional factor [14]. It has been proved that altered *p53* influenced survival of patients with glioma [15].

Sorting out the complex network of signaling proteins that govern neoplastic transformation has opened up a new era in cancer treatment. Modulation or disruption of the major signaling pathways that control the abnormal proliferation and survival of cancer cells seems to be a breakthrough in cancer treatment [16]. By occupying key positions in the highly activated signaling pathways on which cancer cells depend [17], kinases have become attractive targets for inhibition of cancer cell growth and survival.

Modifying the activity of their substrates by reversible phosphorylation on tyrosine and/or serine/threonine residues, protein kinases control various cellular processes:

1)   Metabolism;

2)   Transcription;

3)   Cell cycle progression;

4)   Cytoskeletal rearrangement and cell movement;

5)   Apoptosis;

6)   Differentiation.

Under physiological conditions, kinase activity is tightly controlled and regulated. However, mutations or other genetic alterations result in deregulated kinase activity *via* the perturbation of the normal auto-control mechanisms, thus leading to malignant transformation [18]. Over-expression, activation and mutations of protein kinases, especially protein tyrosine kinases, are connected with pathogenesis of various types of human cancer.

The total number of the revealed kinase genes constitutes about 1.7% of the human genes. The protein tyrosine kinase gene catalog contains 90 tyrosine kinase genes, of which 58 are receptor-type, while 32 are non-receptor-type tyrosine kinases [19].

A large fraction in the group of dominant oncogenes consists of protein tyrosine kinases [18]. The membrane-bound tyrosine kinases, termed as receptor tyrosine kinases (RTK) were among the first kinases to be identified and linked to tumorigenesis [20, 21]. RTKs bind polypeptide ligands which are mostly growth factors (Fig. **1**). Generally, they are activated after binding of the ligand. The activation induces oligomerization, in most cases - dimerization, followed by trans-phosphorylation of tyrosine residues of the intracellular receptor subunits. The phosphotyrosine residues serve as docking sites for proteins bearing Src homology-2 (SH2) or phosphotyrosine-binding (PTB) domains, which mediate further downstream signaling events [22].

Major downstream signaling pathways stimulated by RTKs include the Ras/Raf/MEK/ERK pathway involved in proliferation, and also the PI3K/Akt pathway important for the transduction of survival signals (Fig. **1**). Members of the ErbB family, VEGFR, c-KIT, FLT-3 and PDGFR have been the most extensively studied RTKs linked to malignant cell transformation.

Another large group of tyrosine kinases involved in cancer pathogenesis is comprised of intracellular non-receptor tyrosine kinases. Probably, the most extensively studied member of this group is the Bcr-Abl fusion protein. Bcr-Abl is coded by the bcr-abl chimeric gene generated from the reciprocal chromosome translocation between chromosomes 9 and 22. Abl is a non-receptor tyrosine kinase, expressed in most tissues. Under physiological conditions its activity is strictly regulated. The fusion of Bcr sequences to Abl during the translocation increases the tyrosine kinase activity of Abl. Bcr-Abl operates as an oncoprotein essential for the initiation, maintenance and progression of chronic myeloid leukemia (CML) [23].

Serine/threonine kinases have also been implicated in the pathogeneses of various types of cancer. Among them, mTOR (mammalian target of rapamycin) is responsible for the cell growth promotion and proliferation dependent on the availability of nutrients and energy. mTOR function is also stimulated by the PI3K/Akt pathway. Deregulated PI3K/Akt signaling and subsequent mTOR hyper-activation has been reported in hematological malignancies as well as in solid tumors. mTOR signaling was also activated in response to hypoxia and the expression of VEGF, suggesting that mTOR could mediate tumor angiogenesis [24, 25].

Integrins are heterodimeric cell surface adhesion receptors that consist of two non-covalently associated alpha and beta subunits. They function as receptors for various extracellular matrix proteins such as fibronectin, laminins, collagens, and vitronectin. Cellular protein kinases are indirectly or transiently connected to integrins (Fig. **1**). Ligand binding to the extracellular domain of integrin receptors results in receptor activation followed by transduction of signals essential for cell adhesion, migration, proliferation, differentiation, and survival. In addition, integrins mediate transfer of information on the status of the cells for the efficient remodeling of extracellular environment [26]. The integrins $\alpha v\beta 3$ and $\alpha v\beta 5$ appear to be particularly important in the process of angiogenesis and are expressed in a variety of malignancies. The critical role of integrins in angiogenesis and association with tumor progression make them an attractive target for anti-cancer therapy [27].

TARGETED ANTI-CANCER THERAPY

Various approaches for recovering p53 function have been evaluated (Fig. **1**):

1)   To activate wt p53;

2)   To reactivate mutant p53 or selectively kill cancer cells with mutant p53;

3)   To temporarily inhibit wt p53 for normal cell protection [28].

Gene therapy using human wt p53, delivered by replication-defective adenovirus (Ad-p53), under the brand name of Gendicine, or Advexin (Table 1), has been in clinical use in China since 2003 [29] and in phase 1 to 3 clinical trial in the United States [30]. Gendicine/Advexin is well tolerated by patients and is particularly efficacious in the treatment of head and neck cancer and lung cancer, as a single agent or in combination with chemotherapy or radiation therapy [31, 32]. Another p53-related gene therapy is the use of an E1B-deleted adenovirus, designated as ONYX-015, which selectively replicates in p53-deficient cancer cells and subsequently lyse the cells [33]. ONYX-015 had a marginal anti-cancer activity when administered alone, but a significant effect was obtained in combination with standard chemotherapies [31, 34, 35].

RITA (Reactivation of p53 and induction of cancer cell apoptosis) binds to p53 at the N-terminal domain with a high affinity and suppresses cancer cell growth by inducing massive apoptosis in a p53-dependent manner [36]. RITA-activated p53 causes the transcriptional repression of anti-apoptotic proteins, including Mcl-1, Bcl-2, survivin, and MAP4, down-regulates oncogenic proteins, c-Myc, cyclin E, and β-catenin, and blocks the AKT pathway at multiple levels [37].

Temporary blockage of p53 activation in normal cells during the treatment of p53-deficient tumors should reduce these adverse effects [38]. Two classes of small molecules have been identified, Pifithrin (PFT)-α and PFT-μ which target either p53 transcriptional activity or p53-mitochondrial binding activity, respectively [39].

There are also other therapeutic possibilities relying on reactivation of p53 mutants. The rescue strategies vary, dependent on the mutation types. CDB3 is a short synthetic nine-residue peptide, derived from p53-binding protein 2 that interacts with the p53 core domain and up-regulates p53-dependent trans-activation [40]. CDB3 restores the sequence-specific DNA binding to various p53 mutants by stabilizing them in a bioactive conformation [41]. Furthermore, CDB3 induces the accumulation of wt p53 and sensitizes cancer cells to radiation [42].

CP-31398 is small molecule that changes p53 conformation from mutant to wild type. CP-31398 stabilizes the core domain and enhances transcriptional activity of p53 [43], but the detailed mechanism of action of CP-31398 remains elusive. CP-31398 seems to have other targets in addition to p53 because it could induce cell death in both p53-dependent and -independent manners [44].

PRIMA-1 (p53 reactivation and induction of massive apoptosis) (Table **1**) and MIRA-1 (mutant p53 reactivation and induction of rapid apoptosis) are two classes of compounds with unique chemical structures [45, 46]. The compounds have been found to restore the sequence-specific DNA binding and change the mutant p53 conformation to wild type, leading to trans-activation of p53 target genes [45, 46]. Furthermore, PRIMA-1 has been found to be active against p53-null cancer cell lines through a mechanism involving the JNK pathway and heat shock protein 90 [47, 48].

Ellipticine changes the p53 conformation from mutant to wild type and activates mutant p53 to induce p53 target genes, p21 and Mdm2 [49]. Ellipticine also increases nuclear localization of both wt and mutant p53 in a manner independent of DNA damage [50].

WR-1065 (aminothiol) is an active metabolite of the cytoprotector amifostine and acts as a classic scavenger of reactive oxygen species [51]. WR-1065 has been found to activate both wt and mutant p53 and increase the expression of p53 target genes in a manner independent of DNA damage [51, 52].

Application of chemical compounds that selectively kill human cancer cells harboring a mutant p53 would be of major significance since 50% of human malignancies possess mutated p53. These drugs should have, in theory, minimal adverse effects, because normal cells do not contain a p53 mutation. Paclitaxel, an inhibitor of microtubule polymerization [53] has been identified as selective killer of cells with mutant p53. It is speculated that microtubule-associated protein 4, a p53 transcriptional repressed target, may mediate the sensitivity of cells lacking p53 activity to paclitaxel [54]. Another drug that selectively inhibits p53-deficient cancer cell growth is metformin, a diabetic drug that activates AMP kinase and inhibits oxidative phosphorylation [55].

Interestingly, cardiac glycoside drugs, such as digoxin and ouabain, reduce *de novo* synthesis of p53 protein [56].

Another effective approach to activate wt p53 is to inhibit its negative regulators. The best-known naturally occurring p53 inhibitor is its downstream target, Mdm2 [57]. Several classes of structurally distinctive compounds have been reported to disrupt Mdm2-p53 binding [58, 59]. These compounds include Nutlins (Table **1**), benzodiazepinediones (BDAs), and an Mdm2 inhibitor (MI) series of spiro-oxindoles derivatives, including MI-63, MI-219, and MI-43 [58-64].

The new generation of anti-cancer therapeutics includes two major forms of molecular entities, targeted monoclonal antibodies (mAbs) and small molecule tyrosine kinase inhibitors (TKI). In contrast to the use of mAbs, cell-penetrating small molecule TKIs can be equally effective against both membrane-bound and cytoplasmic targets. Gefitinib targets the intracellular kinase domain of the EGFR by blocking ATP binding and consequently auto-phosphorylation of the receptor [65]. Erlotinib and lapatinib are second generation inhibitors of EGFR and EGFR/HER2, respectively (Fig. **1**, Table **1**).

Bcr-Abl TKI imatinib (Glivec, STI571), currently the first-line therapy for CML, induces a complete cytogenetic response in most patients, especially those in the chronic phase of the disease (Table **1**). Imatinib is quite selective for Bcr-Abl, but it also inhibits other targets such as some RTKs (c-kit and PDGF-R) (Fig. **1**). Due to the extensive occurrence of imatinib resistant refractory leukemia, several novel Bcr-Abl inhibitors have been developed and are already in clinical use, such as the imatinib derivative compound nilotinib or the structurally unrelated dasatinib [66] (Table **1**).

Sunitinib is a multi-targeted TKI (Fig. **1**) that inhibits PDGFR, VEGFR, c-Kit, FMS-like TK-3 receptor and the glial cell-line derived neurotrophic factor receptor in an ATP-competitive manner [67]. Sunitinib is approved for the treatment of advanced renal cell carcinoma and imatinib-resistant gastrointestinal

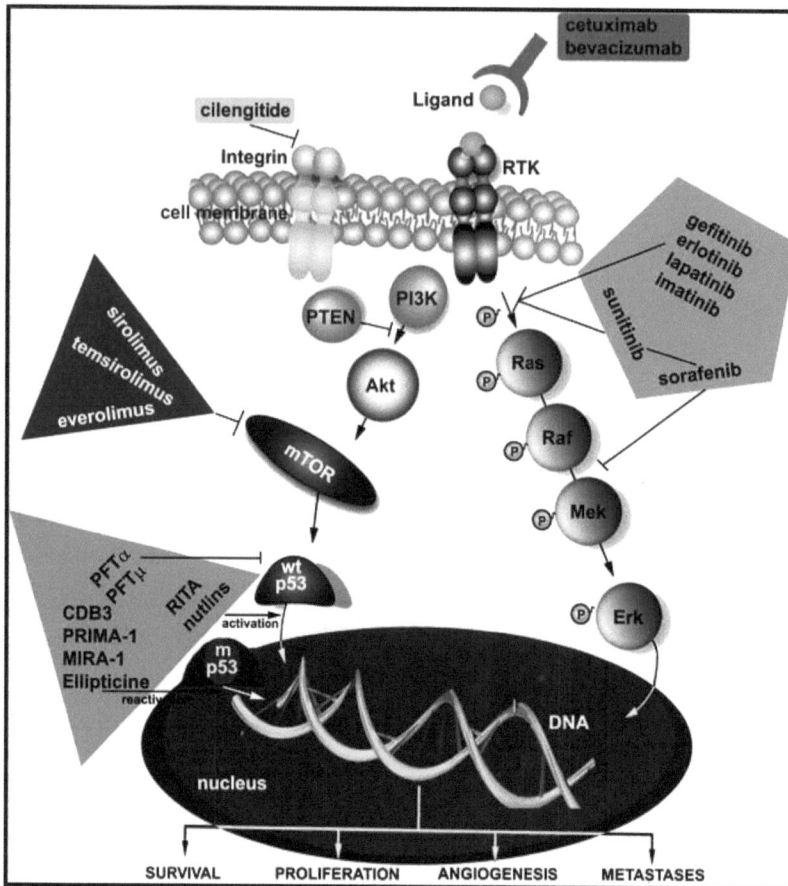

Fig. (1). Activated signaling pathways in cancer and associated molecularly targeted agents. A variety of mechanisms contribute to cancer chemoresistance including tumor hypoxia, expression of DNA repair enzymes and abrogation of apoptotic effector pathways by altered expression of genes such as *p53*. Also, a number of key signaling pathways are deregulated in cancer providing an opportunity for pharmacological intervention with targeted agents. RTK - receptor tyrosine kinase; wtp53 - wild-type p53; mp53 - mutated p53; Cilengitide inhibits the integrins αvβ3 and αvβ5, cetuximab acts as ligand for EGFR while bevacizumab acts as ligand for VEGFR. Gefitinib and erlotinib inhibit the tyrosine kinase part of EGFR, lapatinib inhibits EGFR/HER2, imatinib inhibits c-KIT, PDGFR, Bcr-Abl. Sunitinib and sorafenib inhibit c-KIT, FLT-3, PDGFR and VEGFR. Sirolimus, everolimus, temsirolimus inhibit mTOR. Pifithrin (PFT)-α and PFT-μ inhibit either p53 transcriptional activity or p53-mitochondrial binding activity, respectively. RITA (reactivation of p53 and induction of cancer cell apoptosis) binds to p53 and induces massive apoptosis in a p53-dependent manner while nutlins disrupt Mdm2-p53 binding. CDB3 up-regulates p53-dependent trans-activation, p53 PRIMA-1 (reactivation and induction of massive apoptosis) and MIRA-1 (mutant p53 reactivation and induction of rapid apoptosis) restore the sequence-specific DNA binding and change the mutant p53 conformation to wild type. Ellipticine changes the p53 conformation from mutant to wild type and activates mutant p53 to induce p53 target genes, p21 and Mdm2.

stromal tumors (Table **1**). Sorafenib is a multi-kinase inhibitor with a similar target kinase spectrum (Fig. **1**) approved for the treatment of patients with advanced renal cell carcinoma and hepatocellular carcinoma [68] (Table **1**).

Rapamycin (sirolimus), a naturally occurring compound isolated from the soil bacterium *Streptomyces hydroscopius*, was originally used as an antifungal and immunosuppressive agent [69]. Subsequent discovery of mTOR as the target of rapamycin and the drug's inherent anti-proliferative properties led to investigation of this compound as an anti-cancer agent (Fig. **1**, Table **1**). Limitations in the solubility and pharmacokinetic properties of rapamycin resulted in the development of the first generation of rapamycin analogs (rapalogs), including temsirolimus (CCI-779, Wyeth, NJ), everolimus (RADD001, Novartis, Basel, Switzerland), and ridaforolimus (AP23573, Ariad Pharmaceuticals, MA) (Table **1**).

Cilengitide (EMD 121974), a cyclic Arg-Gly-Glu (RGD) peptide is a potent and selective inhibitor of the integrins $\alpha v \beta 3$ and $\alpha v \beta 5$ [70]. Cilengitide has been well tolerated, with no significant toxicities, but with a modest anti-cancer activity (Table **1**).

ACQUIRED RESISTANCE TO TARGETED THERAPY

Since drugs are usually given systemically, their fate in the body is subject to individual variations of absorption, metabolism, and delivery to target tissues. In order to accumulate in cancer cells, they must pass through the membranes into diverse body compartments. Therefore, various membrane transporter proteins may modulate their accumulation at tumor site and into the cancer cells. In general, drugs may loose their desired activity due to systemic or cellular mechanisms [71].

The major limitation in the successful treatment of cancer patients with targeted therapies is the development of resistance to chemotherapeutic drugs. Experts for drug interactions usually focus on resistance mechanisms that are directly related to the specific target modulation. However, active efflux, mediated by MDR-ABC transporters, should also be considered as a major impediment to the successful clinical use of targeted therapeutics [9].

At least 12 out of the 48 human ABC proteins have been documented to contribute to the emergence of MDR [72]. Selection with cytotoxic drugs has been shown to induce the over-expression of endogenous ABCA2, ABCB1, ABCC1, ABCC2, ABCC4 and ABCG2. The major MDR-ABC proteins that are widely accepted to be responsible for the MDR phenotype of cancer cells are ABCB1/MDR1/P-gp, ABCC1/MRP1 and ABCG2/BCRP/MXR/ABCP. They are promiscuous transporters that overlap in substrate recognition [73].

The molecular background of the promiscuous substrate recognition is still unidentified [74]. MDR-ABC complex xenobiotic defense machinery has recently been referred to as a 'chemoimmunity system' based on characteristic features shared with the classical immune system [73]. In this manner, MDR-ABC transporters, the xenobiotic metabolizing enzymes, and the related xenobiotic sensor mechanisms (nuclear receptors) form a defense system similar to the classical immune system.

Tyrosine kinases play key role in tumor progression by promoting cell division, enhancing tumor angiogenesis or inhibiting apoptotic processes through the constitutive hyper-activation of downstream signaling cascades [16]. Poor response to TKI therapies due to acquired resistance is recognized as a major weakness of this anti-cancer strategy [65]. Although TKIs increase progression-free survival, they rarely result in complete eradication of malignant cells.

Several mechanisms of TKI resistance have been shown to appear in recurrent tumors:

1)   Alterations of the target kinases (mutations, altered protein levels);

2)   Changes in gene expression that control cell cycle or apoptosis;

3)   Enhanced DNA repair;

4)   Increased drug metabolism;

5)   Increased expression of MDR-ABC transporters, which leads to cross resistance towards a huge cluster of structurally and functionally unrelated chemotherapeutic drugs [75].

Chronic myeloid leukemia (CML) is a stem cell disease where Bcr-Abl oncogenic tyrosine kinase plays a fundamental role in promoting malignant transformation and suppressing apoptotic processes in leukemic cells [76]. According to the long-term follow-up studies, Bcr-Abl TKI imatinib (Glivec, STI571), which is currently the first-line therapy for CML, is unable to eradicate complete Bcr-Abl expressing leukemic stem cell population, and resistance develops in many cases [77]. This problem prompted the clinical use of novel Bcr-Abl inhibitors: imatinib derivative compound nilotinib and structurally unrelated dasatinib [66].

In the last few years, significant advances have been made in understanding the role of mTOR in cancer development and progression. Increased mTOR signaling in cancers often occurs because of mutations in pathways closely related to mTOR. Up-regulation of the PI3K/Akt pathway through mutations can constitutively activate mTOR signaling [69]. Furthermore, loss or inactivation of phosphatase and tensin homolog - PTEN or p53 can also result in mTOR activation [78]. It has been shown that combined inactivation of *p53* and *PTEN* could be used as an adverse prognostic factor for NSCLC patients' outcome and that it identifies a subgroup of patients with a particularly aggressive disease [79]. Also, aberrant *p16* and altered *PTEN* cooperate in NSCLC pathogenesis [80]. Recently, activating mutations of mTOR itself have been identified [81].

Molecular inhibition of mTOR leads to a significant decrease in proliferation of cancer cells and attenuates cell cycle progression [82, 83]. It is known that in a complex with the small protein FKBP12 rapamycin irreversibly binds to the FKBP12-rapamycin domain of mTORC1 and inhibits its kinase activity [84]. Interestingly, increased apoptosis in rapamycin-resistant colorectal cancer cells has been observed after knockdown of mTOR complex 2 (mTORC2), but not mTORC1 [85].

The chemical modifications made in the development of rapalogs preserves their interactions with FKBP12 and mTOR, thus maintaining a mechanism of action similar to rapamycin [84], but prolonged exposure to these drugs blocks mTORC2 assembly and subsequently inhibits Akt signaling [85]. The sensitivity of mTORC2 to rapalogs has been demonstrated in a clinical setting where treatment with temsirolimus or everolimus of patients with acute myeloid leukemia not only inhibited mTORC1, but also blocked Akt activation *via* inhibition of mTORC2 formation [86].

Overall, rapalogs are relatively well tolerated in cancer patients. However, only limited benefits from rapalog therapy have been observed in clinical trials. A number of mechanisms for the resistance to rapalogs have been proposed:

1) Rapalog inhibition of mTORC1 is incomplete [87] or at least insufficient to effectively block activity of mTORC1 kinase towards its substrate 4E-BP1;

2) Rapalog's inability to effectively inhibit mTORC2 [88];

3) The existence of feedback loops counteracting the action of rapalogs, particularly S6K-mediated negative feedback loops [84, 89];

4) Independent of the mTOR pathway - PI3K and Akt may drive tumorigenesis by regulating proteins involved in cell cycle, such as FOXO proteins, cyclinD1, and p27, or proteins of apoptotic response such as MDM2 and caspase-9 [89].

Limitations of rapamycin-based therapies in the clinical setting have led to development of a second generation of mTOR inhibitors known as ATP-competitive mTOR kinase inhibitors (TKIs). They inhibit the kinase activity of both the TORC1 and TORC2 and the feedback activation of PI3K/Akt signaling [90]. Numerous TKIs have been developed, including Torin1, Torin 2, PP242, PP30, KU0063794, WAY-600, WYE-687, WYE-354, OSI-027, AZD-8055, KU-BMCL-200908069-1, Wyeth-BMCL-200908069-2, XL-388, INK-128, and AZD-2014. Recently developed dual PI3K/mTOR inhibitors include NVP-BEZ235, BGT226, XL765/SAR245409, SF1126, GDC-0980, PI-103, PF-04691502, PKI-587, and GSK2126458. These inhibitors target the p110a, b, and c isoforms of PI3K as well as the ATP-binding sites of mTORC1 and mTORC2, completely suppressing PI3K/Akt signaling even in cancers with activating mutations in this pathway.

Although a number of cancers respond to mono-therapy treatment with rapalogs, TKIs and dual PI3K/mTOR, resistance remains a major concern [88].

INTERACTION OF TARGETED THERAPEUTICS WITH ABC TRANSPORTERS

The application of targeted therapy in cancer is a promising modern strategy for the treatment of this incurable disease. A further break through (breakthrough) in this field with more specific and more effective agents is expected. Unfortunately, resistance against all new anti-cancer agents seems to be a persistent problem. They may fail to kill cancer cells for a variety of reasons. Therefore, there is an increasing demand for new molecular markers that would improve targeted cancer therapy [91, 92].

The finding that ABCB1 transcription is induced by some p53 mutants but is repressed by wild-type p53 should be considered in application of new therapeutics [93, 94]. However, rare studies have investigated the interaction between MDR-ABC transporters and p53-targeted therapy.

It has been shown that PRIMA-1, p53 reactivating agent, able to change the mutant p53 conformation to wild-type, is not a substrate for ABCB1 [95]. Contrary to this, nutlin-3 interferes with ABCB1 function as an ABCB1 substrate. Nontoxic nutlin-3 concentrations have been known to strongly sensitize different p53-mutated, ABCB1-expressing cell lines to vincristine and other structurally non-related ABCB1 substrates [96]. Nutlin-3 also interferes with ABCC1 activity. Notably, nutlin-3a is an enantiomer that inhibits MDM2, whereas nutlin-3b does not [97]. However, both enantiomers similarly interfere with ABCB1, indicating that the underlying structure-activity relationships differ from those defined for MDM2 inhibition [96].

However, interaction between TKIs and MDR-ABC transporters may be complex. First, TKIs may be extruded at the cellular membrane barriers by the MDR-ABC transporters. At the same time, TKIs may inhibit these transporters, thus inducing a chemo-sensitizing effect and increasing the activity of other anti-cancer drugs (Fig. **2**). It is important to emphasize that the same TKI compound may behave both as a substrate and an inhibitor of a given transporter, depending on the concentration range applied. It has been shown that active extrusion occurs at low TKI concentrations, while at higher TKI concentrations transporter inhibition becomes dominant [98].

Imatinib is transported by both ABCB1 and ABCG2, but only in a narrow concentration range, whereas at higher concentrations imatinib efficiently inhibits the function of these proteins [98]. Both nilotinib and dasatinib have been shown to interact with ABCB1 and ABCG2 [99]. At higher concentrations, both nilotinib and dasatinib are able to inhibit the function of these transporters (Fig. **2**). Interestingly, bosutinib, a Bcr-Abl inhibitor TKI currently in clinical trials, has been shown to inhibit ABCB1- and ABCG2, but bosutinib is not a transported substrate for either of these transporters in the therapeutic concentration range [98].

It is confirmed that gefitinib, an efficient EGFR inhibitor, is actively transported by ABCB1 and ABCG2 at lower concentrations [100], while at higher doses, MDR-ABC transporters are no more capable of extruding gefitinib [101] (Fig. **2**). Second generation inhibitors of EGFR and EGFR/HER2, erlotinib and lapatinib, also interact with both ABCB1 and ABCG2, and like gefitinib, are transported only within a narrow concentration range [102, 103] (Fig. **2**). Recent reports have shown that multi-TKIs sunitinib and sorafenib are recognized, bound and effluxed by ABCB1 and ABCG2 [104] (Fig. **2**).

In vitro screening using various model cell lines with MDR phenotype has confirmed that imatinib efficiently reverses resistance to mitoxantrone [105], topotecan and SN-38 [106], vincristine, paclitaxel and etoposide [107]. Nilotinib resensitizes cells to mitoxantrone, doxorubicin, colchicine, vincristine and paclitaxel [108]. Gefitinib has been shown to reverse SN-38, vincristine [109], topotecan and mitoxantrone resistance [105]. Combination with erlotinib results in increased cytotoxic effect of vincristine and paclitaxel [110], mitoxantrone and flavopiridol [111]. Lapatinib sensitizes cancer cells to mitoxantrone, doxorubicin and topotecan [102]. Sunitinib co-treatment reverses topotecan and SN-38 resistance [112].

In addition to combining a TKI with a conventional chemotherapeutic drug, combinations of different TKIs may also improve treatment outcomes on a similar basis (Fig. **2**). The increase in anti-cancer effect by co-treatment with imatinib and nilotinib has been observed [113]. This was due to an increase in the intracellular accumulation of nilotinib through MDR-ABC transporter inhibition by imatinib [114]. To increase the cytotoxic effect of the targeted EGFR inhibitors, multiple combination therapies are under clinical development [115]. The effects of combination of gefitinib with 5-fluorouracil, leucovorin and irinotecan were evaluated by Veronese *et al.* in patients with colorectal cancer [116] Combination therapy with imatinib plus cytarabine has recently been studied in newly diagnosed CML patients. This treatment strategy was associated with a high rate of complete molecular responses [117]. Clinical studies have also been reported that both imatinib and dasatinib enhance intracellular accumulation of the multi-drug transporter substrates cyclophosphamide as well as tamoxifen [118].

In this regard, pharmacokinetic and pharmacodynamic drug interactions that also affect the clinical outcome should be considered. Indeed, recent studies have shown that gefitinib enhanced the oral bioavailability and anti-cancer activity of irinotecan [119], increased the bioavailability and decreased the clearance of topotecan [100], and enhanced topotecan penetration of gliomas in mice [120].

To date, limited data are available regarding the involvement of MDR-ABC transporters in TKI biodistribution and toxicity in patients. Such studies usually deal with the influence of the ABCB1 or ABCG2 polymorphic variants. Genotype-specific influence of ABCB1 and ABCG2 on pharmacokinetics of imatinib and gefitinib were described by Dulucq *et al.* in 2005 and Cusatis G *et al.* in 2006 [121, 122]. ABCB1 1236C/T and 2677G/T polymorphisms altered imatinib plasma levels and, as a consequence, decreased the response to standard-dose treatment [121].

All FDA-approved TKIs have been shown to undergo extensive metabolism by the enzymes of the CYP3A family [123, 124]. Generation of phase II conjugated organic anion metabolites have been described for imatinib and erlotinib [125, 126]. Coordinately, TKI metabolites should be considered as interacting substrates and/or inhibitors of MDR-ABC transporters that recognize detoxified metabolites [127].

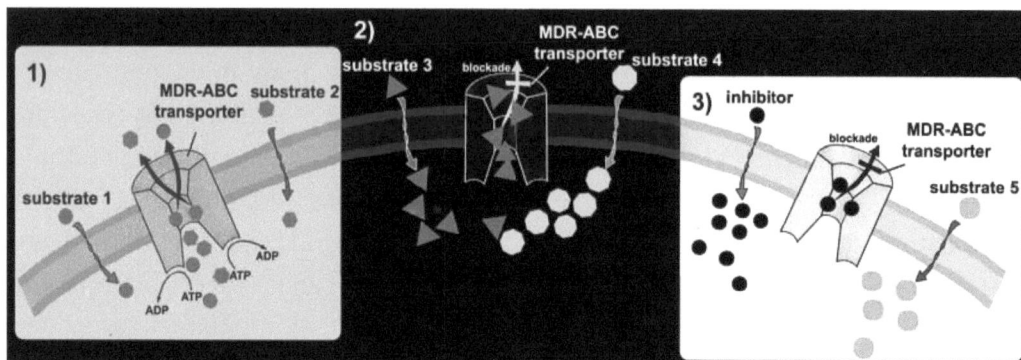

Fig. (2). The illustration of the combinations of small molecule anti-cancer agents depending on their interaction with MDR-ABC transporters. Beside enhanced anti-cancer activity by acting through different pathways, combined treatment could block MDR-ABC transporters and increase the intracellular concentration of co-administered drugs resulting in the overcoming of the MDR phenotype. In addition, in the presence of MDR, high dose is needed for single drug treatment which results in toxicity to the normal cells. Combined treatment is able to reduce the dose of each single drug through synergistic action and thereby decrease the toxicity.

The accumulation of small molecule anti-cancer agents in the cancer cells may be modified by MDR-ABC transporter function:

1) Two anti-cancer agents applied in combination may be both MDR-ABC transporter substrates (substrate 1 and 2). In this case, the MDR-ABC transporter directly extrudes both drugs in an ATP-dependent fashion and such drugs may not reach its (their) intracellular target.

2) At higher concentrations, the MDR-ABC substrate 3 may act as inhibitor of the MDR-ABC function, allowing eventual accumulation of substrate 3 and 4 in the cell.

3) Small molecule anti-cancer agent may be direct MDR-ABC inhibitor and therefore the MDR-ABC transporters cannot prevent the cellular entry of either inhibitor or substrate 5.

When administered in combination with other anti-cancer compounds, the MDR-ABC substrates and/or inhibitors may influence the interaction of the transporter with the substrate drugs, and modify their cellular entry and pharmacological fate.

A recent study has shown that rapamycin could reverse the MDR phenotype in cancer cells by modulating both the expression and function of ABCB1 as effectively as verapamil [128]. Although, as a potential inhibitor of ABCB1, rapamycin decreased the rate of ATP hydrolysis with respect to the basal rate, it did not completely inhibit the ABCB1 activity. Hence, rapamycin can be classified as a substrate transported by ABCB1 [129]. Consequently, tumors over-expressing ABCB1 may be resistant to rapamycin [130].

It seems that everolimus could be considered at the same time as substrate and inhibitor of ABCB1. A recent study has emphasized the necessity of a therapeutic monitoring of everolimus combined with an inhibitor of the ABCB1 and CYP 450 in future cancer treatments [7]. Contrary to this, other authors have shown that everolimus efficiently modulated vandetanib (a kinase inhibitor of a number of cell receptors, mainly the vascular endothelial growth factor receptor (VEGFR), the epidermal growth factor receptor (EGFR), and the RET-tyrosine kinase) brain penetration due to the inhibition of ABCB1 in blood-brain barrier [131]. However, no significant affect on vandetanib brain uptake was observed following temsirolimus co-administration.

Accordingly, combination therapeutic strategies may provide a way for overcoming the resistance to mTOR targeting agents and improve their efficacy. Rapalogs have been tested in combination with standard chemotherapy, receptor tyrosine kinase targeted therapies, and angiogenesis inhibitors [67]. Combinations of dual PI3K/mTOR inhibitors with the receptor tyrosine kinase inhibitors such as sorafenib have also demonstrated enhanced anti-cancer activity [132, 133].

It has been suggested that cilengitide, a selective inhibitor of the integrins $\alpha v \beta 3$ and $\alpha v \beta 5$ is a substrate for several ABC transporters, including ABCB1. An inconsistent relationship between ABCB1 genotype and pharmacokinetic phenotype has been reported for most drugs. In a pharmacogenomic study, a suggestive relationship between ABCB1 genotype, specifically exon 26 single nucleotide polymorphism C to T, and cilengitide systemic and renal clearance has been shown. It is important to further investigate the interaction between cilengitide and ABCB1 transporter because the authors concluded that patients with the TT polymorphism could have an increased exposure to cilengitide [134].

PROBLEMS WITH THE EFFICACY OF MDR MODULATORS

Classical mechanism of MDR confers to the enhanced activity of ATP-binding cassette (ABC)-transporters. These membrane embedded transport proteins act as

Table 1.   Examples of Targeted Therapies Currently in Clinical Trials and their Interactions with ABC Transporters

Target	Drug	Cancer	ABC Transporters
EGFR	Gefitinib/Iressa/ZD1839	NSCLC	ABCB1 and ABCG2 substrate/inhibitor
EGFR	Erlotinib/Tarceva/OSI-774	NSCLC	ABCB1 and ABCG2 substrate/inhibitor
EGFR/HER2	Lapatinib/GW572016	LFT	ABCB1 and ABCG2 substrate/inhibitor
EGFR/HER2	EKB-569	CC, NSCLC	
EGFR/HER2	HKI-272 (neratinib)	BC, NSCLC	ABCB1 inhibitor
PanErbB	CI-1033 (Canertinib)	BC, NSCLC	ABCG2 substrate
PanErbB	PF00299804	ST	
c-KIT	Imatinib/Gleevec/STI-571	LFT	ABCB1 and ABCG2 substrate/inhibitor
c-KIT	Nilotinib/AMN107	GIST, CML, AML	ABCB1 and ABCG2 substrate/inhibitor
c-KIT	Dasatinib/BMS-354825	GIST	ABCB1 and ABCG2 substrate/inhibitor
c-KIT/PDGFR/VEGFR	Sunitinib/SU11248	ALL, GC,, AML, PC	ABCB1 substrate; ABCB1 and ABCG2 inhibitor
c-KIT/PDGFR/VEGFR	Sorafenib/BAY-43-9006	AML, ALL	ABCB1 substrate; ABCB1 and ABCG2 inhibitor
VEGFR	AMG 706	NSCLC, RC, CC, PC, EC, TC	
VEGFR	BIBF 1120	ASM	ABCB1 inhibitor
EGFR/VEGFR	AEE788	ASM, Glioblastoma	
EGFR/VEGFR/RET	Vandetanib/ZD6474	ASM, MM, NSCLC	ABCB1 and ABCG2 inhibitor
Bcr-Abl	Imatinib/Gleevec/STI-571	CML, ST	ABCB1 and ABCG2 substrate/inhibitor
Bcr-Abl/Src kinases	Bosutinib/SKI-606	CML, ABC, PC, Glioblastoma	ABCB1 and ABCG2 inhibitor
Bcr-Abl/Lyn	Bafetinib/INNO-406	CML, ALL, BCCLL	ABCB1 and ABCG2 substrate
Abl/Src kinases	Saracatinib/AZD0530	ST	ABCB1 inhibitor
Bcr-Abl (T315I)	MK-0457/VX-680	CML, ALL	/
mTOR	Rapamycin/Sirolimus	ASM, BC	ABCB1 and ABCG2 substrate/inhibitor
	Temsirolimus/CCI-779	CC, Leukemia, Lymphoma, RCC	
	Everolimus/RAD-001	BC, GIST, Glioblastoma, PC, NSCLC	ABCB1 and ABCG2 substrate/inhibitor

(Table 1) contd.....

Target	Drug	Cancer	ABC Transporters
	Deferolimus/AP23573	HM, PC, Sarcoma, BC, EC, NSCLC, Glioma, RCC	
p53	Nutlin	Cancer	ABCB1 substrate
	Advexin/Gendicine	HNC, BC, BLC, LC, OC	
	JNJ-26854165	ST	
	APR-246 (PRIMA-1 analog)	HM; PC	/
αvβ3 and αvβ5 integrins	Cilengitide	BCNST, AST, AML, AML, ANSCLC, HM	ABCB1 substrate

NSCLC:Non-small cell lung cancer; LFT: Liver function tests; CC: Colorectal cancer; BC: Breast cancer; ST: Solid tumors; GIST: Gastrointestinal stromal tumors; CML: Chronic myelogenous (or myeloid) leukemia; AML: Acute myeloid leukemia; ALL: Acute lymphoblastic leukemia; GC: Gastrointestinal cancer; PC: Prostate cancer; RC: Rectal cancer; EC: Esophageal cancer; TC: Thyroid cancer; ASM: Advanced solid malignancies; MM: Multiple myeloma; ABC: Advanced breast cancer; BCCLL: B-cell chronic lymphoid leukemia; RCC: Renal cell carcinoma; HM: Hematologic malignancies; EC: Endometrial cancer; HNC: Head and Neck Cancer; BLC: Bladder cancer; LC: Liver Cancer; OC: Ovarian Cancer; BCNST: Brain and Central Nervous System Tumors; ANSCLC: Advanced NSCLC;

energy-dependent drug extrusion pumps. Because of their activity, the intracellular concentration of drugs decrease and cannot reach the level necessary for the killing of cancer cells [135].

The drug extrusion pump ABCB1 is the most extensively studied ABC transporter. ABCB1 is characterized by unusually wide substrate specificity. It transports mainly hydrophobic compounds across the membrane lipid bilayer and removes them directly from the membrane. Actually, ABCB1 has been referred to as molecular "vacuum cleaner" [136]. However, the phenomenon of MDR cannot be explained merely by the over-expression of ABC transporters. Alternative forms of MDR, known as atypical MDR: the change in drug targets (*e.g.,* decreased activity of Topoisomerase II), better elimination of drugs due to the increase in the levels of glutathione and related enzymes, alterations in the repair of DNA damage and inability to initiate apoptosis could be developed within cancer cell [74, 135]. These mechanisms of drug resistance may coexist, leaving cancer cells unaffected by drugs with single target [137].

The search for nontoxic anti-cancer agents able to overcome MDR has been a great challenge in the area of drug design and discovery for many years. There are two main approaches in combating the problem of MDR in cancer:

1)   Development of agents able to preserve cytotoxic activity toward MDR cancer cells;

2)   Development of compounds able to restore the cytotoxicity of classic anti-cancer drugs [138].

The agents interfering with either the expression of the transporter proteins or their function are referred to as MDR modulators. ABCB1 over-expression in cancer cells has become a therapeutic target for circumventing MDR. The classical pharmacological strategy for achieving this goal involves the co-administration of ABCB1 inhibitor and cytotoxic agent that is a substrate of ABCB1. The reversal of MDR by modulators is usually achieved through their direct interaction with ABCB1. Various mechanisms are responsible for the inhibition of anti-cancer drug efflux in cancer cells overexpressing ABCB1. These mechanisms include the blockage of the drug binding sites, the inhibition of ATP hydrolysis, and the alteration of the integrity of cell membrane lipids [139, 140]. As competitive inhibitors, MDR modulators prevent binding of anti-cancer drug by ABCB1 and eventually its extrusion, while noncompetitive inhibitors attenuate the ATPase activity of ABCB1. Modulation of ABCB1 through interactions with membrane phospholipids, thus changing the physicochemical properties of the membrane and perturbing the lipid environment of ABCB1, is also considered as a promising reversal strategy [141].

A number of MDR modulators, from synthetic or natural origin, have been reported to overcome drug resistance *in vitro*. Nevertheless, even though some of them were in clinical trials, they are not approved in clinical practice yet. A wide series of compounds has been studied as ABCB1 inhibitors. First-generation reversal agents are drugs already in clinical use for other indications (*e.g.,* verapamil, cyclosporin A, and quinidine) and they have limited selectivity toward ABCB1. Second-generation agents are analogues of the first generation drugs (*e.g.,* dexverapamil, valspodar, and cinchonine) with evidently higher selectivity and activity. Both first- and second- generation inhibitors compete with the cytotoxic drug as substrates for transport by the ABCB1 [142]. The third-generation compounds comprise molecules that have been developed using quantitative structure-activity relationship studies and combinatorial chemistry.

Their specific physico-chemical characteristics (*e.g.,* lipophilicity, positive charge at neutral pH, and presence of aromatic rings) are considered as a potential for overcoming the limitations of two previous generations of MDR modulators [143]. Particularly, they bind with high affinity to ABCB1 and act through noncompetitive inhibition [139]. Although several ABCB1 inhibitors have been tested in controlled clinical trials, no satisfactory results have been obtained so far [144].

The development of an effective modulator has been hampered by various limiting factors such as toxicity and pharmacokinetic interactions [141, 143, 145]. ABCB1 co-expression with other ABC transporters in MDR cancer cells and its presence in normal tissues caused difficulties in the development of agents that selectively target MDR. First-generation of ABCB1 modulators are intrinsically toxic at normal tissue levels due to their pharmacological activities other than ABCB1 inhibition. That is the reason why further investigation after phase I clinical trials were not allowed [146]. Despite having a more favorable toxicological profile, second-generation compounds are characterized by several factors that have limited their clinical use. Beside ABCB1, they also inhibit other ABC transporters (*e.g.,* MRP2 also named non-bile acid organic anion transporter/cMOAT) [147]. Consequently, adverse effects (neutropenia and other myelotoxic effects) occurred when second-generation compounds were combined with ABCB1 substrate anti-cancer agents [148]. In addition, these compounds are substrates of cytochrome P-450 (CYP) and compete with anti-cancer drugs for CYP-mediated oxidative reactions. This inhibition of anti-cancer drug metabolism resulted in pharmacokinetic interactions that led to host intoxication with cytotoxic drug [149].

Combined application of third generation ABCB1 modulators with chemotherapeutic agents did not show pharmacokinetic alterations, suggesting a lack of significant interaction with CYP or other ABC transporters [150]. Results from phase I-II trials with third-generation inhibitors (*e.g.,* zosuquidar, tariquidar, laniquidar, *etc.*) were published by Lee CH *et al.* in 2010 [142]. Some of the few phase III studies carried out with third-generation compounds have been stopped due to toxicity [142] or failed to demonstrate an advantage of the arm including the ABCB1 inhibitor over that with the cytotoxic agent alone [151].

So far, no overall satisfactory results have been obtained in clinical trials targeting ABCB1. The main limitations were the enrollment of patient population (*e.g.,* cancer patients without laboratory proof of MDR) and difficulties in the diagnosis of clinical MDR [152]. Other possible reasons for failure of ABCB1 inhibitors may be alternative mechanisms of resistance and empirical dose reduction of chemotherapy [74]. Polymorphisms of ABCB1 gene have also been suggested as a reason for the variability in the action of ABCB1 inhibitors and anti-cancer agents. The most studied ABCB1 single nucleotide polymorphisms (SNPs) in relation to possible effects on pharmacokinetics and therapeutic outcome of cancer patients, is the C3435T variant at exon 26 [153].

NEW MDR REVERSAL STRATEGIES

In recent years, the need for synthesis of ABCB1 inhibitors using a rational approach has been emphasized. Due to ABCB1 strong impact on MDR and pharmacokinetics, a number of experimental and computational studies have been carried out in order to reveal its drug-binding interactions and why it possesses such a broad substrate specificity. A few confusing factors in the prediction of ABCB1 substrate specificity have been proposed:

1) The discrepancy between the ABCB1 substrate specificity values obtained in different assays;

2) The uncertainty which compound is a substrate and which is an inhibitor;

3) The dilemma about lipophilicity and amphiphilicity of ABCB1 substrates;

4) And how to describe specific relationships when ABCB1 has no binding sites, but shows high ligand specificity [154].

A series of different computational methods and models including ligand-based models as well as structure-based models [155] have been employed to identify substrates and non-substrates of ABCB1 within a large series of compounds (from 100 to 2.000 compounds). The knowledge about the structure of this transporter protein has been improved by the determination of the X-ray crystal structure of mouse ABCB1, which shares 87% sequence identity with human ABCB1, at 3.8

AÚ resolution [156]. It is the highest resolution of a mammalian transporter protein to date. The structure analysis confirmed the "hydrophobic vacuum cleaner" model proposed for ABCB1 function [136] and is expected to help in designing more potent and safer MDR modulators.

Alternative approaches to circumvent ABCB1-mediated MDR have been tested in experimental cancer models. They include specific monoclonal antibodies for ABCB1, the use of antisense oligonucleotides and transcriptional regulators of ABCB1 gene expression. The encapsulation of ABCB1 substrate drugs in liposomes or nanoparticles is already used in clinical setting. These approaches have been summarized in a series of comprehensive reviews [99, 157]. The development of anti-cancer drugs that are not substrates of ABCB1 is another important strategy for overcoming MDR. To date, many compounds with different chemical structures and mechanisms of action have been developed with this purpose (Fig. **3**). They include:

1)   Microtubule stabilizing agents which promote polymerization of tubulin to microtubules and prevent depolymerization (*e.g.,* epothilones, second- and third-generation taxanes) [158-161] (Fig. **3**);

It is worth mentioning that some favorable anti-cancer characteristics of paclitaxel (Fig. **3**), such as decrease of vascular endothelial growth factor (VEGF) secretion, were retained even in the presence of MDR [162]

2)   Microtubule destabilizing agents which prevent polymerization of tubulin and promote depolymerization of filamentous microtubule (*e.g.,* cryptophycins, halichondrins (Fig. **3**), hemiasterlins, and STX140) [163, 164];

3)   Inhibitors of topoisomerase I (*e.g.,* lipophilic camptothecins, homocamptothecins (Fig. **3**), and dibenzonaphthyridinones) [165];

4)   Inhibitors of topoisomerase II (*e.g.,* lipophilic anthracyclines) [166] (Fig. **3**);

5)   Compounds whose activity is potentiated by the expression of ABCB1 [167].

Recently, it has been shown that MDR cancer cells cross-resistant to structurally and functionally unrelated drugs are paradoxically hypersensitive to certain compounds [145]. This phenomenon is referred to as "collateral sensitivity" and described in several studies [74, 167, 168]. The cell growth inhibition effect of NSC73306, an isatin-β-thiosemicarbazone derivative (Fig. **3**), was shown to be positively correlated with the level of ABCB1 expression [169]. Although NSC73306 is neither a substrate nor inhibitor of ABCB1, further investigations have shown that this compound is a substrate for another ABC transporter (ABCG2, known as breast cancer resistance protein - BCRP) [170].

The effects of some old drugs such as purine nucleoside and nucleotide analogs include the reversion of MDR during cancer treatment. In view of their considerable efficacy and moderate toxicity these drugs are suitable for combining with other chemotherapeutic agents. Their impact on ABCB1 expression and the accumulation of chemotherapeutics qualify purine analogs as useful agents for MDR reversion [171, 172].

After three decades of searching for the efficient way to overcome the MDR in cancer, innovative strategies, such as the fallback to natural products, the design of peptidomimetics and dual activity ligands emerged as a fourth generation of ABCB1 inhibitors [173].

Plants play an important role in drug discovery. Specifically, 60% of the chemotherapeutic agents currently in clinical practice originate from nature. The wide structural diversity of plants' secondary metabolites is an extremely valuable source of bioactive compounds for rational drug design [174, 175].

In the last two decades, considerable attention has been focused on Euphorbia species (Euphorbiaceae), as a source of several biologically active compounds [176-178]. Euphorbia species, commonly named spurge, range from annual or perennial herbs, woody shrubs, trees and succulent plants. Their latex has been used in traditional medicine to treat tumors and warts [179, 180]. However, the use of Euphorbia species has been impeded by the occurrence of skin irritation and tumor-promotion by their latex. The compounds responsible for this toxicity are polycyclic diterpenoids, named "phorboids", with tigliane, ingenane or daphanane skeletons.

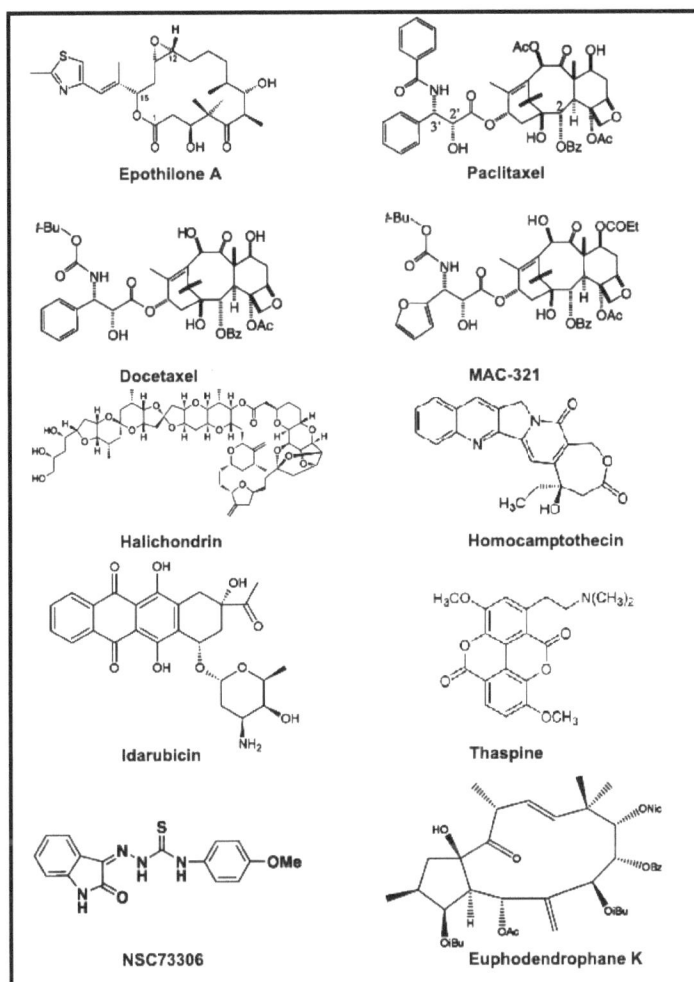

Fig. (3). Many compounds (natural products and artificially generated agents) with different chemical structures and mechanisms of action have been developed in order to overcome MDR. Epithilone A (natural product) is a microtubule stabilizing agent which promotes the polymerization of tubulin as well as paclitaxel and docetaxel (first generation taxanes). MAC-321 (third generation taxane) is chemically modified docetaxel with minimal affinity for ABCB1 transporter. Halichondrin B (natural compound) is a potent tubulin inhibitor, but poor substrate for ABCB1, an efficient alternative for Vinca alkaloids. Homocamptothecin is a camptothecin homolog (Topoisomerase I inhibitor) with no affinity for MDR-ABC transporters. Idarubicin, a second-generation anthracycline (Topoisomerase II inhibitor) has high lipophilicity and high cellular uptake. Thaspine (natural product) is dual Topoisomerase I and II inhibitor that evades the activity ABCB1 transporter. NSC73306, an isatin-β-thiosemicarbazone derivative that is neither a substrate nor an inhibitor of ABCB1, exploits the presence of ABCB1 over-expression in a unique way of action and preferentially kills MDR cancer cells. Euphodendrophane K completely blocks ABCB1 transporter and demonstrates higher inhibitory activity than third-generation MDR modulator-tariquidar.

Nevertheless, Euphorbia genus has been subjected to extensive phytochemical research because of structurally unique macrocyclic diterpenes: jatrophanes and lathyranes characterized by a 5:11:3 and 5:12 fused ring systems, respectively. These compounds have in common a very flexible macrocyclic ring with several acylating groups. Great attention has been paid to these compounds due to their structural complexity and biogenetic relevance, as well as biological properties [177, 178]. The first reported investigations that showed jatrophane and lathyrane diterpenes as promising modulators of MDR in cancer cells were carried out by Hohmann *et al.* [181-183] and Corea *et al.* [184, 185]. Recently, other jatrophane and lathyrane diterpenes have been isolated from E. dendroides and E. helioscopia [186-189]. The majority of these compounds were found to be strong inhibitors of ABCB1 in various MDR cancer cells (Euphodendrophane K, Fig. **3**). Furthermore, new anti-cancer characteristics of jatrophanes were described for the first time: beside ABCB1 inhibition, jatrophane diterpenes from E. dendroides caused G2/M arrest, cell killing and anti-angiogenic activity [190].

CONCLUDING REMARKS

Acquired resistance to chemotherapy is an increasing problem of the novel targeted anti-cancer approaches. Target-independent resistance mechanisms may include:

1)   Altered CYP function;

2)   Decreased drug uptake;

3)   Increased drug efflux;

4)   Activation of salvage pathways;

5)   Resistant clone selection;

6)   Existence of cancer stem cells [191].

The most relevant mechanism of target-independent resistance is the over-expression of MDR-ABC transporters that contributes to intensive drug extrusion from cancer cells. A clinical example of a patient with acquired resistance to gefitinib without any mutation in the EGFR gene but a massive over-expression of the ABCG2 protein was reported by Usuda J. *et al.* [192]. In addition, chronic imatinib treatment induced the expression of the ABCB1, ABCC1, ABCC2 and the ABCG2 transporters [193].

Consequently, more coherent data and statistically powered studies to correlate functional expression of MDR-ABC transporters with treatment efficacy are definitely warranted. Development of MDR could be considered as innate chemo-immunity response [9]. The induction of high expression levels of MDR-ABC transporters in the intestine, liver and kidney may significantly affect the bioavailability of orally administered small molecule mass drugs. Similarly, a passage through the sanctuary barriers, such as blood-brain-barrier, may disrupt the local effects of drug [194]. In addition, both the expression levels and the functional activity of the MDR-ABC transporters may differ between individuals due to genetic polymorphisms or pathological conditions. Therefore, a major inter-individual difference in the pharmacokinetic behavior of the same drug may be expected to occur.

As a conclusion, each FDA-approved small molecular mass drug could be an interacting partner of at least one of the MDR-ABC transporters. Accordingly, novel anti-cancer therapies should equally focus on the effectiveness of target inhibition and exploration of potential interactions of the designed molecules by membrane transporters. Thus, targeted hydrophobic small molecule compounds should be screened to evade chemo-immunity cellular mechanisms.

Besides, the newly discovered activity of drug as an inhibitor or substrate of an MDR-ABC transporter requires serious consideration during the development of this drug. Findings about synergisms between new drug and other cytotoxic drugs may be reanalyzed concerning the role of MDR-ABC transporters.

ACKNOWLEDGEMENTS

Declared none.

CONFLICT OF INTEREST

The authors confirm that this chapter contents have no conflict of interest.

REFERENCES

[1]   O'Connor R. The pharmacology of cancer resistance. Anticancer Research 2007; 27: 1267-1272.

[2]   Pérez-Tomás R. Multidrug Resistance: Retrospect and Prospects in Anti-Cancer Drug Treatment. Current Medicinal Chemistry 2006; 13: 1859-1876.

[3]   Nobili, S., Landini, I., Mazzei, T., and Mini, E. Overcoming tumor multidrug resistance using drugs able to evade P-glycoprotein or to exploit its expression. Med Res Rev 2012; 32: 1220-62.

[4]   Roninson IB, Abelson HT, Housman DE, Howell N, Varshavsky A. Amplification of specific DNA sequences correlates with multi-drug resistance in Chinese hamster cells. Nature 1984; 309: 626-8.

[5]   Riordan JR, Ling V. Genetic and biochemical characterization of multidrug resistance. Pharmacol Ther 1985; 28: 51-7.

[6]   Gros P, Ben Neriah YB, Croop JM, Housman DE. Isolation and expression of a complementary DNA that confers multidrug resistance. Nature 1986; 323: 728-31.

[7]   Chu C, Abbara C, Noël-Hudson MS, Thomas-Bourgneuf L, Gonin P, Farinotti R, Bonhomme-Faivre L. Disposition of everolimus in mdr1a-/1b- mice and after a pre-treatment of lapatinib in Swiss mice. Biochem Pharmacol 2009; 77: 1629-34.

[8]   Guo J, Anderson MG, Tapang P, Palma JP, Rodriguez LE, Niquette A, Li J, Bouska JJ, Wang G, Semizarov D, Albert DH, Donawho CK, Glaser KB, Shah OJ. Identification of genes that confer tumor cell resistance to the aurora B kinase inhibitor, AZD1152. Pharmacogenomics J 2009; 9: 90-102.

[9]   Brózik A, Hegedüs C, Erdei Z, Hegedus T, Özvegy-Laczka C, Szakács G and Sarkadi B. Tyrosine kinase inhibitors as modulators of ATP binding cassette multidrug transporters: substrates, chemosensitizers or inducers of acquired multidrug resistance? 2011; Expert Opin Drug Met 7: 623-42.

[10]   Di Nicolantonio F, Mercer SJ, Knight LA, Gabriel FG, Whitehouse PA, Sharma S, Fernando A, Glaysher S, Di Palma S, Johnson P, Somers SS, Toh S, Higgins B, Lamont A, Gulliford T, Hurren J, Yiangou C, Cree IA. Cancer cell adaptation to chemotherapy. BMC Cancer 2005; 5: 78.

[11]   Hanahan D, Weinberg RA. The hallmarks of cancer. Cell 2000; 100: 57-70.

[12]   Hollstein M, Rice K, Greenblatt MS, Soussi T, Fuchs R, Sørlie T, Hovig E, Smith-Sørensen B, Montesano R, Harris CC. Database of p53 gene somatic mutations in human tumors and cell lines. Nucleic Acids Res 1994; 22: 3551-5.

[13]   Haupt Y, Maya R, Kazaz A, Oren M. Mdm2 promotes the rapid degradation of p53. Nature 1997; 387: 296-9.

[14]   Freedman DA, Wu L, Levine AJ. Functions of the MDM2 oncoprotein. Cell Mol Life Sci 1999; 55: 96-107.

[15]   Milinkovic V, Bankovic J, Rakic M, Milosevic N, Stankovic T, Jokovic M, Milosevic Z, Skender-Gazibara M, Podolski-Renic A, Pesic M, Ruzdijic S, Tanic N. Genomic instability and p53 alterations in patients with malignant glioma. Exp Mol Pathol 2012; 93: 200-6.

[16]   Sawyers C. Targeted cancer therapy. Nature 2004; 432: 294-7.

[17]   Arslan MA, Kutuk O, Basaga H. Protein kinases as drug targets in cancer. Curr Cancer Drug Targets 2006; 6: 623-34.

[18]   Blume-Jensen P, Hunter T. Oncogenic kinase signalling. Nature 2001; 411: 355-65.

[19]   Robinson DR, Wu YM, Lin SF. The protein tyrosine kinase family of the human genome. Oncogene 2000; 19: 5548-57.

[20]   Gschwind A, Fischer OM, Ullrich A. The discovery of receptor tyrosine kinases: targets for cancer therapy. Nat Rev Cancer 2004; 4: 361-70.

[21]   Sebolt-Leopold JS, English JM. Mechanisms of drug inhibition of signalling molecules. Nature   2006; 441: 457-62.

[22]   Hubbard SR, Miller WT. Receptor tyrosine kinases: mechanisms of activation and signaling. Curr Opin Cell Biol 2007; 19: 117-23.

[23]   Ren R. Mechanisms of BCR-ABL in the pathogenesis of chronic myelogenous leukaemia. Nat Rev Cancer 2005; 5: 172-83.

[24]   Rao RD, Buckner JC, Sarkaria JN. Mammalian target of rapamycin (mTOR) inhibitors as anti-cancer agents. Curr Cancer Drug Targets 2004; 4: 621-35.

[25]   Faivre S, Kroemer G, Raymond E. Current development of mTOR inhibitors as anticancer agents. Nat Rev Drug Discov 2006; 5: 671-88.

[26]   Rüegg C, Postigo AA, Sikorski EE, Butcher EC, Pytela R, Erle DJ. Role of integrin alpha 4 beta 7/alpha 4 beta P in lymphocyte adherence to fibronectin and VCAM-1 and in homotypic cell clustering. J Cell Biol 1992; 117: 179-89.

[27]   Stupp R, Ruegg C. Integrin inhibitors reaching the clinic. J Clin Oncol 2007; 25: 1637-8.

[28]   Wang Z, Sun Y. Targeting p53 for Novel Anticancer Therapy. Transl Oncol 2010; 3: 1-12.

[29]   Pearson S, Jia H, Kandachi K. China approves first gene therapy. Nat Biotechnol 2004; 22: 3-4.

[30]   Vazquez A, Bond EE, Levine AJ, Bond GL. The genetics of the p53 pathway, apoptosis and cancer therapy. Nat Rev Drug Discov 2008; 7: 979-87.

[31]   Bouchet BP, Caron de Fromentel C, Puisieux A, Galmarini CM. p53 as a target for anti-cancer drug development. Crit Rev Oncol Hematol 2006; 58: 190-207.

[32]   Peng Z. Current status of gendicine in China: recombinant human Ad-p53 agent for treatment of cancers. Hum Gene Ther 2005; 16: 1016-27.

[33]   Bischoff JR, Kirn DH, Williams A, Heise C, Horn S, Muna M, Ng L, Nye JA, Sampson-Johannes A, Fattaey A, McCormick F. An adenovirus mutant that replicates selectively in p53-deficient human tumor cells. Science 1996; 274: 373-6.

[34]   Heise C, Lemmon M, Kirn D. Efficacy with a replication-selective adenovirus plus cisplatin-based chemotherapy: dependence on sequencing but not p53 functional status or route of administration. Clin Cancer Res 2000; 6: 4908-14.

[35]   Khuri FR, Nemunaitis J, Ganly I, Arseneau J, Tannock IF, Romel L, Gore M, Ironside J, MacDougall RH, Heise C, Randlev B, Gillenwater AM, Bruso P, Kaye SB, Hong WK, Kirn DH. A controlled trial of intratumoral ONYX-015, a selectively-replicating adenovirus, in combination with cisplatin and 5-fluorouracil in patients with recurrent head and neck cancer. Nat Med 2000; 6: 879-85.

[36]   Issaeva N, Bozko P, Enge M, Protopopova M, Verhoef LG, Masucci M, Pramanik A, Selivanova G. Small molecule RITA binds to p53, blocks p53-HDM-2 interaction and activates p53 function in tumors. Nat Med 2004; 10: 1321-8.

[37]   Grinkevich VV, Nikulenkov F, Shi Y, Enge M, Bao W, Maljukova A, Gluch A, Kel A, Sangfelt O, Selivanova G. Ablation of key oncogenic pathways by RITA-reactivated p53 is required for efficient apoptosis. Cancer Cell 2009; 15: 441-53.

[38]   Gudkov AV, Komarova EA. Dangerous habits of a security guard: the two faces of p53 as a drug target. Hum Mol Genet 2007; 16 Spec No 1: R67-72.

[39]   Green DR, Kroemer G. Cytoplasmic functions of the tumour suppressor p53. Nature 2009; 458: 1127-30.

[40]   Samuels-Lev Y, O'Connor DJ, Bergamaschi D, Trigiante G, Hsieh JK, Zhong S, Campargue I, Naumovski L, Crook T, Lu X. ASPP proteins specifically stimulate the apoptotic function of p53. Mol Cell 2001; 8: 781-94.

[41]   Friedler A, Hansson LO, Veprintsev DB, Freund SM, Rippin TM, Nikolova PV, Proctor MR, Rüdiger S, Fersht AR. A peptide that binds and stabilizes p53 core domain: chaperone strategy for rescue of oncogenic mutants. Proc Natl Acad Sci USA 2002; 99: 937-42.

[42]   Issaeva N, Friedler A, Bozko P, Wiman KG, Fersht AR, Selivanova G. Rescue of mutants of the tumor suppressor p53 in cancer cells by a designed peptide. Proc Natl Acad Sci USA 2003; 100: 13303-7.

[43]   Foster BA, Coffey HA, Morin MJ, Rastinejad F. Pharmacological rescue of mutant p53 conformation and function. Science 1999; 286: 2507-10.

[44]   Selivanova G, Wiman KG. Reactivation of mutant p53: molecular mechanisms and therapeutic potential. Oncogene 2007; 26: 2243-54.

[45]   Bykov VJ, Issaeva N, Selivanova G, Wiman KG. Mutant p53-dependent growth suppression distinguishes PRIMA-1 from known anticancer drugs: a statistical analysis of information in the National Cancer Institute database. Carcinogenesis 2002; 23: 2011-8.

[46]   Bykov VJ, Issaeva N, Zache N, Shilov A, Hultcrantz M, Bergman J, Selivanova G, Wiman KG. Reactivation of mutant p53 and induction of apoptosis in human tumor cells by maleimide analogs. J Biol Chem 2005; 280: 30384-91.

[47]   Li Y, Mao Y, Brandt-Rauf PW, Williams AC, Fine RL. Selective induction of apoptosis in mutant p53 premalignant and malignant cancer cells by PRIMA-1 through the c-Jun-NH2-kinase pathway. Mol Cancer Ther 2005; 4: 901-9.

[48]   Rehman A, Chahal MS, Tang X, Bruce JE, Pommier Y, Daoud SS. Proteomic identification of heat shock protein 90 as a candidate target for p53 mutation reactivation by PRIMA-1 in breast cancer cells. Breast Cancer Res 2005; 7: R765-74.

[49]   Peng Y, Li C, Chen L, Sebti S, Chen J. Rescue of mutant p53 transcription function by ellipticine. Oncogene 2003; 22: 4478-87.

[50]   Xu GW, Mawji IA, Macrae CJ, Koch CA, Datti A, Wrana JL, Dennis JW, Schimmer AD. A high-content chemical screen identifies ellipticine as a modulator of p53 nuclear localization. Apoptosis 2008; 13: 413-22.

[51]   Grdina DJ, Shigematsu N, Dale P, Newton GL, Aguilera JA, Fahey RC. Thiol and disulfide metabolites of the radiation protector and potential chemopreventive agent WR-2721 are linked to both its anti-cytotoxic and anti-mutagenic mechanisms of action. Carcinogenesis 1995; 16: 767-74.

[52]   North S, El-Ghissassi F, Pluquet O, Verhaegh G, Hainaut P. The cytoprotective aminothiol WR1065 activates p21waf-1 and down regulates cell cycle progression through a p53-dependent pathway. Oncogene 2000; 19: 1206-14.

[53]   Weinstein JN, Myers TG, O'Connor PM, Friend SH, Fornace AJ Jr, Kohn KW, Fojo T, Bates SE, Rubinstein LV, Anderson NL, Buolamwini JK, van Osdol WW, Monks AP, Scudiero DA, Sausville EA, Zaharevitz DW, Bunow B, Viswanadhan VN, Johnson GS, Wittes RE, Paull KD. An information-intensive approach to the molecular pharmacology of cancer. Science 1997; 275: 343-9.

[54]   Zhang CC, Yang JM, Bash-Babula J, White E, Murphy M, Levine AJ, Hait WN. DNA damage increases sensitivity to vinca alkaloids and decreases sensitivity to taxanes through p53-dependent repression of microtubule-associated protein 4. Cancer Res 1999; 59: 3663-70.

[55]   Buzzai M, Jones RG, Amaravadi RK, Lum JJ, DeBerardinis RJ, Zhao F, Viollet B, Thompson CB. Systemic treatment with the antidiabetic drug metformin selectively impairs p53-deficient tumor cell growth. Cancer Res 2007; 67: 6745-52.

[56]   Wang Z, Zheng M, Li Z, Li R, Jia L, Xiong X, Southall N, Wang S, Xia M, Austin CP, Zheng W, Xie Z, Sun Y. Cardiac glycosides inhibit p53 synthesis by a mechanism relieved by Src or MAPK inhibition. Cancer Res 2009; 69: 6556-64.

[57]   Wu X, Bayle JH, Olson D, Levine AJ. The p53-mdm-2 autoregulatory feedback loop. Genes Dev 1993; 7: 1126-32.

[58]   Shangary S, Wang S. Targeting the MDM2-p53 interaction for cancer therapy. Clin Cancer Res 2008; 14: 5318-24.

[59]   Bassett EA, Wang W, Rastinejad F, El-Deiry WS. Structural and functional basis for therapeutic modulation of p53 signaling. Clin Cancer Res 2008; 14: 6376-86.

[60]   Vassilev LT, Vu BT, Graves B, Carvajal D, Podlaski F, Filipovic Z, Kong N, Kammlott U, Lukacs C, Klein C, Fotouhi N, Liu EA. *In vivo* activation of the p53 pathway by small-molecule antagonists of MDM2. Science 2004 Feb 6;303(5659):844-8.

[61]   Grasberger BL, Lu T, Schubert C, Parks DJ, Carver TE, Koblish HK, Cummings MD, LaFrance LV, Milkiewicz KL, Calvo RR, Maguire D, Lattanze J, Franks CF, Zhao S, Ramachandren K, Bylebyl GR, Zhang M, Manthey CL, Petrella EC, Pantoliano MW, Deckman IC, Spurlino JC, Maroney AC, Tomczuk BE, Molloy CJ, Bone RF. Discovery and cocrystal structure of benzodiazepinedione HDM2 antagonists that activate p53 in cells. J Med Chem 2005; 48: 909-12.

[62]   Ding K, Lu Y, Nikolovska-Coleska Z, Wang G, Qiu S, Shangary S, Gao W, Qin D, Stuckey J, Krajewski K, Roller PP, Wang S. Structure-based design of spiro-oxindoles as potent, specific small-molecule inhibitors of the MDM2-p53 interaction. J Med Chem 2006; 49: 3432-5.

[63]   Sun SH, Zheng M, Ding K, Wang S, Sun Y. A small molecule that disrupts Mdm2-p53 binding activates p53, induces apoptosis and sensitizes lung cancer cells to chemotherapy. Cancer Biol Ther 2008; 7: 845-52.

[64]   Koblish HK, Zhao S, Franks CF, Donatelli RR, Tominovich RM, LaFrance LV, Leonard KA, Gushue JM, Parks DJ, Calvo RR, Milkiewicz KL, Marugán JJ, Raboisson P, Cummings MD, Grasberger BL, Johnson DL, Lu T, Molloy CJ, Maroney AC. Benzodiazepinedione inhibitors of the Hdm2:p53 complex suppress human tumor cell proliferation *in vitro* and sensitize tumors to doxorubicin *in vivo*. Mol Cancer Ther 2006; 5: 160-9.

[65]   Sierra JR, Cepero V, Giordano S. Molecular mechanisms of acquired resistance to tyrosine kinase targeted therapy. Mol Cancer 2010; 9: 75.

[66]   Bradeen HA, Eide CA, O'Hare T, Johnson KJ, Willis SG, Lee FY, Druker BJ, Deininger MW. Comparison of imatinib mesylate, dasatinib (BMS-354825), and nilotinib (AMN107) in an N-ethyl-N-nitrosourea (ENU)-based mutagenesis screen: high efficacy of drug combinations. Blood 2006; 108: 2332-8.

[67]   Sulkes A. Novel multitargeted anticancer oral therapies: sunitinib and sorafenib as a paradigm. Isr Med Assoc J 2010; 12: 628-32.

[68]   Hu S, Chen Z, Franke R, Orwick S, Zhao M, Rudek MA, Sparreboom A, Baker SD. Interaction of the multikinase inhibitors sorafenib and sunitinib with solute carriers and ATP-binding cassette transporters. Clin Cancer Res 2009; 15: 6062-9.

[69]   Alvarado Y, Mita MM, Vemulapalli S, Mahalingam D, Mita AC. Clinical activity of mammalian target of rapamycin inhibitors in solid tumors. Target Oncol 2011; 6: 69-94.

[70]   Reardon DA, Nabors LB, Stupp R, Mikkelsen T. Cilengitide: an integrin-targeting arginine-glycine-aspartic acid peptide with promising activity for glioblastoma multiforme. Expert Opin Investig Drugs 2008; 17: 1225-35.

[71]   Hegedus C, Ozvegy-Laczka C, Szakács G, Sarkadi B. Interaction of ABC multidrug transporters with anticancer protein kinase inhibitors: substrates and/or inhibitors? Curr Cancer Drug Targets. 2009; 9: 252-72.

[72]   Szakács G, Paterson JK, Ludwig JA, Booth-Genthe C, Gottesman MM. Targeting multidrug resistance in cancer. Nat Rev Drug Discov 2006; 5: 219-34.

[73]   Sarkadi B, Homolya L, Szakács G, Váradi A. Human multidrug resistance ABCB and ABCG transporters: participation in a chemoimmunity defense system. Physiol Rev 2006; 86: 1179-236.

[74]   Seeger MA, van Veen HW. Molecular basis of multidrug transport by ABC transporters. Biochim Biophys Acta 2009; 1794: 725-37.

[75]   Hopper-Borge EA, Nasto RE, Ratushny V, Weiner LM, Golemis EA, Astsaturov I. Mechanisms of tumor resistance to EGFR-targeted therapies. Expert Opin Ther Targets 2009; 13: 339-62.

[76]   Valent P. Imatinib-resistant chronic myeloid leukemia (CML): Current concepts on pathogenesis and new emerging pharmacologic approaches. Biologics 2007; 1: 433-48.

[77]   Druker BJ, Guilhot F, O'Brien SG, Gathmann I, Kantarjian H, Gattermann N, Deininger MW, Silver RT, Goldman JM, Stone RM, Cervantes F, Hochhaus A, Powell BL, Gabrilove JL, Rousselot P, Reiffers J, Cornelissen JJ, Hughes T, Agis H, Fischer T, Verhoef G, Shepherd J, Saglio G, Gratwohl A, Nielsen JL, Radich JP, Simonsson B, Taylor K, Baccarani M, So C, Letvak L, Larson RA; IRIS Investigators. Five-year follow-up of patients receiving imatinib for chronic myeloid leukemia. N Engl J Med 2006; 355: 2408-17.

[78]   Wander SA, Hennessy BT, Slingerland JM. Next-generation mTOR inhibitors in clinical oncology: how pathway complexity informs therapeutic strategy. J Clin Invest 2011; 121: 1231-41.

[79]   Andjelkovic T, Bankovic J, Stojsic J, Milinkovic V, Podolski-Renic A, Ruzdijic S, Tanic N. Coalterations of p53 and PTEN tumor suppressor genes in non-small cell lung carcinoma patients. Transl Res 2011; 157: 19-28.

[80]   Andjelkovic T, Bankovic J, Milosevic Z, Stojsic J, Milinkovic V, Pesic M, Ruzdijic S, Tanic N. Concurrent alteration of p16 and PTEN tumor suppressor genes could be

considered as potential molecular marker for specific subgroups of NSCLC patients. Cancer Biomark 2011-2012; 10: 277-86.

[81]   Hardt M, Chantaravisoot N, Tamanoi F. Activating mutations of TOR (target of rapamycin). Genes Cells 2011; 16: 141-51.

[82]   Roulin D, Cerantola Y, Dormond-Meuwly A, Demartines N, Dormond O. Targeting mTORC2 inhibits colon cancer cell proliferation *in vitro* and tumor formation *in vivo*. Mol Cancer 2010; 9: 57.

[83]   Wu WK, Lee CW, Cho CH, Chan FK, Yu J, Sung JJ. RNA interference targeting raptor inhibits proliferation of gastric cancer cells. Exp Cell Res 2011; 317: 1353-8.

[84]   Liu Q, Thoreen C, Wang J, Sabatini D, Gray NS. mTOR Mediated Anti-Cancer Drug Discovery. Drug Discov Today Ther Strateg 2009; 6: 47-55.

[85]   Gulhati P, Cai Q, Li J, Liu J, Rychahou PG, Qiu S, Lee EY, Silva SR, Bowen KA, Gao T, Evers BM. Targeted inhibition of mammalian target of rapamycin signaling inhibits tumorigenesis of colorectal cancer. Clin Cancer Res 2009; 15: 7207-16.

[86]   Zeng Z, Sarbassov dos D, Samudio IJ, Yee KW, Munsell MF, Ellen Jackson C, Giles FJ, Sabatini DM, Andreeff M, Konopleva M. Rapamycin derivatives reduce mTORC2 signaling and inhibit AKT activation in AML. Blood 2007; 109: 3509-12.

[87]   Liu Q, Kang SA, Thoreen CC, Hur W, Wang J, Chang JW, Markhard A, Zhang J, Sim T, Sabatini DM, Gray NS. Development of ATP-competitive mTOR inhibitors. Methods Mol Biol 2012; 821: 447-60.

[88]   Guertin DA, Sabatini DM. The pharmacology of mTOR inhibition. Sci Signal 2009; 2: pe24.

[89]   Efeyan A, Sabatini DM. mTOR and cancer: many loops in one pathway. Curr Opin Cell Biol 2010; 22: 169-76.

[90]   Yu K, Toral-Barza L, Shi C, Zhang WG, Lucas J, Shor B, Kim J, Verheijen J, Curran K, Malwitz DJ, Cole DC, Ellingboe J, Ayral-Kaloustian S, Mansour TS, Gibbons JJ, Abraham RT, Nowak P, Zask A. Biochemical, cellular, and *in vivo* activity of novel ATP-competitive and selective inhibitors of the mammalian target of rapamycin. Cancer Res 2009; 69: 6232-40.

[91]   Markovic J, Stojsic J, Zunic S, Ruzdijic S, Tanic N. Genomic instability in patients with non-small cell lung cancer assessed by the arbitrarily primed polymerase chain reaction. Cancer Invest 2008; 26: 262-8.

[92]   Bankovic J, Stojsic J, Jovanovic D, Andjelkovic T, Milinkovic V, Ruzdijic S, Tanic N. Identification of genes associated with non-small-cell lung cancer promotion and progression. Lung Cancer 2010; 67: 151-9.

[93]   Sampath J, Sun D, Kidd VJ, Grenet J, Gandhi A, Shapiro LH, Wang Q, Zambetti GP, Schuetz JD. Mutant p53 cooperates with ETS and selectively up-regulates human MDR1 not MRP1. J Biol Chem 2001; 276: 39359-67.

[94]   Andjelkovic T, Pesic M, Bankovic J, Tanic N, Markovic ID, Ruzdijic S. Synergistic effects of the purine analog sulfinosine and curcumin on the multidrug resistant human non-small cell lung carcinoma cell line (NCI-H460/R). Cancer Biol Ther 2008; 7: 1024-32.

[95]   Nahi H. P53 guardian of the genome and target for improved treatment of leukemia. Thesis for doctoral degree (Ph.D.) 2007; Karolinska University Hospital, Huddinge. Stockholm, Sweden.

[96]   Michaelis M, Rothweiler F, Klassert D, von Deimling A, Weber K, Fehse B, Kammerer B, Doerr HW, Cinatl J Jr. Reversal of P-glycoprotein-mediated multidrug resistance by the murine double minute 2 antagonist nutlin-3. Cancer Res 2009; 69: 416-21.

[97]   Vassilev LT. MDM2 inhibitors for cancer therapy. Trends Mol Med 2007; 13: 23-31.

[98]   Hegedus C, Ozvegy-Laczka C, Apáti A, Magócsi M, Német K, Orfi L, Kéri G, Katona M, Takáts Z, Váradi A, Szakács G, Sarkadi B. Interaction of nilotinib, dasatinib and bosutinib with ABCB1 and ABCG2: implications for altered anti-cancer effects and pharmacological properties. Br J Pharmacol 2009; 158: 1153-64.

[99]   Dohse M, Scharenberg C, Shukla S, Robey RW, Volkmann T, Deeken JF, Brendel C, Ambudkar SV, Neubauer A, Bates SE. Comparison of ATP-binding cassette transporter interactions with the tyrosine kinase inhibitors imatinib, nilotinib, and dasatinib. Drug Metab Dispos 2010; 38: 1371-80.

[100]   Leggas M, Panetta JC, Zhuang Y, Schuetz JD, Johnston B, Bai F, Sorrentino B, Zhou S, Houghton PJ, Stewart CF. Gefitinib modulates the function of multiple ATP-binding cassette transporters *in vivo*. Cancer Res 2006; 66: 4802-7.

[101]   Nakamura Y, Oka M, Soda H, Shiozawa K, Yoshikawa M, Itoh A, Ikegami Y, Tsurutani J, Nakatomi K, Kitazaki T, Doi S, Yoshida H, Kohno S. Gefitinib ("Iressa", ZD1839), an epidermal growth factor receptor tyrosine kinase inhibitor, reverses breast cancer resistance protein/ABCG2-mediated drug resistance. Cancer Res 2005; 65: 1541-6.

[102]   Dai CL, Tiwari AK, Wu CP, Su XD, Wang SR, Liu DG, Ashby CR Jr, Huang Y, Robey RW, Liang YJ, Chen LM, Shi CJ, Ambudkar SV, Chen ZS, Fu LW. Lapatinib (Tykerb, GW572016) reverses multidrug resistance in cancer cells by inhibiting the activity of ATP-binding cassette subfamily B member 1 and G member 2. Cancer Res 2008; 68: 7905-14.

[103]   Marchetti S, de Vries NA, Buckle T, Bolijn MJ, van Eijndhoven MA, Beijnen JH, Mazzanti R, van Tellingen O, Schellens JH. Effect of the ATP-binding cassette drug transporters ABCB1, ABCG2, and ABCC2 on erlotinib hydrochloride (Tarceva) disposition in *in vitro* and *in vivo* pharmacokinetic studies employing Bcrp1-/-/Mdr1a/1b-/- (triple-knockout) and wild-type mice. Mol Cancer Ther 2008; 7: 2280-7.

[104]   Hu S, Chen Z, Franke R, Orwick S, Zhao M, Rudek MA, Sparreboom A, Baker SD. Interaction of the multikinase inhibitors sorafenib and sunitinib with solute carriers and ATP-binding cassette transporters. Clin Cancer Res 2009; 15: 6062-9.

[105]   Ozvegy-Laczka C, Hegedus T, Várady G, Ujhelly O, Schuetz JD, Váradi A, Kéri G, Orfi L, Német K, Sarkadi B. High-affinity interaction of tyrosine kinase inhibitors with the ABCG2 multidrug transporter. Mol Pharmacol 2004; 65: 1485-95.

[106]   Houghton PJ, Agbedahunsi JM, Adegbulugbe A. Choline esterase inhibitory properties of alkaloids from two Nigerian Crinum species. Phytochemistry 2004; 65: 2893-6.

[107]   Mukai M, Che XF, Furukawa T, Sumizawa T, Aoki S, Ren XQ, Haraguchi M, Sugimoto Y, Kobayashi M, Takamatsu H, Akiyama S. Reversal of the resistance to STI571 in human chronic myelogenous leukemia K562 cells. Cancer Sci 2003; 94: 557-63.

[108]   Tiwari AK, Sodani K, Wang SR, Kuang YH, Ashby CR Jr, Chen X, Chen ZS. Nilotinib (AMN107, Tasigna) reverses multidrug resistance by inhibiting the activity of the ABCB1/Pgp and ABCG2/BCRP/MXR transporters. Biochem Pharmacol 2009; 78: 153-61.

[109]   Yanase K, Tsukahara S, Asada S, Ishikawa E, Imai Y, Sugimoto Y. Gefitinib reverses breast cancer resistance protein-mediated drug resistance. Mol Cancer Ther 2004; 3: 1119-25.

[110] Noguchi K, Kawahara H, Kaji A, Katayama K, Mitsuhashi J, Sugimoto Y. Substrate-dependent bidirectional modulation of P-glycoprotein-mediated drug resistance by erlotinib. Cancer Sci 2009; 100: 1701-7.

[111] Shi Z, Parmar S, Peng XX, Shen T, Robey RW, Bates SE, Fu LW, Shao Y, Chen YM, Zang F, Chen ZS. The epidermal growth factor tyrosine kinase inhibitor AG1478 and erlotinib reverse ABCG2-mediated drug resistance. Oncol Rep 2009; 21: 483-9.

[112] Shukla S, Robey RW, Bates SE, Ambudkar SV. Sunitinib (Sutent, SU11248), a small-molecule receptor tyrosine kinase inhibitor, blocks function of the ATP-binding cassette (ABC) transporters P-glycoprotein (ABCB1) and ABCG2. Drug Metab Dispos 2009; 37: 359-65.

[113] Weisberg E, Catley L, Wright RD, Moreno D, Banerji L, Ray A, Manley PW, Mestan J, Fabbro D, Jiang J, Hall-Meyers E, Callahan L, DellaGatta JL, Kung AL, Griffin JD. Beneficial effects of combining nilotinib and imatinib in preclinical models of BCR-ABL+ leukemias. Blood 2007; 109: 2112-20.

[114] White DL, Saunders VA, Quinn SR, Manley PW, Hughes TP. Imatinib increases the intracellular concentration of nilotinib, which may explain the observed synergy between these drugs. Blood 2007; 109: 3609-10.

[115] Visentin M, Biason P, Toffoli G. Drug interactions among the epidermal growth factor receptor inhibitors, other biologics and cytotoxic agents. Pharmacol Ther 2010; 128: 82-90.

[116] Veronese ML, Sun W, Giantonio B, Berlin J, Shults J, Davis L, Haller DG, O'Dwyer PJ. A phase II trial of gefitinib with 5-fluorouracil, leucovorin, and irinotecan in patients with colorectal cancer. Br J Cancer 2005; 92: 1846-9.

[117] Deenik W, Janssen JJ, van der Holt B, Verhoef GE, Smit WM, Kersten MJ, Daenen SM, Verdonck LF, Ferrant A, Schattenberg AV, Sonneveld P, van Marwijk Kooy M, Wittebol S, Willemze R, Wijermans PW, Beverloo HB, Löwenberg B, Valk PJ, Ossenkoppele GJ, Cornelissen JJ. Efficacy of escalated imatinib combined with cytarabine in newly diagnosed patients with chronic myeloid leukemia. Haematologica 2010; 95: 914-21.

[118] Haouala A, Widmer N, Duchosal MA, Montemurro M, Buclin T, Decosterd LA. Drug interactions with the tyrosine kinase inhibitors imatinib, dasatinib, and nilotinib. Blood 2011; 117: e75-87.

[119] Stewart CF, Leggas M, Schuetz JD, Panetta JC, Cheshire PJ, Peterson J, Daw N, Jenkins JJ 3rd, Gilbertson R, Germain GS, Harwood FC, Houghton PJ. Gefitinib enhances the antitumor activity and oral bioavailability of irinotecan in mice. Cancer Res 2004; 64: 7491-9.

[120] Carcaboso AM, Elmeliegy MA, Shen J, Juel SJ, Zhang ZM, Calabrese C, Tracey L, Waters CM, Stewart CF. Tyrosine kinase inhibitor gefitinib enhances topotecan penetration of gliomas. Cancer Res 2010; 70: 4499-508.

[121] Dulucq S, Bouchet S, Turcq B, Lippert E, Etienne G, Reiffers J, Molimard M, Krajinovic M, Mahon FX Multidrug resistance gene (MDR1) polymorphisms are associated with major molecular responses to standard-dose imatinib in chronic myeloid leukemia. Blood 2008; 112: 2024-7.

[122] Cusatis G, Gregorc V, Li J, Spreafico A, Ingersoll RG, Verweij J, Ludovini V, Villa E, Hidalgo M, Sparreboom A, Baker SD. Pharmacogenetics of ABCG2 and adverse reactions to gefitinib. J Natl Cancer Inst 2006; 98: 1739-42.

[123] Cohen MH, Johnson JR, Chen YF, Sridhara R, Pazdur R. FDA drug approval summary: erlotinib (Tarceva) tablets. Oncologist 2005; 10: 461-6.

[124] Kamath AV, Wang J, Lee FY, Marathe PH. Preclinical pharmacokinetics and *in vitro* metabolism of dasatinib (BMS-354825): a potent oral multi-targeted kinase inhibitor against SRC and BCR-ABL. Cancer Chemother Pharmacol 2008; 61: 365-76.

[125] Gschwind HP, Pfaar U, Waldmeier F, Zollinger M, Sayer C, Zbinden P, Hayes M, Pokorny R, Seiberling M, Ben-Am M, Peng B, Gross G. Metabolism and disposition of imatinib mesylate in healthy volunteers. Drug Metab Dispos 2005; 33: 1503-12.

[126] Ling J, Johnson KA, Miao Z, Rakhit A, Pantze MP, Hamilton M, Lum BL, Prakash C. Metabolism and excretion of erlotinib, a small molecule inhibitor of epidermal growth factor receptor tyrosine kinase, in healthy male volunteers. Drug Metab Dispos 2006; 34: 420-6.

[127] Declèves X, Bihorel S, Debray M, Yousif S, Camenisch G, Scherrmann JM. ABC transporters and the accumulation of imatinib and its active metabolite CGP74588 in rat C6 glioma cells. Pharmacol Res 2008; 57: 214-22.

[128] Pop IV, Pop LM, Ghetie MA, Vitetta ES. Targeting mammalian target of rapamycin to both downregulate and disable the P-glycoprotein pump in multidrug-resistant B-cell lymphoma cell lines. Leuk Lymphoma 2009; 50: 1155-62.

[129] Kerr KM, Sauna ZE, Ambudkar SV. Correlation between steady-state ATP hydrolysis and vanadate-induced ADP trapping in Human P-glycoprotein. Evidence for ADP release as the rate-limiting step in the catalytic cycle and its modulation by substrates. J Biol Chem 2001; 276: 8657-64.

[130] Kurmasheva RT, Huang S, Houghton PJ. Predicted mechanisms of resistance to mTOR inhibitors. Br J Cancer 2006; 95: 955-60.

[131] Minocha M, Khurana V, Qin B, Pal D, Mitra AK. Co-administration strategy to enhance brain accumulation of vandetanib by modulating P-glycoprotein (P-gp/Abcb1) and breast cancer resistance protein (Bcrp1/Abcg2) mediated efflux with m-TOR inhibitors. Int J Pharm 2012; 434): 306-14.

[132] Roulin D, Waselle L, Dormond-Meuwly A, Dufour M, Demartines N, Dormond O. Targeting renal cell carcinoma with NVP-BEZ235, a dual PI3K/mTOR inhibitor, in combination with sorafenib. Mol Cancer 2011; 10: 90.

[133] Gedaly R, Angulo P, Hundley J, Daily MF, Chen C, Koch A, Evers BM. PI-103 and sorafenib inhibit hepatocellular carcinoma cell proliferation by blocking Ras/Raf/MAPK and PI3K/AKT/mTOR pathways. Anticancer Res 2010; 30: 4951-8.

[134] MacDonald TJ, Stewart CF, Kocak M, Goldman S, Ellenbogen RG, Phillips P, Lafond D, Poussaint TY, Kieran MW, Boyett JM, Kun LE. Phase I clinical trial of cilengitide in children with refractory brain tumors: Pediatric Brain Tumor Consortium Study PBTC-012. J Clin Oncol 2008; 26: 919-24.

[135] Lage H. An overview of cancer multidrug resistance: a still unsolved problem. Cell Mol Life Sci 2008; 65: 3145-67.

[136] Raviv Y, Pollard HB, Bruggemann EP, Pastan I, Gottesman MM. Photosensitized labeling of a functional multidrug transporter in living drug-resistant tumor cells. J Biol Chem 1990; 265: 3975-80.

[137] Teodori E, Dei S, Scapecchi S, Gualtieri F. The medicinal chemistry of multidrug resistance (MDR) reversing drugs. Farmaco 2002; 57: 385-415.

[138] Borowski E, Bontemps-Gracz MM, Piwkowska A. Strategies for overcoming ABC-transporters-mediated multidrug resistance (MDR) of tumor cells. Acta Biochim Pol 2005; 52: 609-27.

[139] Yang K, Wu J, Li X. Recent advances in the research of P-glycoprotein inhibitors. Biosci Trends 2008; 2: 137-46.

[140] Ernst R, Kueppers P, Stindt J, Kuchler K, Schmitt L. Multidrug efflux pumps: substrate selection in ATP-binding cassette multidrug efflux pumps--first come, first served? FEBS J 2010; 277: 540-9.

[141] Takara K, Sakaeda T, Okumura K. An update on overcoming MDR1-mediated multidrug resistance in cancer chemotherapy. Curr Pharm Des 2006; 12: 273-86.

[142] Lee CH. Reversing agents for ATP-binding cassette drug transporters. Methods Mol Biol 2010; 596: 325-40.

[143] Mayur YC, Peters GJ, Prasad VV, Lemo C, Sathish NK. Design of new drug molecules to be used in reversing multidrug resistance in cancer cells. Curr Cancer Drug Targets 2009; 9: 298-306.

[144] Fletcher JI, Haber M, Henderson MJ, Norris MD. ABC transporters in cancer: more than just drug efflux pumps. Nat Rev Cancer 2010; 10: 147-56.

[145] Hall MD, Handley MD, Gottesman MM. Is resistance useless? Multidrug resistance and collateral sensitivity. Trends Pharmacol Sci 2009; 30: 546-56.

[146] Robert J, Jarry C. Multidrug resistance reversal agents. J Med Chem 2003; 46: 4805-17.

[147] Krishna R, Mayer LD. Multidrug resistance (MDR) in cancer. Mechanisms, reversal using modulators of MDR and the role of MDR modulators in influencing the pharmacokinetics of anticancer drugs. Eur J Pharm Sci 2000; 11: 265-83.

[148] Lhommé C, Joly F, Walker JL, Lissoni AA, Nicoletto MO, Manikhas GM, Baekelandt MM, Gordon AN, Fracasso PM, Mietlowski WL, Jones GJ, Dugan MH. Phase III study of valspodar (PSC 833) combined with paclitaxel and carboplatin compared with paclitaxel and carboplatin alone in patients with stage IV or suboptimally debulked stage III epithelial ovarian cancer or primary peritoneal cancer. J Clin Oncol 2008; 26: 2674-82.

[149] Kang MH, Figg WD, Ando Y, Blagosklonny MV, Liewehr D, Fojo T, Bates SE. The P-glycoprotein antagonist PSC 833 increases the plasma concentrations of 6alpha-hydroxypaclitaxel, a major metabolite of paclitaxel. Clin Cancer Res 2001; 7: 1610-7.

[150] Cnubben NH, Wortelboer HM, van Zanden JJ, Rietjens IM, van Bladeren PJ. Metabolism of ATP-binding cassette drug transporter inhibitors: complicating factor for multidrug resistance. Expert Opin Drug Metab Toxicol 2005; 1: 219-32.

[151] Cripe LD, Uno H, Paietta EM, Litzow MR, Ketterling RP, Bennett JM, Rowe JM, Lazarus HM, Luger S, Tallman MS. Zosuquidar, a novel modulator of P-glycoprotein, does not improve the outcome of older patients with newly diagnosed acute myeloid leukemia: a randomized, placebo-controlled trial of the Eastern Cooperative Oncology Group 3999. Blood 2010; 116: 4077-85.

[152] Gottesman MM, Fojo T, Bates SE. Multidrug resistance in cancer: role of ATP-dependent transporters. Nat Rev Cancer 2002; 2: 48-58.

[153] Lepper ER, Nooter K, Verweij J, Acharya MR, Figg WD, Sparreboom A. Mechanisms of resistance to anticancer drugs: the role of the polymorphic ABC transporters ABCB1 and ABCG2. Pharmacogenomics 2005; 6: 115-38.

[154] Didziapetris R, Japertas P, Avdeef A, Petrauskas A. Classification analysis of P-glycoprotein substrate specificity. J Drug Target 2003; 11: 391-406.

[155] Demel MA, Krämer O, Ettmayer P, Haaksma EE, Ecker GF. Predicting ligand interactions with ABC transporters in ADME. Chem Biodivers 2009; 6: 1960-9.

[156] Aller SG, Yu J, Ward A, Weng Y, Chittaboina S, Zhuo R, Harrell PM, Trinh YT, Zhang Q, Urbatsch IL, Chang G. Structure of P-glycoprotein reveals a molecular basis for poly-specific drug binding. Science 2009; 323: 1718-22.

[157] Dong X, Mumper RJ. Nanomedicinal strategies to treat multidrug-resistant tumors: current progress. Nanomedicine (Lond) 2010; 5: 597-615.

[158] Lazo JS, Reese CE, Vogt A, Vollmer LL, Kitchens CA, Günther E, Graham TH, Hopkins CD, Wipf P. Identifying a resistance determinant for the antimitotic natural products disorazole C1 and A1. J Pharmacol Exp Ther 2010; 332: 906-11.

[159] Galmarini CM. Sagopilone, a microtubule stabilizer for the potential treatment of cancer. Curr Opin Investig Drugs 2009; 10: 1359-71.

[160] Ferlini C, Ojima I, Distefano M, Gallo D, Riva A, Morazzoni P, Bombardelli E, Mancuso S, Scambia G. Second generation taxanes: from the natural framework to the challenge of drug resistance. Curr Med Chem Anticancer Agents 2003; 3: 133-8.

[161] Gross M, Pendergrass K, Leitner S, Leichman G, Pugliese L, Silberman S. TPI 287, a thirdgeneration taxane, is active and well tolerated as 2nd line therapy after failure of docetaxel in hormone refractory prostate cancer (HRPC). J Clin Oncol (ASCO Annu Meet Proc) 2008; 26: 16130.

[162] Podolski-Renić A, Andelković T, Banković J, Tanić N, Ruždijić S, Pešić M. The role of paclitaxel in the development and treatment of multidrug resistant cancer cell lines. Biomed Pharmacother 2011; 65: 345-53.

[163] Ismael GF, Rosa DD, Mano MS, Awada A. Novel cytotoxic drugs: old challenges, new solutions. Cancer Treat Rev 2008; 34: 81-91.

[164] Newman SP, Foster PA, Stengel C, Day JM, Ho YT, Judde JG, Lassalle M, Prevost G, Leese MP, Potter BV, Reed MJ, Purohit A. STX140 is efficacious *in vitro* and *in vivo* in taxane-resistant breast carcinoma cells. Clin Cancer Res 2008; 14: 597-606.

[165] Teicher BA. Next generation topoisomerase I inhibitors: Rationale and biomarker strategies. Biochem Pharmacol 2008; 75: 1262-71.

[166] Chhikara BS, Mandal D, Parang K. Synthesis, anticancer activities, and cellular uptake studies of lipophilic derivatives of doxorubicin succinate. J Med Chem 2012; 55: 1500-10.

[167] Blagosklonny MV. Targeting cancer cells by exploiting their resistance. Trends Mol Med 2003; 9: 307-12.

[168] Türk D, Szakács G. Relevance of multidrug resistance in the age of targeted therapy. Curr Opin Drug Discov Devel 2009; 12: 246-52.

[169] Ludwig JA, Szakács G, Martin SE, Chu BF, Cardarelli C, Sauna ZE, Caplen NJ, Fales HM, Ambudkar SV, Weinstein JN, Gottesman MM. Selective toxicity of NSC73306 in MDR1-positive cells as a new strategy to circumvent multidrug resistance in cancer. Cancer Res 2006; 66: 4808-15.

[170] Wu CP, Shukla S, Calcagno AM, Hall MD, Gottesman MM, Ambudkar SV. Evidence for dual mode of action of a thiosemicarbazone, NSC73306: a potent substrate of the multidrug resistance linked ABCG2 transporter. Mol Cancer Ther 2007; 6: 3287-96.

[171] Pesic M, Andjelkovic T, Bankovic J, Markovic ID, Rakic L, Ruzdijic S. Sulfinosine enhances doxorubicin efficacy through synergism and by reversing multidrug resistance in the human non-small cell lung carcinoma cell line (NCI-H460/R). Invest New Drugs 2009; 27: 99-110.

[172] Pesic M, Podolski A, Rakic L, Ruzdijic S. Purine analogs sensitize the multidrug resistant cell line (NCI-H460/R) to doxorubicin and stimulate the cell growth inhibitory effect of verapamil. Invest New Drugs 2010; 28: 482-92.

[173] Palmeira A, Sousa E, Vasconcelos MH, Pinto MM. Three decades of P-gp inhibitors: skimming through several generations and scaffolds. Curr Med Chem 2012; 19: 1946-2025.

[174] Newman DJ, Cragg GM. Natural products as sources of new drugs over the last 25 years. J Nat Prod 2007; 70: 461-77.

[175] Jones M, Barrett B, Bell C, Brown E, Feng L, Emerson D. TPI 287, a third-generation taxanederivative, functionally modulates the MDR1 P-glycoprotein drug transport pump and is active in resistant tumor cells. Proc AACR-NCI-EORTC Int Conf Mol Targets Cancer Ther 2007; 128: (Abstr. A192).

[176] Ferreira MJU, Duarte N, Lage H, Molnár J. Reversal of Multidrug Resistance by Macrocyclic and Polycyclic Diterpenoids from *Euphorbia* species. In: Geetanjali K, Govil JN, Eds. Recent Progress in Medicinal Plants, Vol 32-Ethnomedicine and Therapeutic Validation. Studium Press LLC, U.S.A., 2012; pp. 193-213.

[177] Shi QW, Su XH, Kiyota H. Chemical and pharmacological research of the plants in genus Euphorbia. Chem Rev 2008; 108: 4295-327.

[178] Jassbi AR. Chemistry and biological activity of secondary metabolites in Euphorbia from Iran. Phytochemistry 2006; 67: 1977-84.

[179] Hartwell J. Plants used against cancer. A survey. Lloydia 1969; 32: 153-205.

[180] Judd W, Campbell C, Kellog E, Stevens P, Donoghue M. Plant Systematics. A Phylogenetic Approach. 3rd Ed. Massachusetts: Sinauer Associated, Inc. Sunderland 2002; pp. 355-359.

[181] Hohmann, J., Evanics, F., Dombi, G., Molnár, J. and Szabo, P. 2001. Euphosalicin, a new diterpene polyester with multidrug resistance reversing activity from *Euphorbia salicifolia*. *Tetrahedron* 57: 211-215.

[182] Hohmann J, Molnár J, Rédei D, Evanics F, Forgo P, Kálmán A, Argay G, Szabó P. Discovery and biological evaluation of a new family of potent modulators of multidrug resistance: reversal of multidrug resistance of mouse lymphoma cells by new natural jatrophane diterpenoids isolated from Euphorbia species. J Med Chem 2002; 45: 2425-31.

[183] Hohmann J, Rédei D, Forgo P, Molnár J, Dombi G, Zorig T. Jatrophane diterpenoids from Euphorbia mongolica as modulators of the multidrug resistance of L5128 mouse lymphoma cells. J Nat Prod 2003; 66: 976-9.

[184] Corea G, Fattorusso E, Lanzotti V, Taglialatela-Scafati O, Appendino G, Ballero M, Simon PN, Dumontet C, Di Pietro A. Jatrophane diterpenes as Pglycoprotein inhibitors. First insights of structure-activity relationships and discovery of a new, powerful lead. J Med Chem 2003; 46: 3395-3402.

[185] Corea G, Fattorusso E, Lanzotti V, Motti R, Simon PN, Dumontet C, Di Pietro A. Jatrophane diterpenes as modulators of multidrug resistance. Advances of structure-activity relationships and discovery of the potent lead pepluanin A. J Med Chem 2004; 47: 988-92.

[186] Jadranin M, Pešić M, Aljančić IS, Milosavljević SM, Todorović NM, Podolski-Renić A, Banković J, Tanić N, Marković I, Vajs VE, Tešević VV. Jatrophane diterpenoids from the latex of Euphorbia dendroides and their anti-P-glycoprotein activity in human multi-drug resistant cancer cell lines. Phytochemistry 2012; doi: 10.1016/j.phytochem.2012.09.003.

[187] Aljancić IS, Pesić M, Milosavljević SM, Todorović NM, Jadranin M, Milosavljević G, Povrenović D, Banković J, Tanić N, Marković ID, Ruzdijić S, Vajs VE, Tesević VV.

Isolation and biological evaluation of jatrophane diterpenoids from Euphorbia dendroides. J Nat Prod 2011; 74: 1613-20.

[188]   Jiao W, Dong W, Li Z, Deng M, Lu R. Lathyrane diterpenes from Euphorbia lathyris as modulators of multidrug resistance and their crystal structures. Biorganic and Medicinal Chemistry 2009; 17: 4786-4792.

[189]   Barile E, Lanzotti V. Biogenetical related highly oxygenated macrocyclic diterpenes from sea spurge *Euphorbia paralias*. Organic Letters 2007; 9: 3603-3606.

[190]   Pesic M, Bankovic J, Aljancic IS, Todorovic NM, Jadranin M, Vajs VE, Tesevic VV, Vuckovic I, Momcilovic M, Markovic ID, Tanic N, Ruždijic S. New anti-cancer characteristics of jatrophane diterpenes from Euphorbia dendroides. Food Chem Toxicol 2011; 49: 3165-73.

[191]   Agrawal M, Garg RJ, Cortes J, Quintás-Cardama A. Tyrosine kinase inhibitors: the first decade. Curr Hematol Malig Rep 2010; 5: 70-80.

[192]   Usuda J, Ohira T, Suga Y, Oikawa T, Ichinose S, Inoue T, Ohtani K, Maehara S, Imai K, Kubota M, Tsunoda Y, Tsutsui H, Furukawa K, Okunaka T, Sugimoto Y, Kato H. Breast cancer resistance protein (BCRP) affected acquired resistance to gefitinib in a "never-smoked" female patient with advanced non-small cell lung cancer. Lung Cancer 2007; 58: 296-9.

[193]   Burger H, van Tol H, Brok M, Wiemer EA, de Bruijn EA, Guetens G, de Boeck G, Sparreboom A, Verweij J, Nooter K. Chronic imatinib mesylate exposure leads to reduced intracellular drug accumulation by induction of the ABCG2 (BCRP) and ABCB1 (MDR1) drug transport pumps. Cancer Biol Ther 2005; 4: 747-52.

[194]   Daood M, Tsai C, Ahdab-Barmada M, Watchko JF. ABC transporter (P-gp/ABCB1, MRP1/ABCC1, BCRP/ABCG2) expression in the developing human CNS. Neuropediatrics 2008; 39: 211-8.

Frontiers in Anti-Cancer Drug Discovery, 2014, 3, 151-190 151

CHAPTER 4

Understanding Tumor Metabolism and its Potential as a Target for the Treatment of Cancer

Ana Carolina Santos de Souza[*,1], Alexandre Donizeti Martins Cavagis[2], Carmen Veríssima Ferreira[3] and Giselle Zenker Justo[4]

[1]Center of Natural Sciences and Humanities, Federal University of ABC, Rua Santa Adélia, 166, 09210-170, Santo André, SP, Brazil; [2]Department of Physics, Chemistry and Mathematics, Federal University of São Carlos (UFSCar), campus Sorocaba, Rodovia João Leme dos Santos, Km 110, CEP 18052-780, Sorocaba, SP, Brazil; [3]Laboratory of Bioassays and Signal Transduction, Institute of Biology, State University of Campinas, Cidade Universitária Zeferino Vaz, s/n, CP 6109, 13083-970, Campinas, SP, Brazil; [4]Department of Biochemistry (Campus São Paulo) and Department of Biological Sciences (Campus Diadema), Federal University of São Paulo, 3 de Maio, 100, 04044-020, São Paulo, SP, Brazil

Abstract: The role played by oncogenes and tumor suppressors in the genesis of cancer is well established. Considering that cancer cells are a product of genetic disorders that alter crucial intracellular signaling pathways associated with the regulation of survival, proliferation, differentiation and death mechanisms it is not surprising that traditional antitumor approaches target specific molecular players whose action/expression is altered in cancer cells. However, because the physiology of normal cells is controlled by the same signaling pathways that are disturbed in cancer cells many cancer therapies also cause important side effects and multidrug resistance, the main causes of therapy failure. Since the pioneering work of Otto Warburg, over 80 years ago, the subversion of normal cellular metabolism by cancer cells has been highlighted by many studies. In recent years, the study of tumor metabolism has received considerable attention because metabolic transformation is now recognized as a crucial cancer hallmark and a direct consequence of disturbances in oncogenes and tumor suppressors. Far from being a completely understood phenomenon, metabolic transformation constitutes a challenge for researchers and a potential target for cancer therapies. In this chapter, we describe the anabolic and catabolic pathways of cancer cell metabolism, compare their functions and regulation with those of non-tumor cell metabolism and discuss some of the major questions in this field of investigation. We also discuss tumor metabolism and metabolic transformations from the perspective of oncogenes, tumor suppressors, miRNAs and protein signaling pathways. Finally, recent attempts to target metabolism as a treatment for cancer are discussed.

*Address correspondence to Ana Carolina Santos de Souza: Center of Natural Sciences and Humanities, Federal University of ABC, Rua Santa Adélia, 166, 09210-170, Santo André, SP, Brazil; Tel: +55-11-4996-8376; Fax: +55-11-4996-0090; E-mail: ana.galvao@ufabc.edu.br

Keywords: Metabolic therapy, metabolic transformation, oncogenes, tumor metabolism, tumor suppressors, Warburg effect.

INTRODUCTION

Cancer cells are the product of genetic disorders that affect oncogenes, tumor suppressors and genes associated with mechanisms of DNA repair. But how is the expression of many genes affected during malignant transformation? In a seminal review, Hanahan and Weinberg [1] indicated that the malignant transformation of a cell involves the acquisition of six hallmarks: sustained proliferative signaling, evasion of growth suppressors, resistance to cell death, acquisition of replicative immortality, induction of angiogenesis and activation of invasion and metastasis. More recently, these authors added an additional emerging hallmark to this list: the reprogramming of energy metabolism [2]. Although the subversion of normal metabolism by cancer cells has been known since the pioneering studies of Otto Warburg over 80 years ago [3], this field of cancer biology has, until recently, received little attention. Indeed, with the discovery of the roles played by oncogenes and tumor suppressors in cancer genesis, many researchers have focused their efforts on the search for such genes and on investigating their actions in crucial intracellular signaling pathways related to the regulation of cell survival, proliferation, differentiation and death mechanisms. Furthermore, much attention has been given to the study of cancer cell metabolism, primarily because of recent discoveries showing that many of the mutations responsible for activating oncogenes and inhibiting tumor suppressors also control metabolic changes associated with tumorigenesis, while metabolic enzymes have been identified as human tumor suppressors or oncogenes [4].

The recent interest in tumor cell metabolism has created an exciting and promising field of cancer research. However, relatively little is still known about the details of the metabolic circuitry of cancer cells at the molecular level, despite the fact that initial studies in this field demonstrated important differences in relation to the metabolism of normal proliferating cells. Nevertheless, despite this incomplete understanding of cancer cell metabolism, several studies *in vitro* and *in vivo* have attempted to exploit our current knowledge of this field to improve the treatment of cancer by using strategies referred to as "metabolic therapies". In this chapter we discuss the function and regulation of the major metabolic pathways in cancer cells and the role of oncogenes, tumor suppressors and miRNAs in malignant metabolic transformation. We also compare cancer metabolism with the metabolism of normal proliferating cells. Finally, we discuss potential molecular targets for metabolic therapy and comment on the future of this field based on the results of recent clinical trials with metabolic modulators.

METABOLISM IN CANCER CELLS

The Warburg Effect: Glucose as an Essential Source of Carbon Atoms, ATP and Reducing Power for Proliferating Cells

Like other rapidly proliferating cells, cancer cells have a high demand for ATP and carbon atoms to meet the energy and catabolic requirements for cell growth and division. For this reason, it was initially hard for those working in this field at the time to understand the findings of Nobel Prize winner Otto Warburg, who showed that rapidly proliferating ascites tumor cells were predisposed to consume glucose at a surprisingly high rate compared to normal cells and that glucose was converted to lactate, even at normal O_2 tension, a phenomenon known as the "Warburg effect" [3, 5, 6]. Since the metabolism of glucose to lactate generates only two ATPs per molecule of glucose, whereas oxidative phosphorylation generates up to 36 ATPs through the complete oxidation of one glucose molecule, why do cancer cells, even in the presence of sufficient oxygen, "prefer" to obtain the ATP necessary for growth and proliferation through a less efficient form of metabolism (in terms of the number of ATP molecules produced)? According to Warburg, this peculiarity of cancer cells metabolism resulted from irreversible damage to mitochondrial respiration followed by an increase in glycolysis to replace the ATP lost through defective oxidative phosphorylation. This shift from oxidative phosphorylation to glycolysis was the trigger to turn highly differentiated cells into undifferentiated cells that proliferated as cancer cells. Interestingly, numerous studies in subsequent years demonstrated that, while the Warburg effect is a hallmark of many cancer cell types, this event develops independently of the functional status of mitochondria. Indeed, many studies have shown that, in most tumors, mitochondria are not dysfunctional and oxygen consumption by these cells is not reduced when compared to normal cells [7, 8]. In addition, the Warburg effect is not peculiar to cancer cells since normal proliferating cells also show this phenomenon [9]. Overall, the Warburg effect involves crucial metabolic reprogramming that allows normal and cancer cells to obtain the energy, building blocks and reducing power necessary for the synthesis of biomolecules required during cell growth [10]. However, while in normal cells this phenomenon is regulated by coordinated signaling pathways, in tumors such reprogramming is a direct consequence of oncogene activation and the loss of tumor suppressors.

Although the decrease in glucose oxidation caused by this metabolic shift is initially puzzling, the key to understanding the importance of the Warburg effect in proliferating cells is to remember that cell growth requires much more than energy in the form of ATP. Indeed, cell growth demands a source of NADPH and molecular intermediates to sustain the continuous synthesis of macromolecular building blocks needed to drive the increase in cellular biomass and duplication of genetic material. Consequently, it is reasonable to suppose that cells rescue glucose molecules from mitochondrial metabolism and drive them to the glycolytic and pentose phosphate pathways. Indeed, glycolytic intermediates are important precursors for the synthesis of non-essential amino acids, lipids and nucleic acids, while the accumulation of glycolytic intermediates and their channeling to the pentose phosphate pathway generate ribose-5-phosphate for nucleic acid synthesis and NADPH as a reducing source for fatty acid and cholesterol biosynthesis [11, 12] (Fig. **1**).

The Warburg Effect in Neoplastic Cells and its Association with Cancer Progression, Resistance to Cell Death and Aggressiveness

As indicated above, the Warburg effect represents a fundamental metabolic adaptation for any proliferating cell. Apart from the advantages of using aerobic glycolysis during proliferation, do cancer cells reap any other benefits from this metabolic reprogramming? Given the transformed nature of these cells, is it possible that the structure, function and regulation of metabolic pathways differ significantly from those of normal proliferating cells? There is considerable evidence indicating an association between the Warburg effect and the degree of tumor malignancy, as well as the existence of differences between normal and cancer cells in the molecular mechanisms of this metabolic reprogramming.

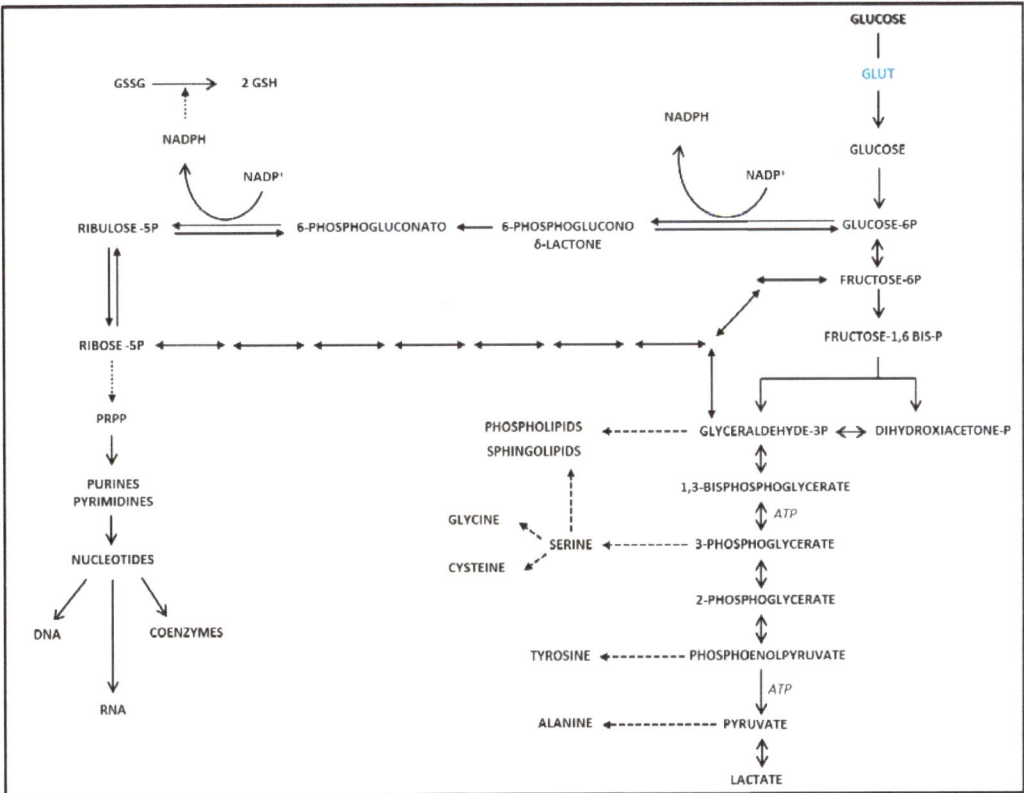

Fig. (1): Increased glycolysis and the pentose phosphate pathway supply cancer cells with precursors for biomolecules. As a result of oncogene activation and tumor suppressor inhibition, cancer cells increase their consumption and metabolism of glucose. The rapid transformation of glucose *via* the glycolytic pathway generates ATP very quickly while the accumulation of glycolytic intermediates supplies the cells with molecular precursors for biosynthesis. Furthermore, the high influx of glucose into the glycolytic pathway stimulates the pentose phosphate pathway, leading to an increase in ribose 5-phosphate levels, a precursor for nucleotide synthesis and NADPH production; the latter provides the reducing power that allows cancer cells to synthesize their macromolecules and, at the same time, protects them against damage caused by oxidative species. The enhanced glucose metabolism of cancer cells thus supplies their bioenergetic and anabolic requirements. GLUT: glucose transporter, GSH: reduced glutathione; GSSG: oxidized glutathione, PRPP: phosphoribosylpyrophosphate.

Compared to normal proliferating cells, aerobic glycolysis is faster in cancer cells. Indeed, cancer cells have a greater capacity to take up glucose from the blood and metabolize it than do normal cells. This increased glucose consumption is a direct consequence of the overexpression of glucose transporters (GLUT1, GLUT3 and/or GLUT12) and also mainly of isoform M2 of pyruvate kinase (PK-M2), one of the principal regulators of glycolysis that is frequently overexpressed in transformed cells. In addition, virtually all enzymes of the glycolytic pathway appear to be overexpressed as a consequence of oncogene activation [13-15]. The overexpression and/or overactivation of hexokinase (HK), phosphofructokinase (PFK) and PK, the main enzymes controlling the glycolytic pathway, has been described for a number of tumors [8, 14, 15]. Interestingly, tumor cells have been suggested to use isoforms of glycolytic enzymes that differ from those used to metabolize glycolysis in normal cells, although there is still insufficient data to confirm this [16, 17].

The high glycolytic rate of tumor cells has been related to their resistance to chemo- and radiotherapy [18, 19]. Indeed, the metabolic transformation that accompanies a malignant transformation apparently provides the means by which tumor cells can prevent death and progress towards more aggressive and metastatic phenotypes. This scenario turns lactate, an apparently disposable byproduct, into a fundamental molecule for the motility and metastatic ability to cancer cells. The excess lactate derived from the high rate of glycolysis and overexpression of lactate dehydrogenase A (LDH-A) in cancer cells is secreted by plasma membrane monocarboxylate transporters (MCTs) that co-transport H^+. Thus, lactate secretion establishes an acidic environmental in which cathepsins and metalloproteinases can be activated, leading to the degradation of extracellular matrix and an increase in the susceptibility of the endothelial basal membrane to proteolytic attack [20-22]. Moreover, the modification of the local environmental caused by lactate can suppress anticancer immune effectors by inhibiting immune cell proliferation, cytokine production and cytolytic activity of cytotoxic T lymphocytes [23].

In addition to driving the proliferation of cancer cells, high glycolytic rates also protect these cells from different types of cell death, such as that induced by the withdrawal of growth factors. Under normal glucose levels, the removal of IL-3 targets the anti-apoptotic protein Mcl-1 for proteasome degradation, leading to cell death. Interestingly, leukemic cells that overexpress hexokinase 1 and GLUT1 are more protected against IL-3 withdrawal. When glucose levels are high, Mcl-1 is more stable and prevents cancer cell death [24, 25]. Enhanced glycolytic activity also inhibits the expression or activity of several pro-apoptotic

BH3-only proteins and leads to an increase in cFLIP levels. Thus, the "glucose addiction" of cancer cells contributes to their resistance to apoptotic cell death at the level of the mitochondria and death receptors [26, 27].

This enhanced resistance to cell death has been related to alterations in normal mitochondrial physiology caused by the non-enzymatic functions of glycolytic enzymes and/or by the accumulation of glycolytic intermediates [28, 29]. One of these alterations involves HK2 which, in cancer cells, often translocates to mitochondria. According to Pastorino and Hoek [30], in mitochondria HK2 can compete with proteins of the Bcl2 family for binding to the voltage-dependent anion channel (VDAC) in a process that alters the balance of pro- and anti-apoptotic proteins which in turn controls the permeabilization of the outer mitochondrial membrane. After an apoptotic stimulus, pro-apoptotic proteins of the Bcl2 family, such as Bax and Bak, oligomerize in the outer mitochondrial membrane to form a channel through which pro-apoptotic proteins and cytochrome c are released. Once in the cytosol, cytochrome c associates with Apaf-1, dATP and procaspase-9 to form the apoptosome, which is responsible for the execution phase of apoptosis by stimulating caspase activation. The binding of HK2 to the VDAC displaces the anti-apoptotic protein Bcl-XL and makes it available for interaction with Bax and Bak, thereby inhibiting their pro-apoptotic effects that cause outer membrane permeabilization. HK2 binding also reduces VDAC permeability by closing the channel, thereby preventing cytochrome c release. Finally, HK2 antagonizes the pro-apoptotic effects of the protein Bid that activates Bax and Bak [31].

The high glycolytic rate of cancer cells is advantageous for growth and proliferation. However, this characteristic also challenges tumor cells to deal with increased mitochondrial metabolism and higher amounts of reactive oxygen species (ROS). Once more, glycolytic pathway components can alter the structure and function of mitochondria to prevent the activation of programmed cell death. Indeed, cancer cells exposed to high glucose concentrations can repress oxidative metabolism, a phenomenon known as the Crabtree effect [32]. The precise mechanism by which the Crabtree effect is triggered is unknown, although several possibilities have been proposed. Diaz-Ruiz and collaborators [29] demonstrated that the glycolytic intermediate fructose 1,6-bisphosphate inhibits the activity of cytochrome c oxidase, leading to inhibition of the mitochondrial respiratory chain and to a decreased production of ROS. Furthermore, the inhibition of cytochrome c oxidase also favors the maintenance of cytochrome c in its reduced state, disabling it to trigger programmed cell death. Interestingly, in addition to preventing massive ROS production by mitochondria, the high glycolytic rate also protects cancer cells against cellular oxidative damage in a more direct way. As explained before, increased glucose consumption leads to the accumulation of glycolytic intermediates and stimulation of the pentose phosphate pathway that produces NADPH. Higher levels of intracellular NADPH, in turn, increase the amounts of reduced glutathione (GSH), a major non-enzymatic antioxidant, which helps tumor cells to detoxify antineoplastic drugs or antagonize their effects, thereby contributing to the development of more aggressive and resistant phenotypes [22, 33].

Finally, high glycolytic metabolism has been associated with increased expression of P-glycoprotein (P-gp), a member of the ABC (ATP binding cassette) transporters [34]. The ABC family of transmembrane proteins acts as efflux pumps by efficiently removing structurally unrelated chemotherapeutic drugs from within tumor cells; the resulting decrease in the concentration of the drug to a level below the effective intracellular concentrations results in multidrug resistance (MDR). These findings indicate that the inhibition of glycolysis could improve traditional antineoplastic therapies by sensitizing cancer cells to programmed cell death and reversing the MDR phenotype.

The Tricarboxylic Acid Cycle and Glutamine: Meeting the Energy and Molecular Precursor Requirements of Cancer Cells

Although the Warburg effect provides highly proliferating cancer cells with many advantages, a crucial question remains, namely, how does one identify the main source of energy for these cells, given the relative inefficiency of the glycolytic pathway in generating ATP when compared with the complete oxidization of glucose *via* mitochondrial oxidative phosphorylation? For some researchers, ATP production by glycolysis is (apparently) a problem only if nutritional resources are scarce. Indeed, some studies have been demonstrated that anaerobic glycolysis can provide cells with high ratios of ATP/ADP and NADH/NAD$^+$, with the advantage of generating such products faster than by mitochondrial metabolism [9, 35, 36]. Furthermore, it is estimated that only 10% of the pyruvate generated by the glycolytic pathway actually feeds into the tricarboxylic acid cycle (TCA) and mitochondrial metabolism, which suggests a secondary role for these pathways in energy production by cancer cells. Indeed, cancer cell metabolism appears adapted to drive glucose carbons away from mitochondrial metabolism through multiple mechanisms. The first adaptation involves increased expression of PK-M2, the enzyme that catalyzes the last step of glycolysis and transfers phosphate from phosphoenolpyruvate (PEP) to ADP to generate ATP. Unlike PK-M1, the PK isoform that predominates in most normal cells, PK-M2 is negatively regulated by tyrosine-phosphorylated proteins and can exist as a dimer or tetramer, a characteristic that enables this enzyme to oscillate between a low activity form (dimeric) and a high activity form (tetrameric). In cancer cells, the activation of oncogenes leads to a predominance of dimeric PK-M2 with low activity, thereby allowing glycolytic intermediates to be siphoned off for biosynthesis or other conversions through the pentose phosphate pathway [37]. The glucose molecules that escape from anabolic pathways and are converted into pyruvate then face two more obstacles before reaching the mitochondria, namely, LDH-A activity and the partial blockade of pyruvate transport to mitochondria. In cancer cells, the conversion of pyruvate to lactate is stimulated through the overexpression of LDH-A which helps to prevent the entrance of pyruvate into mitochondria. Moreover, pyruvate molecules that escape LDH-A have to overcome the problem of transport into mitochondria; this transport is considered to be slower than in non-tumor cells [38-40]. Finally, since pyruvate molecules that reach mitochondria can return to the cytosol, the complete oxidation of glucose must involve the rapid conversion of pyruvate into acetyl-CoA through catalysis *via* the pyruvate dehydrogenase complex (PDC). However, PDC is phosphorylated by pyruvate dehydrogenase kinases (PDKs) and its activity is diminished in tumor cells, a factor that contributes to the diversion of glucose carbons from the TCA cycle and mitochondrial metabolism [9].

Although glucose carbons are diverted from the TCA cycle, most cancer cells depend upon the delivery of pyruvate to mitochondria and on the proper functioning of mitochondrial respiration for survival [41]. Pyruvate is the main source of carbon atoms that, once incorporated into the TCA cycle as acetyl-CoA, drives the *de novo* synthesis of lipids and proteins [42]. The TCA cycle has a central role as a source of metabolic intermediates for anabolic pathways (lipid, protein and nucleic acid biosynthesis) in growing cells and shows enhanced activity in a variety of tumor cells, despite the low supply of pyruvate [43] (Fig. **2**). The functions of the TCA cycle in cancer cells are still not completely understood, although it is clear that the high use of glutamine by most of these cells is fundamental for the activity of their metabolic pathways. Glutamine has been identified as a critical nutrient for cancer cells and, like glucose, its metabolism is strongly associated with the supply of building blocks and energy for anabolic pathways [44, 45]. During glutaminolysis, the metabolic pathway responsible for the conversion of glutamine into lactate, the TCA cycle is fed with α-ketoglutarate, which ensures the provision of biomolecule precursors and reduced coenzymes. The production of oxaloacetate also allows the entry of glucose carbons into the TCA cycle (in the form of acetyl-CoA) and leads to the synthesis of citrate which can participate in the TCA reaction or, alternatively, translocate to the cytosol to promote fatty acid synthesis. Glutamine-dependent transamination also provides nitrogen for the synthesis of non-essential amino acids [45-47].

Like glycolysis, the glutaminolytic pathway contributes to a more aggressive and resistant phenotype in cancer cells through the activation of oncogenes such as Myc, which stimulates glutaminolysis through transcriptional regulation [46, 48]. As with the metabolism of glucose *via* the pentose phosphate pathway, glutaminolysis produces NADPH *via* malic enzyme, an $NADP^+$-specific malate dehydrogenase. The amount of NADPH supplied by malic enzyme for cellular metabolism is the same as that provided by the pentose phosphate pathway, which further highlights the importance of glutamine in generating the redox potential required for anabolic processes in cell growth and protection against oxidative stress and cell death [42, 49]. Glutamine metabolism in cancer cells also produces a significant amount of lactate that results in a more acidic cellular environment and influences cell motility, metastatic capacity and the ability to evade the immune system.

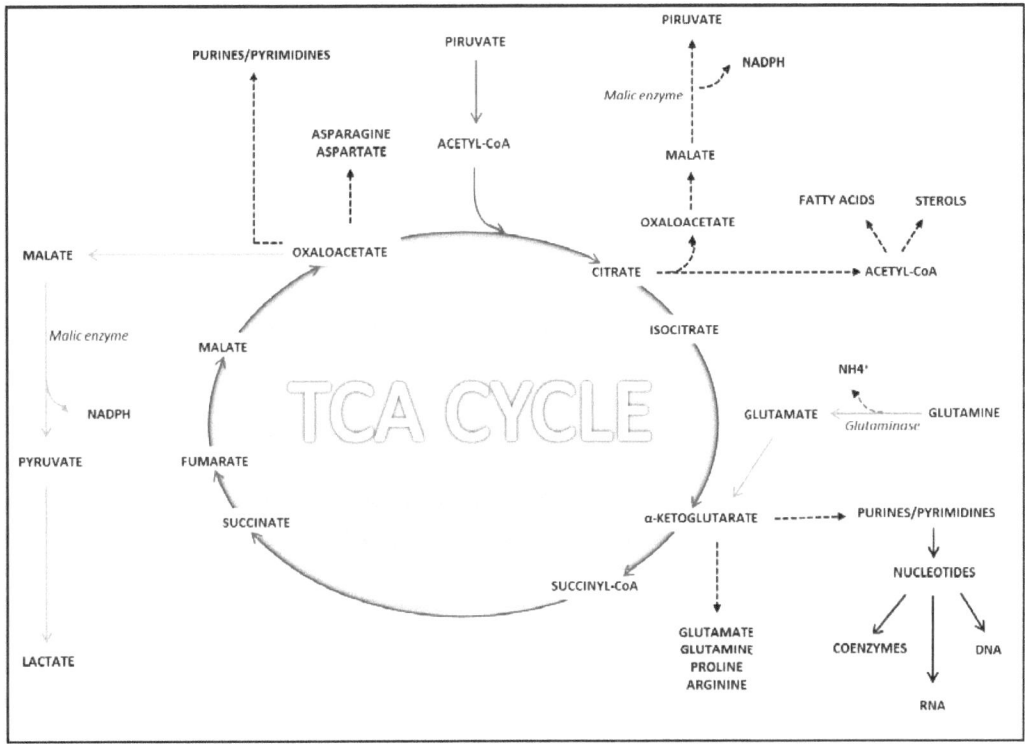

Fig. (2): TCA cycle intermediates and glutamine metabolism cooperate to supply the catabolic requirements of cancer cells. Although the extent to which the TCA cycle and glutaminolysis (reactions shown in red arrows) contribute to the energy needs of cancer cells is still not well understood, both pathways nevertheless have a crucial role in supplying molecular precursors and reducing power during cell growth and proliferation.

The high consumption of glutamine by cancer cells and the association between glutaminolysis and the TCA cycle are new pieces in the puzzle that understanding cancer cell metabolism represents: since the metabolism of glutamine fuels the TCA cycle to sustain the production of NADH and $FADH_2$, could glutamine stimulate the electron transport chain, a very important source of mitochondrial ATP for cancer cells? In addition, could glutamine metabolism be a more important source of ATP for cancer cells than glycolysis? Although these questions still cannot be answered, in many cancer cells the demand for glutamine far exceeds the requirement for nucleotide synthesis or maintenance of the non-essential amino acid pool, a further indication of the importance of this amino acid as an energy substrate.

Any discussion of the energy sources for cancer cells must take into account that cells are frequently exposed to fluctuations in glucose and nutrient availability and that this may alter their metabolic status over time. In particular, depending on their specific location within the tumor mass, cancer cells face restrictions in nutrient and oxygen availability without a corresponding increase in the existing vasculature. Specific metabolic adaptations can therefore occur in different populations of cells, a situation that contributes to metabolic heterogeneity in the tumor mass. Consequently, the potential influence of the surrounding environment on the metabolic adaptation of cancer cells and the existence of short-term mechanisms that enable these cells to continuously alter the functional status of the TCA cycle and mitochondrial respiration must be considered. Finally, the activation of oncogenes and inhibition of tumor suppressors can alter the mechanisms of metabolic regulation in cancer cells when compared with the corresponding pathways in normal proliferating cells. Together, these findings indicate that metabolic regulation in cancer cells differs significantly from that of normal cells. A better knowledge of these differences would be useful in developing more efficient anti-cancer therapies.

ONCOGENES AND TUMOR SUPPRESSORS ARE KEY PLAYERS IN METABOLIC TRANSFORMATION

In normal cells, growth and proliferation are finely regulated processes that occur only when signals received by the cells indicate that the overall state of the organism is permissive. Such signaling prevents cell proliferation when resources are scarce and avoids excessive proliferation when nutrient availability exceeds the levels needed to support cell division. Alterations in or a lack of such crosstalk between metabolic pathways and organism signals is a fundamental cause in the development of cancer and a key point for understanding metabolic transformation.

There is increasing evidence that many of the genetic alterations that activate oncogenes and inhibit tumor suppressors also control the metabolic changes associated with tumorigenesis. Such alterations may overcome the dependence on growth factors, alter the functional status of metabolic pathways and stimulate the uptake of nutrients, particularly glucose and glutamine [36, 50-52]. This is the case of the PI3K/Akt signaling pathway, which acts downstream of various growth factor receptors and angiogenesis inducers. This pathway plays a critical role in promoting growth under normoxic and hypoxic conditions. PI3K/Akt signaling is frequently overactive in cancer cells, leading to increased glucose and glutamine consumption, accelerated glycolysis, high lactate production, increased lipid production, the biosynthesis of important biomolecules and the suppression of macromolecular degradation [9, 53, 54]. Activation of the PI3K/Akt/mTOR pathway also integrates signals from the PI3K/Akt complex and information on the nutritional status to regulate cell growth and proliferation, thereby enhancing many of the metabolic activities associated with the increase in cancer cell biomass [54]. In addition, this pathway increases the expression of nutrient transporters (GLUT 1, GLUT 3) at the cell surface, thereby enhancing the uptake of glucose, amino acids and other nutrients. Similarly, the expression and/or activity of various glycolytic enzymes, including HK1 and 2, PFK1 and 2, aldolases A and C, GAPDH, PGK1, enolase 1 and PK-M2, are stimulated to promote glucose phosphorylation as well as glucose retention and metabolic transformation by the cell [9, 36, 55]. Many of these enzymes are activated even in the presence of oxygen, a finding that reflects the ability of PI3K/Akt/mTOR to activate hypoxia-inducible factor 1 (HIF-1), c-Myc and sterol response element binding protein-1 (SREBP-1) [4, 56]. The transcription factor SREBP-1 induces the expression of lipogenic genes, such as ATP-citrate lyase (ACL), acetyl-CoA carboxylase-1 (ACC) and fatty acid synthase (FAS), as well as several enzymes in the oxidative branch of the pentose phosphate pathway. HIF-1 is a transcription factor complex; the upregulation and stabilization of the HIF-1α subunit result from the activation of mTOR and inhibition of the forkhead transcription factor 3a (FOXO3a). Indeed, HIF-1 is a critical player in the metabolic shift towards glycolysis in cancer cells through its ability to modulate the expression of PK-M2 and inhibit mitochondrial metabolism by increasing the expression of the regulatory enzyme pyruvate dehydrogenase kinase 1 (PDK1), which phosphorylates and inactivates PDC. This phosphorylation leads to the transcriptional activation of BNIP3 that encodes a member of the Bcl2 family which, in turn, triggers selective mitochondrial autophagy [11, 57]. Mitochondrial autophagy may promote cancer cell survival by removing damaged mitochondria, which are potential sources of ROS [58]. A recent study demonstrated that PK-M2 promotes the transcriptional activity of HIF-1 by direct binding, thus highlighting the close relationship between this transcription factor and the regulation of glycolysis [59]. Finally, PI3K/Akt also contributes to resistance to cell death by inducing the translocation of HK2 to the outer mitochondrial membrane where it binds to VDAC, thereby inhibiting permeabilization of the mitochondrial membrane and the consequent induction of apoptosis [22, 60], as explained earlier.

AMP-activated protein kinase (AMPK), a "sensor" of the cellular energy status, counteracts the effects of PI3K/Akt/mTOR signaling. Under conditions of stress, such as hypoxia and nutrient deprivation, intracellular ATP levels decrease and AMPK is activated through phosphorylation by tumor suppressor liver kinase B1 (LKB1). Once activated, AMPK can directly phosphorylate two important components of the mTOR complex 1 (mTORC1) to inhibit the downstream effects of this complex on protein translation and cell growth [61]. The LKB1/AMPK pathway opposes the actions of PI3K/Akt/mTOR signaling by inhibiting HIF-1 and downregulating glycolysis through the phosphorylation of PFK2 and a reduction in GLUT1 and HK2 expression [62, 63]. Activated AMPK also phosphorylates and inhibits acetyl-CoA carboxylase and HMG-CoA reductase, thereby reducing the fatty acid and cholesterol synthesis [64].

In order to proliferate, cells need to progress in the cell cycle and adapt their metabolism to increase their biomass (cell growth) and duplicate their genetic material. The Myc family of genes (c-Myc, L-Myc, S-Myc and N-Myc) has a fundamental role in these activities since these genes encode transcription factors that regulate a variety of cellular processes, including cell growth and proliferation, cell cycle progression, energy metabolism, differentiation, apoptosis and cell motility. In agreement with this, enhanced Myc expression is seen in 70% of all human cancers and the suppression of this expression may lead to tumor regression [65-67]. The association between Myc and metabolic transformations was recently highlighted by Hu and collaborators [68] who showed that changes in a model of c-Myc-driven oncogenesis preceded tumor formation and were modulated by inactivation of c-Myc. Myc expression often shortens G1 as cells enter the cell cycle; Myc is also essential for the G0/G1 to S phase progression since Myc expression in G1 facilitates cell entry into S, partly by activating the expression of cyclins and CDK4 [69]. Myc is a strong inducer of glucose consumption and metabolism and its effects on cancer cells metabolism are very similar to those of PI3K/Akt signaling pathway and HIF. Indeed, c-Myc binds directly to many promoters regulated by HIF-1. Myc increases the expression of most of the glycolytic and glucose transporter genes, such as LDH-A, GLUT1, HK2, PFK, hexosephosphate isomerase (HPI), GAPDH, PGK and enolase 1 [19]. Interestingly, Myc promotes the expression of PK-M2 during the alternative splicing that determines the expression of this enzyme or its analog, PK-M1. The alternative splicing in favor of PKM2 is mediated by three heterogeneous nuclear ribonucleoproteins (hnRNP1, hnRNPA1 and hnRNPA2) that are regulated by c-Myc [70].

Myc shares molecular targets with HIF and contributes to the Warburg effect, even under adequate oxygen tension [46, 71, 72]. Myc also boosts oxidative phosphorylation by stimulating glutamine metabolism and mitochondrial biogenesis [73, 74]. Myc upregulates glutamine transporter genes (SCT2 and SLC7A25) and increases glutaminase protein levels *via* post-transcriptional regulatory mechanisms [46, 48]. As a consequence of enhanced glutamine metabolism, the TCA cycle is supplied with α-ketoglutarate, which contributes to the anabolic role of this cycle [46, 75]. Myc stimulates protein synthesis by driving the transcription of RNA polymerases I (for rRNA transcription) and III (for tRNA and small RNA transcription), together with RNA polymerase II, thereby inducing ribosome synthesis. Myc also controls the expression of multiple components of the protein synthesis machinery, including ribosomal proteins, tRNA and key factors involved in translation, initiation and elongation, such as eIF4F (subunits eIF4AI and eIF4GI) [46, 76, 77].

The protein p53, encoded by the tumor suppressor gene p53, is the most frequently mutated gene in human tumors. As a transcription factor, this protein mediates cellular adaptation to a variety of stress conditions, inducing cell cycle arrest, senescence and apoptosis. Importantly, p53 also coordinates the function of metabolic pathways by triggering stress-induced transcriptional programs in order to maintain energy homeostasis [78]. The phosphorylation and stabilization of p53 by AMPK demonstrate an interaction between these proteins in controlling cell metabolism, especially at the catabolic level. p53 decelerates glycolysis by diminishing the levels of fructose 2,6-bisphosphate, an allosteric activator of PFK-1, as a consequence of enhanced expression of the gene TIGAR (TP53-induced glycolysis and apoptosis regulator) [79]. p53 also suppresses the expression of phosphoglycerate mutase which leads to the diversion of carbon atoms towards the pentose phosphate pathway and increases mitochondrial respiration by upregulating the expression of SCO_2 (synthesis of cytochrome oxidase 2), an enzyme required for the assembly of cytochrome c oxidase [9, 80]. These actions of p53 can reduce glycolytic intermediates and affect mitochondrial metabolism, leading to the catabolism of other nutrients. p53 can also contribute to catabolic processes by enhancing the β-oxidation of fatty acids through the action of carnitine palmitoyl-transferase and can boost macroautophagy through upregulation of the damage-regulated autophagy modulator (DRAM) gene [81, 82]. As with Myc, p53 enhances glutamine use by upregulating glutaminase 2 [83, 84]. Given the importance of the functional status of p53 as an indicator of cancer prognosis, recent findings on the roles of this protein in metabolic transformation reinforce its critical function in cancer genesis and progression.

Our current knowledge based on the studies discussed above indicates that there is a strong relationship between metabolic transformation and oncogenic transformation: in general, oncogenic pathways, such as those mediated by PI3K/Akt or Myc, promote glycolysis, whereas tumor suppressors, such as p53 and AMP, inhibit this process (Fig. **3**).

META-REGULATION OF CANCER CELLS METABOLISM BY microRNAs

Nearly 20 years ago, studies performed using the nematode *Caenorhabditis elegans* showed for the first time that the small RNA lin-4 could regulate the expression of lin-14 in this organism. This finding marked the beginning of a major shift in biological research demonstrating that RNA molecules could be more than "simple" intermediates between DNA and proteins playing important roles in gene regulation [85]. After the discovery of lin-4, a number of small regulatory RNAs have expanded dramatically. One important class of such RNA molecules are microRNAs (miRNAs), small non-coding RNA molecules that

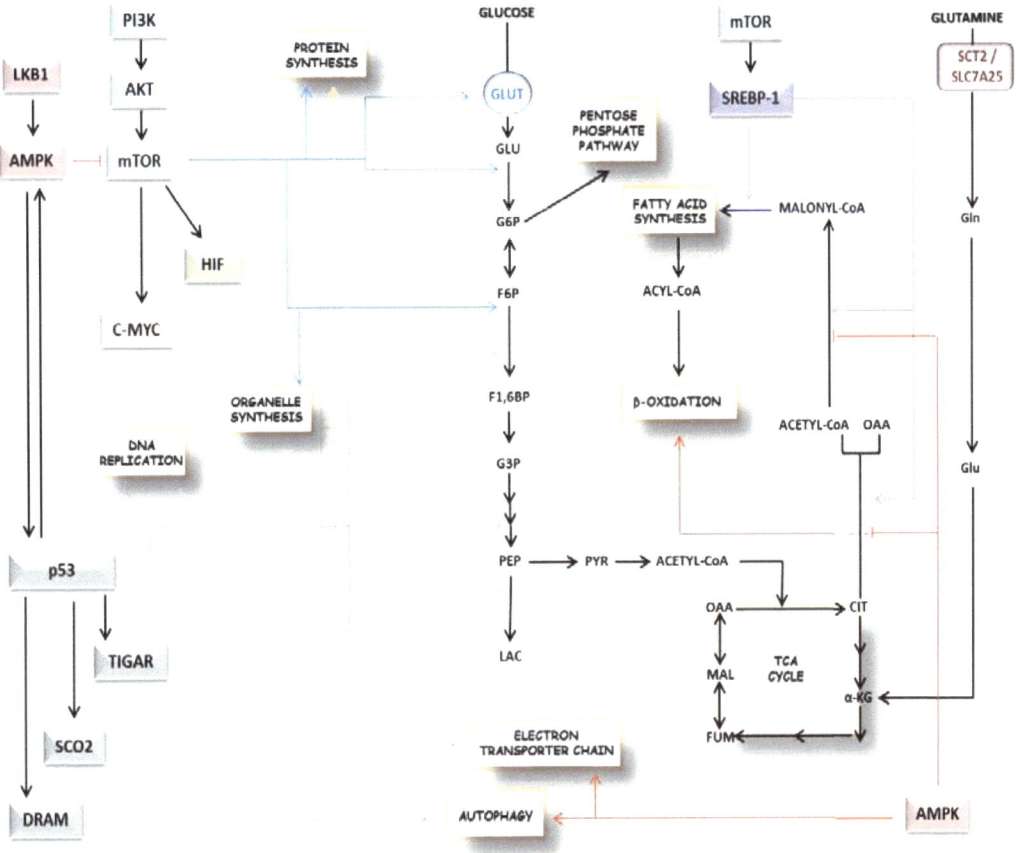

Fig. (3): Roles of oncogenes and tumor suppressors in the regulation of cancer cell metabolism. Whereas normal cells proliferate only when stimulated by growth factors, cancer cells proliferate freely because of oncogene activation or the loss of tumor suppressors required to promote the metabolic transformation needed to sustain growth and division. In general, oncogenic pathways, such as those mediated by PI3K/Akt or Myc, promote glycolysis, whereas tumor suppressors, such as p53 and AMP, inhibit this process and stimulate oxidative phosphorylation. CIT: citrate; F1,6BP: fructose 1,6-bisphosphate; F2,6BP: fructose 2,6-bisphosphate; F6P: fructose-6-phosphate; FUM: fumarate; G3P: glyceraldehyde 3-phosphate; G6P: glucose-6-phosphate; Gln: glutamine; GLU: glucose; Glu: glutamate; GLUT: glucose transporter; LAC: lactate; MAL: malate; OAA: oxaloacetate; PEP: phosphoenolpyruvate; PYR: pyruvate; SCT2 and SLC7A25: glutamine transporters; α-KG: α-ketoglutarate.

contain around 19-30 nucleotides (on average 20 nucleotides) and regulates genes expression through binding to mRNAs inducing either translational repression or decreased mRNA stability [86] (Fig. **4**). In general microRNAs are believed to target about one-third of human mRNAs and a single miRNA targeting

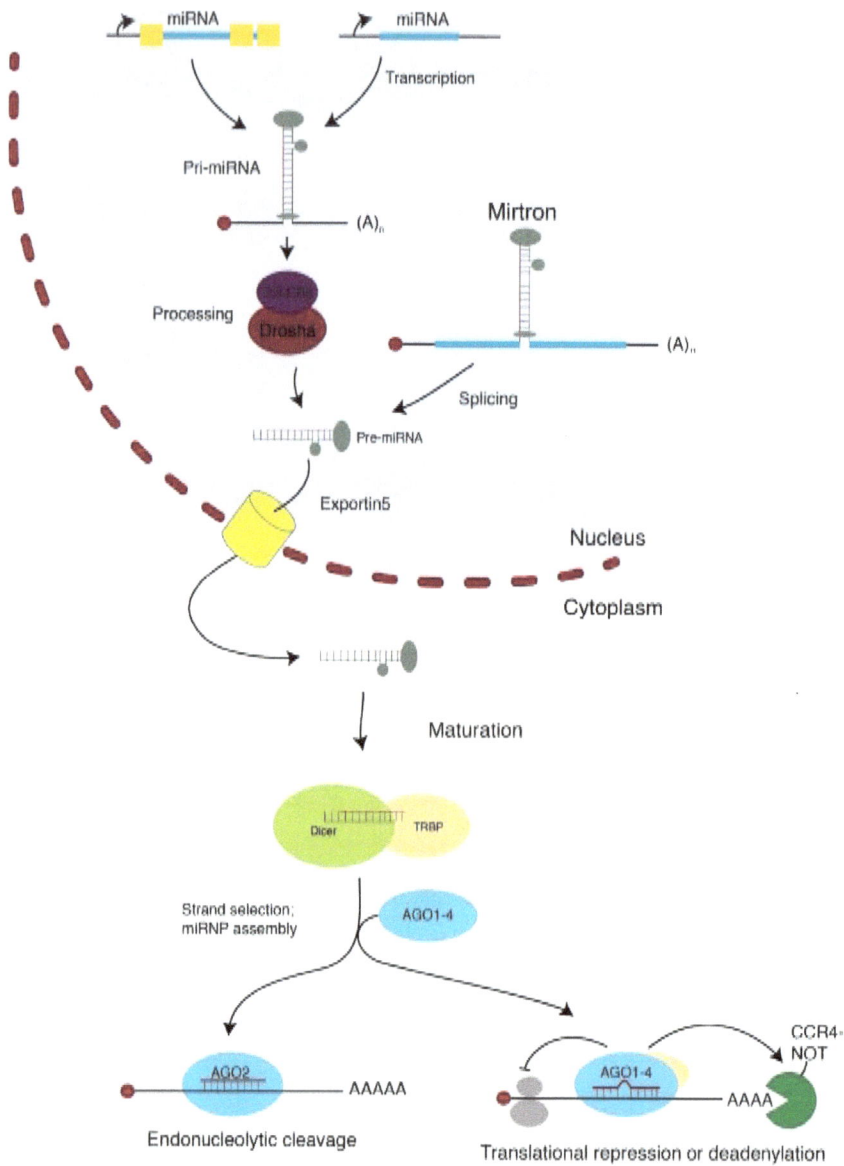

Fig. (4): Biogenesis and mechanism of action of microRNA. Pre-miRNAs generated by the canonical or non-canonical pathways are transported by an exportin 5 and RAN-GTP-dependent process from nucleus to the cytosol. The precursors are further processed by the Dicer and transactivation-response RNA-binding protein (TRBP) RNase III enzyme complex to form the mature double-stranded microRNA. Next, argonaute proteins facilitate incorporation of the mature miRNA-targeting strand into the AGO-containing RNA-induced silencing complex (RISC). The RISC-microRNA assembly is then guided to specific target sequences in mRNAs resulting either in translational repression or decreased mRNA stability.

approximately 200 transcripts simultaneously [87-89]. Therefore, microRNAs have been implicated in almost every biological process, including development, cell cycle regulation, cell growth and differentiation, stress response, and apoptosis. In addition, miRNAs play a role in a variety of diseases and in particular in cancer [90].

MicroRNAs can influence the development and progression of malignancy. Since around 50% of human microRNAs are located in fragile chromosomal regions, which may exhibit DNA amplifications, deletions or translocations during tumor development, their expression is frequently deregulated in cancer [91, 92]. Besides, it has been observed that cellular transformation and tumorigenesis can be promoted by suppression of the key components of microRNA processing machinery. The widespread dowregulation of microRNAs is often detected in human cancers such as breast, ovarian, pancreas and prostate. In general microRNAs can function either as tumor suppressors or as oncogenes (oncomirs) and initiate tumor growth, invasion, metastases, as well as regulate the overall stemness of cancer cells [93].

Taking into account the role of microRNA in regulating the expression of a set of proteins, it is conceivable to think that the capacity of cancer cells to reprogramming their metabolism for consuming either higher glucose or glutamine, could be at least in part, due to microRNAs function. Below we will focus on microRNAs that control glutamine and glucose metabolism.

microRNAs That Control Glutaminase in Tumor Cells

The mechanisms controlling glutaminase in cancer cells are poorly understood but it has recently emerged that microRNAs regulate glutaminase-mediated glutamine metabolism. The study performed by Gao´s group showed that c-Myc transcriptionally represses miR-23a and miR-23b, which target glutaminase mRNA, resulting in higher expression of this mitochondrial protein in human P-493 B lymphoma and PC3 prostate cancer cells [48].

Another important transcription factor, NFκB p65, essential for inducing survival and proliferation of primary and leukemic cells [94], appears as a potent modulator of microRNA-23. Recently, Rathore and collaborators have shown that cells growing in glutamine increase NFκB p65 translocation to the nucleus where it controls glutamine metabolism by downregulating microRNA-23a levels, which leads to an increased glutamine expression [95]. Interestingly, those authors also observed that Jurkat cells overexpressing NFκB p65 show increase basal glutaminase expression and proliferate faster than control cells when culturing in medium with glutamine. Accordingly, overexpressing microRNA-23a in leukemic cells impaired glutamine use and induces mitochondrial dysfunction (loss of potential and increased sensitivity towards reactive oxygen species) leading to cell death.

microRNAs Control Glucose Uptake

Glucose transporters (GLUTs) are present in all plasma membrane that facilitate monosaccharide, *e.g.,* glucose, fructose and galactose, uptake to supply growing and dividing cells [96]. GLUT1 and GLUT4 have been targeted by microRNAs. For instance, in renal cell carcinoma microRNA199a, microRNA138, microRNA150 and microRNA532-5p downregulate GLUT1 expression, whereas microRNA130b, microRNA19a/b and microRNA301a increase GLUT1 expression [97]. It was also detected that microRNA150 dowregulates GLUT4 in rat and human peripheral blood with type 2 diabetes. Notably, microRNAs such as microRNA301 and microRNA130b are highly expressed in pancreatic tumors, and their role in regulating GLUT1 expression could explain the increased glucose uptake that is observed in pancreatic adenocarcinoma [98, 99].

Regulation of Glycolysis and Tricarboxylic Acid Cycle by microRNAs

microRNAs provide switches for the regulation of glycolysis, turning on and off in response to tumor demands, therefore small RNAs are key molecules responsible for providing cancer cell highly capacity of plasticity, such as producing ATP more rapidly from glucose through lactate formation and also various building blocks, such as fatty acids, lipids, nucleotides and proteins. Some reports have shown that miRNAs not only regulate the irreversible steps in glycolysis, but also other important intermediates of the pathway. For instance, microRNA-143 which is located in fragile chromosomal region often deleted in cancers has been found downregulated in a number of cancers. Furthermore, microRNA-143 overexpression has been demonstrated to have a growth inhibitory effect in several cell lines (prostate, leukemia, colorectal and liposarcoma), indicating that loss of miR-143 expression could contribute to the development of cancer [100-106]. Gregersen and collaborators have used a microarray-based approach to identify microRNA-143 targets. These authors reported that miR-143 targets and downregulates the glycolytic enzyme hexokinase 2 in colon cancer cell lines. In addition, when this microRNA was delivered into colon cancer cell lines a decrease in lactate secretion was observed which indicates that microRNA-143-mediated downregulation of hexokinase 2 impairs the efficiency of glycolysis. Therefore, the fact that cancer cell lines usually display low level of microRNA-143 provide those cells a growth advantage due to increase glycolytic flux by promoting the first step of glycolysis [107]. In addition to hexokinase, microRNA103/107, which is crucial for pancreatic tumorigenesis, has been shown to regulate PDK4, a critical inactivator of pyruvate dehydrogenase enzymatic activity [108].

METABOLIC TARGETS FOR CANCER THERAPY

As discussed earlier, mTOR signaling is aberrantly activated in most cancers and is intricately linked to the PI3K/Akt survival pathway, which is also associated with neoplasia and favors survival and proliferation. The LKB1/AMPK pathway opposes the actions of PI3K/Akt/mTOR signaling in regulating cellular growth. Thus, it is not surprising that the central roles of AMPK and mTOR in energy metabolism and cellular functions have attracted considerable attention as prominent drug targets. Indeed, an increased knowledge of these pathways has been a stimulus to develop news drugs and to improve therapeutic strategies.

The serine/threonine kinase mTOR is a central integrator of environmental signals and regulates multiple cellular functions, such as protein and lipid metabolism, growth and proliferation; this protein therefore has a major impact on cellular homeostasis. mTOR controls cellular processes *via* two distinct complexes: mTOR complex 1 (mTORC1) and 2 (mTORC2), which have six and seven protein components, respectively, as well as different sensitivities to rapamycin [109]. Apart from mTOR itself, other proteins that are part of these complexes include the mammalian lethal with sec-13 protein 8 (mLST8, also known as GβL) [110, 111], DEP domain containing mTOR-interacting protein (DEPTOR) [112] and Tti1/Tel2 complex [113]. mTORC1 specifically includes regulatory-associated protein of mammalian target of rapamycin (Raptor) [114, 115] and proline-rich Akt substrate (PRAS40) [116], whereas rapamycin-insensitive companion of mTOR (Rictor) [117], mammalian stress-activated MAP kinase-interacting protein 1 (mSin1) [118] and protein observed Rictor 1 and 2 (Protor1/2) [119] are part of mTORC2. Rapamycin, a macrolide produced by the bacteria *Streptomyces hygroscopicus*, binds to the intracellular 12 kDa FK506-binding protein (FKBP12) and this complex in turn binds to and inhibits the mTOR subunit of mTORC1 [120, 121] but not mTORC2. In addition, rapamycin may interfere with the structural integrity of mTORC1 [115] or allosterically reduce the activity of the kinase domain [122]. Although rapamycin does not inhibit mTORC2 directly, prolonged administration may impair its action in several tumor cell types [123]. mTORC1 is modulated by several upstream stimuli, such as amino acids, growth factors, energy status and cellular stress, all of which influence protein and lipid biosynthesis and autophagy. In contrast, mTORC2 is apparently stimulated only by growth factors and regulates cytoskeletal reorganization, as well as cell survival and metabolism [109, 124].

AMPK has been regarded as an energy sensor that coordinates multiple metabolic pathways to balance cellular energy levels. However, AMPK also affects other cellular functions, such as the regulation of mitochondrial biogenesis and disposal, autophagy, cell polarity and cell growth and proliferation. AMPK is activated by LKB1 phosphorylation, which was initially identified as a tumor suppressor [125-128]. mTOR signaling is a major downstream pathway of AMPK. Initially, AMPK phosphorylates tuberous sclerosis 2 (TSC2) and activates the TSC1/TSC2 complex which in turn inhibits mTOR/Raptor by maintaining the mTORC1 activator Ras homolog enriched in brain (Rheb) inactive [129, 130]. mTORC1 plays a major role in protein biosynthesis by activating ribosomal protein S6 kinase (S6K) and inhibiting the eukaryotic initiation factor 4E-binding protein (4E-BP), thereby activating eukaryotic initiation factor 4E (eIF4E) to induce protein translation [131].

mTORC1 stimulates lipogenesis, glycolysis and the oxidative part of the pentose phosphate pathway to promote tumorigenesis [132]. Furthermore, mTORC1 inhibits autophagy through phosphorylation of the kinase complex ULK1/Atg13/FIP200 (unc-51-like kinase 1/mammalian autophagy-related gene/focal adhesion kinase family-interacting protein of 200 kDa) [133] and stimulates angiogenesis through HIF-1α stabilization [134]. Amplification of the gene encoding for the p110α subunit of PI3K *PIK3CA*, the loss or inactivation of phosphatase and tensin homolog (*PTEN*), the classic inhibitor of PI3K, as well as mutations in *TSC1* and *TSC2*, *P53* and *LKB1*, also activate mTOR signaling [124, 135, 136].

In view of the central roles of AMPK and mTOR in modulating cellular nutrient responses and energy homeostasis there has been considerable interest in mTOR inhibitors and AMPK activators as potential drugs for the treatment of cancer.

AMPK Activators

Metformin, a biguanide, is a prototype drug that stimulates AMPK. Since its approval by the Food and Drug Administration (FDA) in the 1970s, metformin has been used to treat type 2 diabetes mellitus and other metabolic disorders [137]. The finding that metformin is associated with significant reductions in breast, prostate and pancreatic cancers has generated interest in this compound as an anticancer agent [138, 139]. Metformin acts mainly as an activator of AMPK, although AMPK-independent mechanisms have been identified [139, 140]. Metformin exerts its effects by inhibiting the mitochondrial respiratory chain complex I, which increases the AMP/ATP ratio and leads to the phosphorylation and activation of AMPK by LKB1 [141, 142].

The anti-proliferative and anti-invasive activities of metformin and its ability to induce apoptosis have been associated with its antitumor activity. These effects are mediated by the inhibition of IGF-1 signaling, downregulation of Bcl-2 proteins and modulation of MAP kinases, such as the inhibition of ERK and stimulation of JNK/p38 MAPK [143-149]. Metformin also potentiates the beneficial effects of chemotherapy when used in combination therapy [150-153]. The effects of metformin in animal models vary, depending on the tumor type (*e.g.*, pancreas, breast, ovarian, colon, lung) and its metabolic status [143, 153-159]. In contrast, clinical evidence of metformin activity is restricted to a few recent studies [160, 161], although a number of trials are currently investigating the therapeutic potential of this compound in combination with hormone therapy or traditional chemotherapy (www.clinicaltrials.gov).

Other potential AMPK activators include thiazolidinediones [162, 163] and statins [164-166] that also increase the AMP/ATP ratio by inhibiting mitochondrial ATP synthesis. 5-Aminoimidazole-4-carboxamide ribonucleoside (AICAR) is a cell-permeating drug that can activate AMPK after intracellular conversion to an AMP mimetic [166]. Several natural products can also affect tumor cell growth by activating AMPK signaling. One of these, resveratrol, inhibits cell growth and induces apoptosis in chemoresistant HT-29 colon cancer cells by a mechanism that involves AMPK activation and the generation of reactive oxygen species [167]. Finally, another very interesting example of AMPK activator is pemetrexed (PMX), a multi-targeted antifolate cytotoxic agent that inhibits several key folate-dependent enzymes in the thymidine and purine biosynthetic pathways, including thymidylate synthase. Currently, the use of PMX is approved by FDA for use in patients with non-small cell lung cancer (NSCLC) in both first- and second-line settings and in the treatment of malignant mesothelioma. PMX treatment of CCRF-CEM ALL and a number of solid tumor cell lines resulted in marked accumulations of the second folate-dependent enzyme of *de novo* purine synthesis, aminoimidazolecarboxamide ribonucleotide formyltransferase (AICARFT) substrate, ZMP, an AMP mimetic and activator of AMPK [168, 169].

Rapamycin and Rapalogs

The involvement of the mTOR signaling pathway in cancer and the discovery that mTOR is a target of rapamycin (sirolimus) have stimulated studies of this compound as an anticancer drug. The fact that rapamycin is an FDA-approved drug that has been used for many years as an immunosuppressor in organ transplantation has also contributed to the renewed interest in this compound. Efforts to improve the pharmacokinetic properties of rapamycin led to the development of the first generation of rapamycin analogs (rapalogs), including temsirolimus (CCI-779, Pfizer), everolimus (RAD001, Novartis) and ridaforolimus (AP23573, Ariad Pharmaceuticals). Clinical trials demonstrating the efficacy of temsirolimus against renal cell carcinoma (RCC), with an improvement in the overall survival of patients with metastatic disease [170] led to the approval of this drug by the FDA in 2007. Similarly, the efficacy of everolimus against RCC was demonstrated in a placebo-controlled phase III trial [171] and led to its approval by the FDA in 2009. Current clinical trials are investigating the efficacy of these rapalogs in other cancers, particularly those refractory to conventional chemotherapy [reviewed in 172]. Despite the initial enthusiasm, rapalogs have shown only modest efficacy in tumors for which important benefits were expected. A major cause of failure is that these compounds only partially inhibit 4E-BP phosphorylation and therefore incompletely block mTORC1-induced protein synthesis [173, 174]. Resistance to rapalogs is also attributed to the existence of feedback loops in the mTOR pathway that drive PI3K, mTORC2 and ERK signalling; these pathways oppose the effects of rapalogs on protein synthesis and the cell cycle [175-178].

The finding that rapalogs have limited substrate specificity and activate oncogenic pathways suggested that the inhibition of both mTORC1 and mTORC2 may have a greater impact on cancer cells. Based on this demonstration, a second generation of mTOR inhibitors, known as ATP-competitive mTOR inhibitors (TOR-KIs), and dual PI3K/mTOR inhibitors (PI3K/TOR-KIs) has been developed.

TOR-KIs and PI3K/TOR-KIs

mTOR kinase inhibitors, including PP30 and PP242 (INK-128, Intellikine) [171], WYE354 and WYE132 (Pfizer) [179], AZD8055 (AstraZeneca) [181] and Torin 1 [181], block the phosphorylation of all downstream targets of mTORC1 and mTORC2, thereby inhibiting cell growth and proliferation with a greater potency than rapalogs. The major mechanism involved in the case of TOR-KIs is suppression of the resistant functions of mTORC1. Unlike rapamycin, these inhibitors impair cap-dependent translation, primarily through the complete inhibition of 4E-BP phosphorylation [182]. Other pathways that are also efficiently inhibited by TOR-KIs include reducing aerobic glycolysis, which leads to the starvation of cancer cells and an improved antitumor effect [172]. Lactate accumulation and acidosis activate HIF-1α/HIF-2α, which stimulates the transcription of glycolytic regulators. TOR-KIs strongly reduce lactate production and the expression of Glut1, HIF-1α/HIF-2α due to the lack of PI3K-driven feedback activation. These effects normalize the cellular response to hypoxia and decrease the production of vascular endothelial growth factor [179]. Interestingly, in contrast to rapamycin, TOR-KIs also induce apoptosis [179] and autophagy [180, 181], probably through the inhibition of Akt. In addition, TOR-KIs and PI3K/TOR-KIs cause cell cycle inhibition and G1 arrest by blocking mTORC1-dependent cyclin D1 translation and Akt-mediated cyclin D1 transcription [179]. These two groups of inhibitors also attenuate lipid biosynthesis, which contributes to the loss of rapidly proliferating cancer cells, and inhibit tumor cell invasion and metastasis [172].

Despite the advantages of TOR-KIs, resistance may still develop through the PI3K- and PDK1-driven phosphorylation of Akt at Thr308, even in the absence of mTORC2-mediated Ser473 phosphorylation [173]. These findings, and the similarity between the catalytic domain of mTOR and class I PI3K, prompted the development of dual PI3K/mTOR inhibitors that include NVP-BEZ35 and BGT226 (Novartis), XL765 (Exelixis), GSK2126458 (GlaxoSmithKline), GDC0980 (Genetech), PF-04691502 and PF-0521384 (Pfizer). These inhibitors completely suppress PI3K/Akt signalling, even in tumors with activating mutations in this pathway. These PI3K/TOR-KIs have shown potential benefits in several cancers *in vivo* [172]. Several studies have shown that NVP-BEZ35, a new imidazo-quinoline-based PI3K/TOR-KI, induces apoptosis and/or autophagy and inhibits angiogenesis [182-185]. NVP-BEZ35 inhibits tumor cell growth in chemoresistant cells, such as KRAS-mutant lung cancer and breast cancer resistant to ErbB2 inhibitors [183, 186, 187]. This PI3K/TOR-KI has entered Phase I/II clinical trials for the treatment of RCC, breast and other solid cancers (www.clinicaltrials.gov).

Despite the great potential of TOR-KIs and PI3K/TOR-KIs as single agents in anticancer therapies, their anticancer activities are limited by parallel signalling, bypass pathway activation and feedback loops. Greater efficacy may be attained by combining the use of these compounds with other pathway inhibitors or standard chemotherapeutics. Reliable biomarkers are urgently needed to maximize patient benefits and safety, and a better understanding of cancer signalling will have a prominent role in future strategies to treat cancer.

Other Potential Metabolic Targets

In addition to metformin and mTOR inhibitors various other molecules have been suggested as potential therapeutic targets, including components of glycolysis and fatty acid synthesis, such as hexokinase, pyruvate kinase, acetyl-CoA carboxylase, fatty acid synthase and choline kinase [reviewed in 22]. For instance, the HK2 inhibitor 3-bromopyruvate induces apoptosis in hepatocellular carcinomas *in vitro* and *in vivo* [188], probably by interrupting the anti-apoptotic interaction between HK2 and VDAC [189]. Another example is the inhibition of PDK1 by dichloroacetate, which leads to the restoration of PDH activity and the induction of apoptosis *in vitro* and *in vivo* [190]. Clearly, the development of enzymatic inhibitors with high specificity for clinical studies will improve the current arsenal of anticancer drugs. Finally, the extracellular acidic pH of solid tumors induces an H^+-electrochemical gradient that increase the affinity and broaden substrate specificity of pH-dependent transport systems promoting selective uptake in cancer cells. In this way, transporters identified as crucial to cancer cell viability due to their roles in nutrient delivery or tumor metabolism could be targeted with specific inhibitors as a novel type of anti-cancer therapy based in the hijack of H^+-coupled transporters that are overexpressed in certain cancers such as PCFT, PepT1, PepT2, MCT1 and MCT4 [191].

CONCLUDING REMARKS

Recent advances in our knowledge of cancer cell metabolism have revealed the intimate relationship between oncogenes, tumor suppressors and metabolic transformation, making the latter event a true hallmark of cancer and potential target for the development of anticancer drugs. Some success has been achieved with metabolic therapies and is apparently related to the increased sensitivity of cancer cells to metabolic anticancer drugs and to the fact that this approach is independent of the specific signaling or epigenetic dysfunctions associated with the origin of cancer. However, some features of cancer metabolism remain incompletely understood, specifically with regard to (a) the real contribution of the TCA cycle to energy production in cancer cells, (b) the primary metabolic differences between highly proliferating cells and cancer cells and (c) how these differences might be used to develop more selective antitumor therapies. Understanding tumor metabolism is certainly a challenging task but is also a promising field in the search for molecular targets that can be used to develop novel therapeutic strategies for treating cancer. Fortunately, more and more researchers start to pay attention to this new research front and more research tools have been developed for this kind of study. A noteworthy example is global metabolomics analysis which has been demonstrated to be a potential tool for drug discovery/development and in cancer biomarker discovery [192-194].

ACKNOWLEDGEMENTS

Our research on this field is supported by Fundação de Amparo à Pesquisa do Estado de São Paulo (FAPESP), Coordenação de Aperfeiçoamento de Pessoal de Nível Superior (CAPES) and Conselho Nacional de Desenvolvimento Científico e Tecnológico (CNPq).

CONFLICT OF INTEREST

The authors confirm that this chapter contents have no conflict of interest.

REFERENCES

[1]   Hanahan D, Weinberg RA. The hallmarks of cancer. Cell 2000; 100(1): 57-70.
[2]   Hanahan D, Weinberg RA. Hallmarks of cancer: the next generation. Cell 2011; 144(5): 646-74.
[3]   Warburg O, Posener K, Negelein E. Über den Stoffwechsel der Karzinomzellen. Biochem Z 1924; 15: 309-44.
[4]   Shaw RJ, Cantley LC. Decoding key nodes in the metabolism of cancer cells: sugar & spice and all things nice. F1000 Biology Reports 2012; 4: 2.
[5]   Warburg O. Über den Stoffwechsel der Carcinomzelle. Klin Wochenschr 1925; 4: 534-536.
[6]   Warburg O. On the origin of cancer cells. Science 1956;123(3191): 309-14.
[7]   Gottlieb E, Tomlinson IP. Mitochondrial tumour suppressors: a genetic and biochemical update. Nature Reviews Cancer 2005; 5(11): 857-66.
[8]   Moreno-Sánchez R, Rodríguez-Enríquez S, Marín-Hernández A, Saavedra E. Energy metabolism in tumor cells. FEBS Journal 2007; 274(6): 1393-418.
[9]   DeBerardinis RJ, Lum JJ, Hatzivassiliou G, Thompson CB. The biology of cancer: metabolic reprogramming fuels cell growth and proliferation. Cell Metabolism 2008; 7(1): 11-20.

[10]   de Souza AC, Justo GZ, de Araújo DR, Cavagis AD. Defining the molecular basis of tumor metabolism: a continuing challenge since Warburg's discovery. Cellular Physiology and Biochemistry 2011; 28(5): 771-92.

[11]   Weinberg F, Chandel NS. Mitochondrial metabolism and cancer. Annals of the New York Academy of Sciences 2009; 1177: 66-73.

[12]   Muñoz-Pinedo C, El Mjiyad N, Ricci JE. Cancer metabolism: current perspectives and future directions. Cell Death & Disease 2012; 12(3): e248.

[13]   Macheda ML, Rogers S, Best JD. Molecular and cellular regulation of glucose transporter (GLUT) proteins in cancer. Journal of Cellular Physiology 2005; 202(3): 654-62.

[14]   Pelicano H, Martin DS, Xu RH, Huang P. Glycolysis inhibition for anticancer treatment. Oncogene 2006; 25(34): 4633-46.

[15]   Díaz-Ruiz R, Uribe-Carvajal S, Devin A, Rigoulet M. Tumor cell energy metabolism and its common features with yeast metabolism. Biochimica et Biophysica Acta 2009; 1796(2): 252-65.

[16]   Hammond KD, Balinsky D. Activities of key gluconeogenic enzymes and glycogen synthase in rat and human livers, hepatomas, and hepatoma cell cultures. Cancer Research 1978; 38(5): 1317-22.

[17]   Zancan P, Sola-Penna M, Furtado CM, Da Silva D. Differential expression of phosphofructokinase-1 isoforms correlates with the glycolytic efficiency of breast cancer cells. Molecular Genetics and Metabolism 2010; 100(4): 372-8.

[18]   Fanciulli M, Bruno T, Giovannelli A, Gentile FP, Di Padova M, Rubiu O, Floridi A. Energy metabolism of human LoVo colon carcinoma cells: correlation to drug resistance and influence of lonidamide. Clinical Cancer Research 2000; 6(4): 1590-7.

[19]   Rodríguez-Enríquez S, Marín-Hernández A, Gallardo-Pérez JC, Carreño-Fuentes L, Moreno-Sánchez R. Targeting of cancer energy metabolism. Molecular Nutrion & Food Research 2009; 53(1): 29-48.

[20]   Gatenby RA, RJ Gillies. Why do cancers have high aerobic glycolysis? Nature Reviews Cancer 2004; 4(11): 891-9.

[21]   Gallagher SM, Castorino JJ, Wang D, Philp NJ. Monocarboxylate transporter 4 regulates maturation and trafficking of CD147 to the plasma membrane in the metastatic breast cancer cell line MDA-MB-231. Cancer Research 2007; 67(9): 4182-9.

[22]   Kroemer G, Pouyssegur J. Tumor cell metabolism: cancer's Achilles' heel. Cancer Cell 2008; 13(6): 472-82.

[23]   Fischer K, Hoffmann P, Voelkl S, Meidenbauer N, Ammer J, Edinger M, Gottfried E, Schwarz S, Rothe G, Renner K, Timischl B, Mackensen A, Kunz-Schughart L, Andreesen R, Krause SW, Kreutz M. Inhibitory effect of tumor cell-derived lactic acid on human T cells. Blood 2007; 109(9): 3812–9.

[24]   Rathmell JC, Fox CJ, Plas DR, Hammerman PS, Cinalli RM, Thompson CB. Akt-Directed Glucose Metabolism Can Prevent Bax Conformation Change and Promote Growth Factor-Independent Survival. Molecular and Cellular Biology 2003; 23(20): 7315–28.

[25]   Zhao Y, Altman BJ, Coloff JL, Herman CE, Jacobs SR, Wieman HL, Wofford JA, Dimascio LN, Ilkayeva O, Reya T, Rathmell JC. Glycogen Synthase Kinase 3{alpha} and 3{beta} Mediate a Glucose-Sensitive Antiapoptotic Signaling Pathway To Stabilize Mcl-1. Molecular and Cellular Biology 2007; 27(12): 4328-39.

[26]   Munoz-Pinedo C, Ruiz-Ruiz C, Ruiz de Almodovar C, Palacios C, Lopez-Rivas A. Inhibition of glucose metabolism sensitizes tumor cells to death receptor-triggered

apoptosis through enhancement of death-inducing signaling complex formation and apical procaspase-8 processing. The Journal of Biological Chemistry 2003; 278(15): 12759-68.

[27]   El Mjiyad N, Caro-Maldonado A, Ramirez-Peinado S, Munoz-Pinedo C. Sugar-free approaches to cancer cell killing. Oncogene 2011; 30(3): 253-64.

[28]   Pastorino JG, Shulga N, Hoek JB. Mitochondrial binding of hexokinase II inhibits Bax-induced cytochrome c release and apoptosis. The Journal of Biological Chemistry 2002; 277(9): 7610-8.

[29]   Díaz-Ruiz R, Avéret N, Araiza D, Pinson B, Uribe-Carvajal S, Devin A, Rigoulet M. Mitochondrial oxidative phosphorylation is regulated by fructose 1,6-bisphosphate. A possible role in Crabtree effect induction? The Journal of Biological Chemistry 2008; 283(40): 26948-55.

[30]   Pastorino JG, Hoek JB. Regulation of hexokinase binding to VDAC. Journal of Bioenergetics and Biomembranes 2008; 40(3): 171-82.

[31]   Majewski N, Nogueira V, Robey RB, Hay N. Akt inhibits apoptosis downstream of BID cleavage *via* a glucose-dependent mechanism involving mitochondrial hexokinases. Molecular and Cellular Biology 2004; 24(2): 730-40.

[32]   Crabtree HG. Observations on the carbohydrate metabolism of tumors. Biochemistry Journal 1929; 23(3): 536-45.

[33]   Ben-Haim S, Ell PJ. 18F-FDG PET and PET/CT in the evaluation of cancer treatment response. The Journal of Nuclear Medicine 2009; 50(1): 88-99.

[34]   Wartenberg M, Richter M, Datchev A, Günther S, Milosevic N, Bekhite MM, Figulla HR, Aran JM, Pétriz J, Sauer H. Glycolytic pyruvate regulates P-glycoprotein expression in multicellular tumor spheroids *via* modulation of the intracellular redox state. Journal of Cellular Biochemistry 2010; 109(2): 434-46.

[35]   Christofk HR, Vander Heiden MG, Wu N, Asara JM, Cantley LC. Pyruvate kinase M2 is a phosphotyrosine-binding protein. Nature 2008; 452(7184): 181-6.

[36]   Vander Heiden MG, Cantley LC, Thompson CB. Understanding the Warburg effect: the metabolic requirements of cell proliferation. Science 2009; 324(4930): 1029-33.

[37]   Chaneton B, Gottlieb E. Rocking cell metabolism: revised functions of the key glycolytic regulator PKM2 in cancer. Trends in Biochemical Sciences 2012; 37(8): 309-16.

[38]   Eboli ML, Paradies G, Galeotti T, Papa S. Pyruvate transport in tumor-cell mitochondria. Biochimica et Biophysica Acta 1977; 460(1): 183-7.

[39]   Paradies G, Capuano F, Palombini G, Galeotti T, Papa S. Transport of pyruvate in mitochondria from different tumor cells. Cancer Research 1983; 43(11): 5068-71.

[40]   Zhang Y, Zhang X, Wang X, Gan L, Yu G, Chen Y, Liu K, Li P, Pan J, Wang J, Qin S. Inhibition of LDH-A by lentivirus-mediated small interfering RNA suppresses intestinal-type gastric cancer tumorigenicity through the downregulation of Oct4. Cancer Letters 2012; 321(1): 45-54.

[41]   Thangaraju M, Carswell KN, Prasad PD, Ganapathy V. Colon cancer cells maintain low levels of pyruvate to avoid cell death caused by inhibition of HDAC1/ HDAC3. Biochemical Journal 2009; 417(1): 379-89.

[42]   DeBerardinis RJ, Sayed N, Ditsworth D, Thompson CB. Brick by brick: metabolism and tumor cell growth. Current Opinion in Genetics & Development 2008;18(1): 54-61.

[43]   Fan TW, Kucia M, Jankowski K, Higashi RM, Ratajczak J, Ratajczak MZ, Lane AN. Rhabdomyosarcoma cells show an energy producing anabolic metabolic phenotype compared with primary myocytes. Molecular Cancer 2008; 7: 79.

[44] Wise DR, Thompson CB. Glutamine addiction: a new therapeutic target in cancer. Trends in Biochemical Sciences 2010; 35(8): 427-33.

[45] Daye D, Wellen KE. Metabolic reprogramming in cancer: Unraveling the role of glutamine in tumorigenesis. Seminars in Cell & Developmental Biology 2012; 23(4): 362-9.

[46] Dang CV, Le A, Gao P: MYC-induced cancer cell energy metabolism and therapeutic opportunities. Clinical Cancer Research 2009; 15(21): 6479-83.

[47] DeBerardinis RJ, Cheng T. Q's next: the diverse functions of glutamine in metabolism, cell biology and cancer. Oncogene 2010; 29(3): 313-24.

[48] Gao P, Tchernyshyov I, Chang TC, Lee YS, Kita K, Ochi T, Zeller KI, De Marzo AM, Van Eyk JE, Mendell JT, Dang CV. c-Myc suppression of miR-23a/b enhances mitochondrial glutaminase expression and glutamine metabolism. Nature 2009; 458(7239): 762-5.

[49] Forbes NS, Meadows AL, Clark DS, Blanch HW. Estradiol stimulates the biosynthetic pathways of breast cancer cells: detection by metabolic flux analysis. Metabolic Engineering 2006; 8(6): 639-52.

[50] Vogelstein B, Kinzler KW. Cancer genes and the pathways they control. Nature Medicine 2004; 10(8): 789-99.

[51] Jones RJ, Thompson CB. Tumor suppressors and cell metabolism: a recipe for cancer growth. Genes & Development 2009; 23(5): 537-48.

[52] Jones NP, Schulze A. Targeting cancer metabolism-aiming at a tumour's sweet-spot. Drug Discovery Today 2012; 17(5-6): 232-41.

[53] Jiang BH, Liu LZ. PI3K/PTEN signaling in angiogenesis and tumorigenesis. Advances in Cancer Research 2009; 102: 19-65.

[54] Sun Q, Chen X, Ma J, Peng H, Wang F, Zha X, Wang Y, Jing Y, Yang H, Chen, R, Chang L, Zhang Y, Goto J, Onda H, Chen T, Wang MR, Lu Y, You H, Kwiatkowski D, Zhang H. Mammalian target of rapamycin up-regulation of pyruvate kinase isoenzyme type M2 is critical for aerobic glycolysis and tumor growth. Proceedings of the National Academy of Sciences of the United States of America 2011; 108(10): 4129-34.

[55] Semenza GL. HIF-1: upstream and downstream of cancer metabolism. Current Opinion in Genetics & Development 2010; 20(1): 51-6.

[56] Duvel K, Yecies JL, Menon S, Raman P, Lipovsky AI, Souza AL, Triantafellow E, Ma Q, Gorski R, Cleaver S, Vander Heiden MG, MacKei gan JP, Fin an PM, Clish CB, Murphy LO, Mannin g BD. Activation of a metabolic gene regulatory network downstream of mTOR complex 1. Molecular Cell 2010; 39(2): 171-83.

[57] Zhang H, Bosch-Marce M, Shimoda LA, Tan YS, Baek JH, Wesley JB, Gonzalez FJ, Semenza GL. Mitochondrial autophagy is a HIF-1-dependent adaptive metabolic response to hypoxia. The Journal of Biological Chemistry 2008; 283(16): 10892-903.

[58] Mathew R, White E. Autophagy, Stress, and Cancer Metabolism: What Doesn't Kill You Makes You Stronger. Cold Spring Harbor Symposia on Quantitative Biology. 2011; 76: 389-96.

[59] Luo W, Hu H, Chang R, Zhong J, Knabel M, O'meally R, Cole RN, Pandey A, Semenza GL. Pyruvate Kinase M2 Is a PHD3-Stimulated Coactivator for Hypoxia-Inducible Factor 1. Cell 2011; 145(5): 732-44.

[60] Robey RB, Hay N. Mitochondrial hexokinases, novel mediators of the antiapoptotic effects of growth factors and Akt. Oncogene 2006; 25(34): 4683-96.

[61] Shackelford DB, Shaw RJ. The LKB1-AMPK pathway: metabolism and growth control in tumour suppression. Nature Reviews Cancer 2009; 9(8): 563-75.

[62]   Clem B, Telang S, Clem A, Yalcin A, Meier J, Simmons A, Rasku MA, Arumugam S, Dean WL, Eaton J, Lane A, Trent JO, Chesney J. Small-molecule inhibition of 6-phosphofructo-2-kinase activity suppresses glycolytic flux and tumor growth. Molecular Cancer Therapeutics 2008; 7(1): 110-20.

[63]   Shackelford DB, Vasquez DS, Corbeil J, Wu S, Leblanc M, Wu CL, Vera DR, Shaw RJ. mTOR and HIF-1alpha mediated tumor metabolism in an LKB1 mouse model of Peutz-Jeghers syndrome. Proceedings of the National Academy of Sciences of the United States of America 2009; 106(27): 11137-42.

[64]   Carling D, Zammit VA, Hardie DG. A common bicyclic protein kinase cascade inactivates the regulatory enzymes of fatty acid and cholesterol biosynthesis. FEBS Letters 1987; 223(2): 217-22.

[65]   Felsher DW, Bishop JM. Reversible tumorigenesis by MYC in hematopoietic lineages. Molecular Cell 1999; 4(2): 199-207.

[66]   Dang CV, O'Donnell KA, Zeller KI, Nguyen T, Osthus RC, Li F. The c-Myc target gene network. Seminars in Cancer Biology 2006; 16(4): 253-64.

[67]   Wokolorczyk D, Gliniewicz B, Sikorski A, Zlowocka E, Masojc B, Debniak T, Matyjasik J, Mierzejewski M, Medrek K, Oszutowska D, Suchy J, Gronwald J, Teodorczyk U, Huzarski T, Byrski T, Jakubowska A, Górski B, van de Wetering T, Walczak S, Narod SA, Lubinski J, Cybulski C. A range of cancers is associated with the rs6983267 marker on chromosome 8. Cancer Research 2008; 68(23): 9982-6.

[68]   Hu S, Balakrishnan A, Bok RA, Anderton B, Larson PEZ, Nelson SJ, Kurhanewicz J, Vigneron DB, Goga A. 13C-Pyruvate imaging reveals alterations in glycolysis that precede c-Myc-induced tumor formation and regression. Cell Metabolism 2011; 14(1): 131-42.

[69]   Hermeking H, Rago C, Schuhmacher M, Li Q, Barrett JF, Obaya AJ, O'Connell BC, Mateyak MK, Tam W, Kohlhuber F, Dang CV, Sedivy JM, Eick D, Vogelstein B, Kinzler KW. Identification of CDK4 as a target of c-MYC. Proceedings of the National Academy of Sciences of the United States of America 2000; 97(5): 2229-34.

[70]   David CJ, Chen M, Assanah M, Canoll P, Manley JL. HnRNP proteins controlled by c-Myc deregulate pyruvate kinase mRNA splicing in cancer. Nature 2010; 463(7279): 364-8.

[71]   Kim JW, Dang CV. Cancer's molecular sweet tooth and the Warburg effect. Cancer Res 2006; 66(18): 8927-30.

[72]   Dang CV, Kim JW, Gao P, Yustein J. The interplay between MYC and HIF in cancer. Nature Reviews Cancer 2008; 8(1): 51-6.

[73]   Li F, Wang Y, Zeller KI, Potter JJ, Wonsey DR, O'Donnell KA, Kim JW, Yustein JT, Lee LA, Dang CV. Myc stimulates nuclearly encoded mitochondrial genes and mitochondrial biogenesis. Molecular and Cellular Biology 2005; 25(14): 6225-34.

[74]   Funes JM, Quintero M, Henderson S, Martinez D, Qureshi U Westwood C, Clements MO, Bourboulia D, Pedley RB, Moncada S, Boshoff C. Transformation of human mesenchymal stem cells increases their dependency on oxidative phosphorylation for energy production. Proceedings of the National Academy of Sciences of the United States of America 2007; 104(15): 6223-8.

[75]   Moreadith RW, Lehninger AL. The pathways of glutamate and glutamine oxidation by tumor cell mitochondria. Role of mitochondrial NAD(P)+-dependent malic enzyme. The Journal of Biological Chemistry 1984; 259(10): 6215-6221.

[76]   Lin CJ, Malina A, Pelletier J. c-Myc and eIF4F constitute a feedforward loop that regulates cell growth: implications for anticancer therapy. Cancer Research 2009; 69(19): 7491-4.

[77]   Ruggero D. The role of Myc-induced protein synthesis in cancer. Cancer Research 2009; 69(23): 8839-43.

[78]   Sermeus A, Michiels C. Reciprocal influence of the p53 and the hypoxic pathways. Cell Death & Disease 2011; 2: e164.

[79]   Bensaad K, Tsuruta A, Selak MA, Vidal MN, Nakano K, Bartrons R, Gottlieb E, Vousden KH. TIGAR, a p53-inducible regulator of glycolysis and apoptosis. Cell 2006; 126(1): 107-20.

[80]   Kondoh H, Lleonart ME, Gil J, Wang J, Degan P, Peters G, Martinez D, Carnero A, Beach D. Glycolytic enzymes can modulate cellular life span. Cancer Research 2005, 65(1): 177-85.

[81]   Buzzai M, Jones RG, Amaravadi RK, Lum JJ, DeBerardinis RJ, Zhao F Viollet B, Thompson CB. Systemic treatment with the antidiabetic drug metformin selectively impairs p53-deficient tumor cell growth. Cancer Research 2007; 67(14): 6745-52.

[82]   Maiuri MC, Galluzzi L, Morselli E, Kepp O, Malik SA, Kroemer G. Autophagy regulation by p53. Current Opinion in Cell Biology 2009; 22(2): 181-5.

[83]   Hu W, Zhang C, Wu R, Sun Y, Levine A, Feng Z. Glutaminase 2, a novel p53 target gene regulating energy metabolism and antioxidant function. Proceedings of the National Academy of Sciences of the United States of America 2010; 107(16): 7455-60.

[84]   Suzuki S, Tanaka T, Poyurovsky MV, Nagano H, Mayama T, Ohkubo S, Lokshin M, Hosokawa H, Nakayama T, Suzuki Y, Sugano S, Sato E, Nagao T, Yokote K, Tatsuno I, Prives C. Phosphate-activated glutaminase (GLS2), a p53-inducible regulator of glutamine metabolism and reactive oxygen species. Proceedings of the National Academy of Sciences of the United States of America 2010; 107(16): 7461-66.

[85]   Gommans WM, Berezikov E. Controlling miRNA regulation in disease. Methods in Molecular Biology 2012; 822: 1-18.

[86]   Esteller M. Non-coding RNAs in human diseases. Nature Reviews Genetics 2011; 12: 861-74.

[87]   Bartel DP. MicroRNAs: genomics, biogenesis, mechanism, and function. Cell 2004; 116(2): 281-97.

[88]   Brennecke J, Stark A, Russell RB, Cohen SM. Principles of microRNA-target recognition. PLoS Biology 2005; 3(3): e85.

[89]   Ebert MS, Sharp PA. Roles for microRNAs in conferring robustness to biological processes. Cell 2012; 149(3): 515-24.

[90]   Mendell JT, Olson EN. MicroRNAs in stress signaling and human disease. Cell 2012; 148(6): 1172-87.

[91]   Bartel, D.P. MicroRNAs: target recognition and regulatory functions. Cell 2009; 136(2): 215-33.

[92]   Yamamoto H, Adachi Y, Taniguchi H, Kunimoto H, Nosho K, Suzuki H, Shinomura Y. Interrelationship between microsatellite instability and microRNA in gastrointestinal cancer. World Journal of Gastroenterology 2012; 18(22): 2745-55.

[93]   Ali AS, Ahmad A, Ali S, Bao B, Philip PA, Sarkar FH. The role of cancer stem cells and miRNAs in defining the complexities of brain metastasis. Journal of Cellular Physiology 2012; 228(1): 36-42.

[94]   Karin M. Nuclear factor-kappaB in cancer development and progression. Nature 2006; 441(7092): 431-6.

[95]   Rathore MG, Saumet A, Rossi JF, de Bettignies C, Tempé D, Lecellier CH, Villalba M. The NF-κB member p65 controls glutamine metabolism through miR-23a. The International Journal of Biochemical Cell Biology 2012; 44(9): 1448-56.

[96]   Thorens, B. and Mueckler, M. Glucose transporters in the 21st Century. American Journal of Physiology, Endocrinology and Metabolism 2011; 298(2): E141-E145.

[97]   Chow TF, ManKaruos M, Scorilas A, Youssef Y, Girgis A, Mossad S, Metias S, Rofael Y, Honey RJ, Stewart R, Pace Kt, Yousef GM. The miR-17-92 cluster is over expressed in and has an oncogenic effect on renal cell carcinoma. Journal of Urology 2010; 183(2): 743-51.

[98]   Szafranska AE, Davison TS, John J, Cannon T, Sipos B, Maghnouj A, Labourier E, Hahn SA. MicroRNA expression alterations are linked to tumorigenesis and non-neoplastic processes in pancreatic ductal adenocarcinoma. Oncogene 2007; 26(30): 4442-52.

[99]   Karolina DS, Armugam A, Tavintharan S, Wong MT, Lim SC, Sum CF, Jeyaseelan K. MicroRNA 144 impairs insulin signaling by inhibiting the expression of insulin receptor substrate 1 in type 2 diabetes mellitus. PLoS ONE 2011; 6(8): e22839.

[100]   Michael MZ, O'Connor SM, van Holst Pellekaan NG, Young GP, James RJ. Reduced accumulation of specific microRNAs in colorectal neoplasia. Molecular Cancer Research 2003; 1(12): 882-91.

[101]   Calin GA, Sevignani C, Dumitru CD, Hyslop T, Noch E, Yendamuri S, Shimizu M, Rattan S, Bullrich F, Negrini M, Croce CM. Human microRNA genes are frequently located at fragile sites and genomic regions involved in cancers. Proceedings of the National Academy of Sciences of the United States of America 2004, 101(9): 2999-3004.

[102]   Akao Y, Nakagawa Y, Kitade Y, Kinoshita T, Naoe T. Downregulation of microRNAs-143 and -145 in B-cell malignancies. Cancer Science 2007, 98(12): 1914-20.

[103]   Porkka KP, Pfeiffer MJ, Waltering KK, Vessella RL, Tammela TL, Visakorpi T. MicroRNA expression profiling in prostate cancer. Cancer Research 2007, 67(13): 6130-5.

[104]   Slaby O, Svoboda M, Fabian P, Smerdova T, Knoflickova D, Bednarikova M, Nenutil R, Vyzula R. Altered expression of miR-21, miR-31, miR-143 and miR-145 is related to clinicopathologic features of colorectal cancer. Oncology 2007, 72(5-6): 397-402.

[105]   Chen X, Guo X, Zhang H, Xiang Y, Chen J, Yin Y, Cai X, Wang K, Wang G, Ba Y, Zhu L, Wang J, Yang R, Zhang Y, Ren Z, Zen K, Zhang J, Zhang CY. Role of miR-143 targeting KRAS in colorectal tumorigenesis. Oncogene 2009; 28(10): 1385-92.

[106]   Ugras S, Brill ER, Jacobsen A, Hafner M, Socci N, Decarolis PL, Khanin R, O'Connor RB, Mihailovic A, Taylor BS, Sheridan R, Gimble JM, Viale A, Crago A, Antonescu CR, Sander C, Tuschl T, Singer S. Small RNA sequencing and functional characterization reveals microRNA-143 tumor suppressor activity in liposarcoma. Cancer Research 2011; 71(17): 5659-69.

[107]   Gregersen LH, Jacobsen A, Frankel LB, Wen J, Krogh A, Lund AH. microRNA-143 down-regulates Hexokinase 2 in colon cancer cells. BMC Cancer 2012; 12(1): 232.

[108]   Wilfred, BR, Wang WX, Nelson PT. Energizing miRNA research: a review of the role of miRNAs in lipid metabolism, with a prediction that miR-103/107 regulates human metabolic pathways. Molecular Genetics and Metabolism 2007; 91(3): 209-17.

[109]   Laplante M, Sabatini DM. mTOR signaling at a glance. Journal of Cell Science 2009; 122(Pt 20): 3589-94.

[110]   Kim DH, Sarbassov DD, Ali SM, Latek RR, Guntur KV, Erdjument-Bromage H, Tempst P, Sabatini DM. GβL, a positive regulator of the rapamycin-sensitive pathway required for

the nutrient-sensitive interaction between raptor and mTOR. Molecular Cell 2003; 11(4): 895-904.

[111]   Jacinto E, Loewith R, Schmidt A, Lin S, Rüegg MA, Hall A, Hall MN. Mammalian TOR complex 2 controls the actin cytoskeleton and is rapamycin insensitive. Nature Cell Biology 2004; 6(11): 1122-8.

[112]   Peterson TR, Laplante M, Thoreen CC, Sancak Y, Kang SA, Kuehl WM, Gray NS, Sabatini DM. DEPTOR is an mTOR inhibitor frequently overexpressed in multiple myeloma cells and required for their survival. Cell 2009; 137(5): 873-86.

[113]   Kaizuka T, Hara T, Oshiro N, Kikkawa U, Yonezawa K, Takehana K, Iemura S, Natsume T, Mizushima N. Tti1 and Tel2 are critical factors in mammalian target of rapamycin complex assembly. Journal of Biological Chemistry 2010; 285(26): 20109-16.

[114]   Hara K, Maruki Y, Long X, Yoshino K, Oshiro N, Hidayat S, Tokunaga C, Avruch J, Yonezawa K. Raptor, a binding partner of target of rapamycin (TOR), mediates TOR action. Cell 2002; 110(2): 177-89.

[115]   Kim DH, Sarbassov DD, Ali SM, King JE, Latek RR, Erdjument-Bromage H, Tempst P, Sabatini DM. mTOR interacts with raptor to form a nutrient-sensitive complex that signals to the cell growth machinery. Cell 2002; 110(2): 163-75.

[116]   Sancak Y, Thoreen CC, Peterson TR, Lindquist RA, Kang SA, Spooner E, Carr SA, Sabatini DM. PRAS40 is an insulin-regulated inhibitor of the mTORC1 protein kinase. Molecular Cell 2007; 25(6): 903-15.

[117]   Sarbassov DD, Ali SM, Kim DH, Guertin DA, Latek RR, Erdjument-Bromage H, Tempst P, Sabatini DM. Rictor, a novel binding partner of mTOR, defines a rapamycin-insensitive and raptor-independent pathway that regulates the cytoskeleton. Current Biology 2004; 14(14): 1296-1302.

[118]   Jacinto E, Facchinetti V, Liu D, Soto N, Wei S, Jung SY, Huang Q, Qin J, Su B. SIN1/MIP1 maintains rictor-mTOR complex integrity and regulates Akt phosphorylation and substrate specificity. Cell 2006; 127(1): 125-37.

[119]   Pearce LR, Huang X, Boudeau J, Pawłowski R, Wullschleger S, Deak M, Ibrahim AF, Gourlay R, Magnuson MA, Alessi DR. Identification of Protor as a novel Rictor-binding component of mTOR complex-2. Biochemical Journal 2007; 405(3): 513-22.

[120]   Brown EJ, Albers MW, Shin TB, Ichikawa K, Keith CT, Lane WS, Schreiber SL. A mammalian protein targeted by G1-arresting rapamycin-receptor complex. Nature 1994; 369(6483): 756-8.

[121]   Sabatini DM, Erdjument-Bromage H, Lui M, Tempst P, Snyder SH. RAFT1: a mammalian protein that binds to FKBP12 in a rapamycin-dependent fashion and is homologous to yeast TORs. Cell 1994; 78(1): 35-43.

[122]   Brown EJ, Beal PA, Keith CT, Chen J, Shin TB, Schreiber SL. Control of p70 s6 kinase by kinase activity of FRAP *in vivo*. Nature 1995; 377(6548): 441-6.

[123]   Sarbassov DD, Ali SM, Sengupta S, Sheen JH, Hsu PP, Bagley AF, Markhard AL, Sabatini DM. Prolonged rapamycin treatment inhibits mTORC2 assembly and Akt/PKB. Molecular Cell 2006; 22(2): 159-68.

[124]   Zoncu R, Efeyan A, Sabatini DM. mTOR: from growth signal integration to cancer, diabetes and ageing. Nature Reviews. Molecular Cell Biology 2011; 12(1): 21-35.

[125]   Hardie DG. AMP-activated/SNF1 protein kinases: conserved guardians of cellular energy. Nature Reviews Molecular Cell Biology 2007; 8(10): 774-85.

[126] Lizcano JM, Göransson O, Toth R, Deak M, Morrice NA, Boudeau J, Hawley SA, Udd L, Mäkelä TP, Hardie DG, Alessi DR. LKB1 is a master kinase that activates 13 kinases of the AMPK subfamily, including MARK/PAR-1. EMBO Journal 2004; 23(4): 833-43.

[127] Bright NJ, Thornton C, Carling D. The regulation and function of mammalian AMPK-related kinases. Acta Physiologica (Oxford) 2009; 196(1): 15-26.

[128] Hardie DG. AMP-activated protein kinase: an energy sensor that regulates all aspects of cell function. Genes Development 2011; 25(18): 1895-1908.

[129] Inoki K, Zhu T, Guan KL. TSC2 mediates cellular energy response to control cell growth and survival. Cell 2003; 115(5): 577-90.

[130] Zhang Y, Gao X, Saucedo LJ, Ru B, Edgar BA, Pan D. Rheb is a direct target of the tuberous sclerosis tumour suppressor proteins. Nature Cell Biology 2003; 5(6): 578-81.

[131] Hara K, Yonezawa K, Kozlowski MT, Sugimoto T, Andrabi K, Weng QP, Kasuga M, Nishimoto I, Avruch J. Regulation of eIF-4E BP1 phosphorylation by mTOR. Journal of Biological Chemistry 1997; 272(42): 26457-63.

[132] Yecies JL, Manning BD. Transcriptional control of cellular metabolism by mTOR signaling. Cancer Research 2011; 71(8): 2815-20.

[133] Jung CH, Jun CB, Ro SH, Kim YM, Otto NM, Cao J, Kundu M, Kim DH. ULK-Atg13-FIP200 complexes mediate mTOR signaling to the autophagy machinery. Molecular Biology of the Cell 2009; 20(7): 1992-2003.

[134] Hudson CC, Liu M, Chiang GG, Otterness DM, Loomis DC, Kaper F, Giaccia AJ, Abraham RT. Regulation of hypoxia-inducible factor 1alpha expression and function by the mammalian target of rapamycin. Molecular and Cellular Biology. 2002; 22(20): 7004-14.

[135] Feng Z, Zhang H, Levine AJ, Jin S. The coordinate regulation of the p53 and mTOR pathways in cells. Proceedings of the National Academy of Science of the United States of America 2005; 102(23): 8204-9.

[136] Laplante M, Sabatini DM. mTOR signaling in growth control and disease. Cell 2012; 149(2): 274-93.

[137] Zhou G, Myers R, Li Y, Chen Y, Shen X, Fenyk-Melody J, Wu M, Ventre J, Doebber T, Fujii N, Musi N, Hirshman MF, Goodyear LJ, Moller DE. Role of AMP-activated protein kinase in mechanism of metformin action. Journal of Clinical Investigation 2001; 108(8): 1167-74.

[138] Papanas N, Maltezos E, Mikhailidis DP. Metformin and cancer: licence to heal? Expert Opinion on Investigational Drugs 2010; 19(8): 913-7.

[139] Viollet B, Guigas B, Sanz Garcia N, Leclerc J, Foretz M, Andreelli F. Cellular and molecular mechanisms of metformin: an overview. Clinical Science (London) 2012; 122(6): 253-70.

[140] Rattan R, Giri S, Hartmann LC, Shridhar V. Metformin attenuates ovarian cancer cell growth in an AMP-kinase dispensable manner. Journal of Cellular and Molecular Medicine 2011; 15(1): 166-78.

[141] El-Mir MY, Nogueira V, Fontaine E, Avéret N, Rigoulet M, Leverve X. Dimethylbiguanide inhibits cell respiration *via* an indirect effect targeted on the respiratory chain complex I. Journal Biological Chemistry 2000; 275(1): 223-8.

[142] Owen MR, Doran E, Halestrap AP. Evidence that metformin exerts its anti-diabetic effects through inhibition of complex 1 of the mitochondrial respiratory chain. Biochemical Journal 2000; 348(Pt 3): 607-14.

[143] Kisfalvi K, Eibl G, Sinnett-Smith J, Rozengurt E. Metformin disrupts crosstalk between G protein-coupled receptor and insulin receptor signaling systems and inhibits pancreatic cancer growth. Cancer Research 2009; 69(16): 6539-45.

[144] Liu B, Fan Z, Edgerton SM, Yang X, Lind SE, Thor AD. Potent anti-proliferative effects of metformin on trastuzumab-resistant breast cancer cells *via* inhibition of erbB2/IGF-1 receptor interactions. Cell Cycle 2011; 10(17): 2959-66.

[145] Wu N, Gu C, Gu H, Hu H, Han Y, Li Q. Metformin induces apoptosis of lung cancer cells through activating JNK/p38 MAPK pathway and GADD153. Neoplasma 2011; 58(6): 482-90.

[146] Malki A, Youssef A. Antidiabetic drug metformin induces apoptosis in human MCF breast cancer *via* targeting ERK signaling. Oncology Research 2011; 19(6): 275-85.

[147] Yasmeen A, Beauchamp MC, Piura E, Segal E, Pollak M, Gotlieb WH. Induction of apoptosis by metformin in epithelial ovarian cancer: involvement of the Bcl-2 family proteins. Gynecologic Oncology 2011; 121(3): 492-8.

[148] Tan BK, Adya R, Chen J, Lehnert H, Sant Cassia LJ, Randeva HS. Metformin treatment exerts antiinvasive and antimetastatic effects in human endometrial carcinoma cells. Journal of Clinical Endocrinology and Metabolism 2011; 96(3): 808-16.

[149] Vakana E, Altman JK, Glaser H, Donato NJ, Platanias LC. Antileukemic effects of AMPK activators on BCR-ABL-expressing cells. Blood 2011; 118(24): 6399-6402.

[150] Kawanami T, Takiguchi S, Ikeda N, Funakoshi A. A humanized anti-IGF-1R monoclonal antibody (R1507) and/or metformin enhance gemcitabine-induced apoptosis in pancreatic cancer cells. Oncology Reports 2012; 27(3): 867-72.

[151] Hanna RK, Zhou C, Malloy KM, Sun L, Zhong Y, Gehrig PA, Bae-Jump VL. Metformin potentiates the effects of paclitaxel in endometrial cancer cells through inhibition of cell proliferation and modulation of the mTOR pathway. Gynecologic Oncology 2012; 125(2): 458-69.

[152] Chen G, Xu S, Renko K, Derwahl M. Metformin inhibits growth of thyroid carcinoma cells, suppresses self-renewal of derived cancer stem cells, and potentiates the effect of chemotherapeutic agents. Journal of Clinical Endocrinology and Metabolism 2012; 97(4): E510-E520.

[153] Rattan R, Graham RP, Maguire JL, Giri S, Shridhar V. Metformin suppresses ovarian cancer growth and metastasis with enhancement of cisplatin cytotoxicity *in vivo*. Neoplasia 2011; 13(5): 483-91.

[154] Anisimov VN, Berstein LM, Egormin PA, Piskunova TS, Popovich IG, Zabezhinski MA, Kovalenko IG, Poroshina TE, Semenchenko AV, Provinciali M, Re F, Franceschi C. Effect of metformin on life span and on the development of spontaneous mammary tumors in HER-2/neu transgenic mice. Experimental Gerontology 2005; 40(8-9): 685-93.

[155] Buzzai M, Jones RG, Amaravadi RK, Lum JJ, DeBerardinis RJ, Zhao F, Viollet B, Thompson CB. Systemic treatment with the antidiabetic drug metformin selectively impairs p53-deficient tumor cell growth. Cancer Research 2007; 67(14): 6745-52.

[156] Phoenix KN, Vumbaca F, Claffey KP. Therapeutic metformin/AMPK activation promotes the angiogenic phenotype in the ERalpha negative MDA-MB-435 breast cancer model. Breast Cancer Research and Treatment 2009; 113(1): 101-11.

[157] Algire C, Amrein L, Zakikhani M, Panasci L, Pollak M. Metformin blocks the stimulative effect of a high-energy diet on colon carcinoma growth *in vivo* and is associated with reduced expression of fatty acid synthase. Endocrine-Related Cancer 2010; 17(2): 351-60.

[158]   Memmott RM, Mercado JR, Maier CR, Kawabata S, Fox SD, Dennis PA. Metformin prevents tobacco carcinogen-induced lung tumorigenesis. Cancer Prevention Research (Philadelphia) 2010; 3(9): 1066-76.

[159]   Phoenix KN, Vumbaca F, Fox MM, Evans R, Claffey KP. Dietary energy availability affects primary and metastatic breast cancer and metformin efficacy. Breast Cancer Research and Treatment 2010; 123(2): 333-44.

[160]   Hosono K, Endo H, Takahashi H, Sugiyama M, Sakai E, Uchiyama T, Suzuki K, Iida H, Sakamoto Y, Yoneda K, Koide T, Tokoro C, Abe Y, Inamori M, Nakagama H, Nakajima A. Metformin suppresses colorectal aberrant crypt foci in a short-term clinical trial. Cancer Prevention Research (Philadelphia) 2010; 3(9): 1077-83.

[161]   Hadad S, Iwamoto T, Jordan L, Purdie C, Bray S, Baker L, Jellema G, Deharo S, Hardie DG, Pusztai L, Moulder-Thompson S, Dewar JA, Thompson AM. Evidence for biological effects of metformin in operable breast cancer: a pre-operative, window-of-opportunity, randomized trial. Breast Cancer Research and Treatment 2011; 128(3): 783-94.

[162]   LeBrasseur NK, Kelly M, Tsao TS, Farmer SR, Saha AK, Ruderman NB, Tomas E. Thiazolidinediones can rapidly activate AMP-activated protein kinase in mammalian tissues. American Journal of Physiology, Endocrinology and Metabolism 2006; 291(1): E175-E181.

[163]   Han S, Roman J. Rosiglitazone suppresses human lung carcinoma cell growth through PPARgamma-dependent and PPARgamma-independent signal pathways. Molecular Cancer Therapeutics 2006; 5(2): 430-7.

[164]   Sun W, Lee TS, Zhu M, Gu C, Wang Y, Zhu Y, Shyy JY. Statins activate AMP-activated protein kinase *in vitro* and *in vivo*. Circulation 2006; 114(24): 2655-62.

[165]   Yang PM, Liu YL, Lin YC, Shun CT, Wu MS, Chen CC. Inhibition of autophagy enhances anticancer effects of atorvastatin in digestive malignancies. Cancer Research 2010; 70(19): 7699-7709.

[166]   Woodard J, Joshi S, Viollet B, Hay N, Platanias LC. AMPK as a therapeutic target in renal cell carcinoma. Cancer Biology and Therapy 2010; 10(11): 1168-77.

[167]   Hwang JT, Kwak DW, Lin SK, Kim HM, Kim YM, Park OJ. Resveratrol induces apoptosis in chemoresistant cancer cells *via* modulation of AMPK signaling pathway. Annals of the New York Academy of Sciences 2007; 1095: 441-8.

[168]   Rothbart SB, Racanelli AC, Moran RG. Pemetrexed indirectly activates the metabolic kinase AMPK in human carcinomas. Cancer Research 2010; 70(24): 10299-309.

[169]   Racanelli AC, Rothbart SB, Heyer CL, Moran RG. Therapeutics by cytotoxic metabolite accumulation: pemetrexed causes ZMP accumulation, AMPK activation, and mammalian target of rapamycin inhibition. Cancer Research 2009; 69: 5467–74.

[170]   Hudes G, Carducci M, Tomczak P, Dutcher J, Figlin R, Kapoor A, Staroslawska E, Sosman J, McDermott D, Bodrogi I, Kovacevic Z, Lesovoy V, Schmidt-Wolf IG, Barbarash O, Gokmen E, O'Toole T, Lustgarten S, Moore L, Motzer RJ; Global ARCC Trial. Temsirolimus, interferon alfa, or both for advanced renal-cell carcinoma. New England Journal of Medicine 2007; 356(22): 2271-81.

[171]   Motzer RJ, Escudier B, Oudard S, Hutson TE, Porta C, Bracarda S, Grünwald V, Thompson JA, Figlin RA, Hollaender N, Urbanowitz G, Berg WJ, Kay A, Lebwohl D, Ravaud A; RECORD-1 Study Group. Efficacy of everolimus in advanced renal cell carcinoma: a double-blind, randomised, placebo-controlled phase III trial. Lancet 2008; 372(9637): 449-56.

[172] Wander SA, Hennessy BT, Slingerland JM. Next-generation mTOR inhibitors in clinical oncology: how pathway complexity informs therapeutic strategy. Journal of Clinical Investigation 2011; 121(4): 1231-41.

[173] Feldman ME, Apsel B, Uotila A, Loewith R, Knight ZA, Ruggero D, Shokat KM. Active-site inhibitors of mTOR target rapamycin-resistant outputs of mTORC1 and mTORC2. PLoS Biology 2009; 7(2): e38.

[174] Choo AY, Blenis J. Not all substrates are treated equally: implications for mTOR, rapamycin-resistance and cancer therapy. Cell Cycle 2009; 8(4): 567-72.

[175] Harrington LS, Findlay GM, Gray A, Tolkacheva T, Wigfield S, Rebholz H, Barnett J, Leslie NR, Cheng S, Shepherd PR, Gout I, Downes CP, Lamb RF. The TSC1-2 tumor suppressor controls insulin-PI3K signaling *via* regulation of IRS proteins. Journal of Cell Biology 2004; 166(2): 213-23.

[176] O'Reilly KE, Rojo F, She QB, Solit D, Mills GB, Smith D, Lane H, Hofmann F, Hicklin DJ, Ludwig DL, Baselga J, Rosen N. mTOR inhibition induces upstream receptor tyrosine kinase signaling and activates Akt. Cancer Research 2006; 66(3): 1500-8.

[177] Julien LA, Carriere A, Moreau J, Roux PP. mTORC1-activated S6K1 phosphorylates Rictor on threonine 1135 and regulates mTORC2 signaling. Molecular and Cellular Biology 2010; 30(4): 908-21.

[178] Carracedo A, Ma L, Teruya-Feldstein J, Rojo F, Salmena L, Alimonti A, Egia A, Sasaki AT, Thomas G, Kozma SC, Papa A, Nardella C, Cantley LC, Baselga J, Pandolfi PP. Inhibition of mTORC1 leads to MAPK pathway activation through a PI3K-dependent feedback loop in human cancer. Journal of Clinical Investigation 2008; 118(9): 3065-74.

[179] Yu K, Toral-Barza L, Shi C, Zhang WG, Lucas J, Shor B, Kim J, Verheijen J, Curran K, Malwitz DJ, Cole DC, Ellingboe J, Ayral-Kaloustian S, Mansour TS, Gibbons JJ, Abraham RT, Nowak P, Zask A. Biochemical, cellular, and *in vivo* activity of novel ATP-competitive and selective inhibitors of the mammalian target of rapamycin. Cancer Research 2009; 69(15): 6232-40.

[180] Chresta CM, Davies BR, Hickson I, Harding T, Cosulich S, Critchlow SE, Vincent JP, Ellston R, Jones D, Sini P, James D, Howard Z, Dudley P, Hughes G, Smith L, Maguire S, Hummersone M, Malagu K, Menear K, Jenkins R, Jacobsen M, Smith GC, Guichard S, Pass M. AZD8055 is a potent, selective, and orally bioavailable ATP-competitive mammalian target of rapamycin kinase inhibitor with *in vitro* and *in vivo* antitumor activity. Cancer Research 2010; 70(1): 288-98.

[181] Thoreen CC, Kang SA, Chang JW, Liu Q, Zhang J, Gao Y, Reichling LJ, Sim T, Sabatini DM, Gray NS. An ATP-competitive mammalian target of rapamycin inhibitor reveals rapamycin-resistant functions of mTORC1. Journal of Biological Chemistry 2009; 284(12): 8023-32.

[182] Cho DC, Cohen MB, Panka DJ, Collins M, Ghebremichael M, Atkins MB, Signoretti S, Mier JW. The efficacy of the novel dual PI3-kinase/mTOR inhibitor NVP-BEZ235 compared with rapamycin in renal cell carcinoma. Clinical Cancer Research 2010; 16(14): 3628-38.

[183] Brachmann SM, Hofmann I, Schnell C, Fritsch C, Wee S, Lane H, Wang S, Garcia-Echeverria C, Maira SM. Specific apoptosis induction by the dual PI3K/mTor inhibitor NVP-BEZ235 in HER2 amplified and PIK3CA mutant breast cancer cells. Proceedings of the National Academy of Sciences of the United States of America 2009; 106(52): 22299-304.

[184] Serra V, Markman B, Scaltriti M, Eichhorn PJ, Valero V, Guzman M, Botero ML, Llonch E, Atzori F, Di Cosimo S, Maira M, Garcia-Echeverria C, Parra JL, Arribas J, Baselga J. NVP-BEZ235, a dual PI3K/mTOR inhibitor, prevents PI3K signaling and inhibits the growth of cancer cells with activating PI3K mutations. Cancer Research 2008; 68(19): 8022-30.

[185] Liu TJ, Koul D, LaFortune T, Tiao N, Shen RJ, Maira SM, Garcia-Echevrria C, Yung WK. NVP-BEZ235, a novel dual phosphatidylinositol 3-kinase/mammalian target of rapamycin inhibitor, elicits multifaceted antitumor activities in human gliomas. Molecular Cancer Therapeutics 2009; 8(8): 2204-10.

[186] Konstantinidou G, Bey EA, Rabellino A, Schuster K, Maira MS, Gazdar AF, Amici A, Boothman DA, Scaglioni PP. Dual phosphoinositide 3-kinase/mammalian target of rapamycin blockade is an effective radiosensitizing strategy for the treatment of non-small cell lung cancer harboring K-RAS mutations. Cancer Research 2009; 69(19): 7644-52.

[187] Brünner-Kubath C, Shabbir W, Saferding V, Wagner R, Singer CF, Valent P, Berger W, Marian B, Zielinski CC, Grusch M, Grunt TW. The PI3 kinase/mTOR blocker NVP-BEZ235 overrides resistance against irreversible ErbB inhibitors in breast cancer cells. Breast Cancer Research and Treatment 2011; 129(2): 387-400.

[188] Ko YH, Smith BL, Wang Y, Pomper MG, Rini DA, Torbenson MS, Hullihen J, Pedersen PL. Advanced cancers: eradication in all cases using 3-bromopyruvate therapy to deplete ATP. Biochemical and Biophysical Research Communications 2004; 324(1): 269-75.

[189] Kim W, Yoon JH, Jeong JM, Cheon GJ, Lee TS, Yang JI, Park SC, Lee HS. Apoptosis-inducing antitumor efficacy of hexokinase II inhibitor in hepatocellular carcinoma. Molecular Cancer Therapeutics 2007; 6(9): 2554-62.

[190] Bonnet S, Archer SL, Allalunis-Turner J, Haromy A, Beaulieu C, Thompson R, Lee CT, Lopaschuk GD, Puttagunta L, Bonnet S, Harry G, Hashimoto K, Porter CJ, Andrade MA, Thebaud B, Michelakis ED. A mitochondria-K$^+$ channel axis is suppressed in cancer and its normalization promotes apoptosis and inhibits cancer growth. Cancer Cell 2007; 11(1): 37-51.

[191] Anderson CM, Thwaites DT. Hijacking solute carriers for proton-coupled drug transport. Physiology (Bethesda) 2010; 25(6): 364-77.

[192] Beauparlant P, Bedard D, Bernier C, Chan H, Gilbert K, Goulet D, Gratton MO, Lavoie M, Roulston A, Turcotte E, Watson, M.) Preclinical development of the nicotinamide phosphoribosyl transferase inhibitor prodrug GMX1777. Anticancer Drugs 2009; 20:346-354.

[193] Watson M, Roulston A, Belec L, Billot X, Marcellus R, Bedard D, Bernier C, Branchaud S, Chan H, Dairi K, Gilbert K, Goulet D, Gratton MO, Isakau H, Jang A, Khadir A, Koch E, Lavoie M, Lawless M, Nguyen M, Paquette D, Turcotte E, Berger A, Mitchell M, Shore GC, Beauparlant P. The small molecule GMX1778 is a potent inhibitor of NAD$^+$ biosynthesis: strategy for enhanced therapy in nicotinic acid phosphoribosyltransferase 1-deficient tumors. Molecular and Cellular Biology 2009; 29:5872-5888.

[194] Sreekumar A, Poisson LM, Rajendiran TM, Khan AP, Cao Q, Yu J, Laxman B, Mehra R, Lonigro RJ, Li Y, Nyati MK, Ahsan A, Kalyana-Sundaram S, Han B, Cao X, Byun J, Omenn GS, Ghosh D, Pennathur S, Alexander DC, Berger A, Shuster JR, Wei JT, Varambally S, Beecher C, Chinnaiyan AM. Metabolomic profiles delineate potential role for sarcosine in prostate cancer progression. Nature 2009; 457: 910-914.

Send Orders for Reprints to reprints@benthamscience.net

Frontiers in Anti-Cancer Drug Discovery, 2014, 3, 191-200   191

CHAPTER 5

Nitric Oxide as an Adjuvant Therapeutic in the Clinical Management of Cancer

Nicole J. Kenote[1], Tysha N. Medeiros[2], Dana M. Jarigese[3], Melissa A. Edwards[4] and Mark A. Brown[*,4,5,6,7]

[1]Department of Environmental and Radiological Health Sciences, Colorado State University, Fort Collins, CO, USA; [2]Department of Biochemistry and Molecular Biology, Colorado State University, Fort Collins, CO, USA; [3]Department of Animal Sciences, Colorado State University, Fort Collins, CO, USA; [4]Cell and Molecular Biology Program, Colorado State University, Fort Collins, CO, USA; [5]Department of Clinical Sciences, Colorado State University, Fort Collins, CO, USA; [6]Department of Ethnic Studies, Colorado State University, Fort Collins, CO, USA; [7]Colorado School of Public Health, Fort Collins, CO, USA

Abstract: The ability of tumors to develop resistance to cytotoxic therapies has been a major obstacle in the clinical management of cancer. In addition, dose-limiting toxicity represents yet another impediment in the application of traditional therapeutics. To enhance the sensitivity of tumors to radio-therapeutics, researchers are increasingly turning to nitric oxide for its potential as a powerful adjuvant to existing therapies. Here, we review the aptitude of nitric oxide to serve as a radio-sensitizing, adjuvant therapeutic for the clinical management of cancer.

Keywords: Adjuvant therapy, cancer, nitric oxide, oncology, radiotherapy, therapeutic delivery.

INTRODUCTION

From its diminutive size and high degree of reactivity as a free radical to its lipophilic nature, nitric oxide (NO) plays central roles in signal transduction associated with key regulatory factors [1-4] and acts as a necessary mediator for the facilitation of cytotoxicity of leukocytes by way of superoxide [5-8]. The physiological impacts of NO vary quite broadly depending upon factors such as

*Address correspondence to Mark A. Brown: Department of Clinical Sciences, Colorado State University, Fort Collins, CO, USA; Tel: (970) 491-3132; Fax: (970) 491-3483; E-mail: M.Brown@colostate.edu

local levels of oxygenation and relative concentration of NO. For instance, although cytotoxicity mediated by NO involves precipitously elevated concentrations [8], aggregation of platelets is regulated by precise localization of exact concentrations of NO [9, 10].

The exceptional simplicity of NO, as it relates to chemical composition, results in a compound that can be both quickly generated as well as rapidly metabolized. It is this quality that makes NO particularly well suited for ephemeral signal responses. Endogenously, NO is produced by NO synthase (NOS) as a by-product in the oxidation of L-arginine to L-citrulline (Fig. **1**) *via* a two-part reaction involving O_2 and nicotinamide adenine dinucleotide phosphate as co-substrates [1, 11, 12]. The outer orbital of the resulting nitric oxide contains an available electron which can either be discharged, thereby bestowing an oxidative impact or it can act in an antioxidant role by the acceptance and, thus, stabilization of an electron donor [13, 14]. Production of NO can also occur *via* reduction of nitrate and nitrite by reductive enzymes.

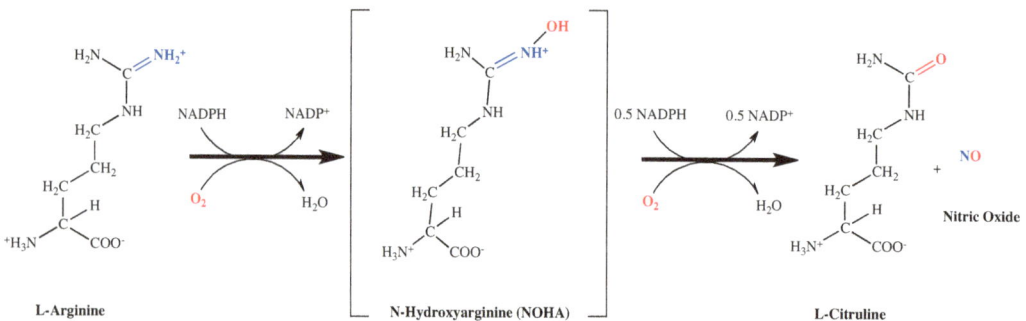

Fig. (1): Production of NO as a by-product in the oxidation of L-arginine to L-citrulline.

Different isoforms of NOS (Fig. **2**) are required to mediate the concentration-specific impacts of NO. Each NOS isoform maintains a unique expression pattern and is capable of a distinct rate of productivity. NOS isoforms include: 1) a calcium-calmodulin regulated form called neuronal NOS (nNOS) involved in signaling within the central nervous system (CNS); 2) endothelial NOS (eNOS) which is also a calcium-calmodulin regulated form that supports cell signaling outside the CNS; and 3) inducible NOS (iNOS) that is central to immunological functions and has the ability to produce rapid, highly concentrated bursts of NO [1, 11].

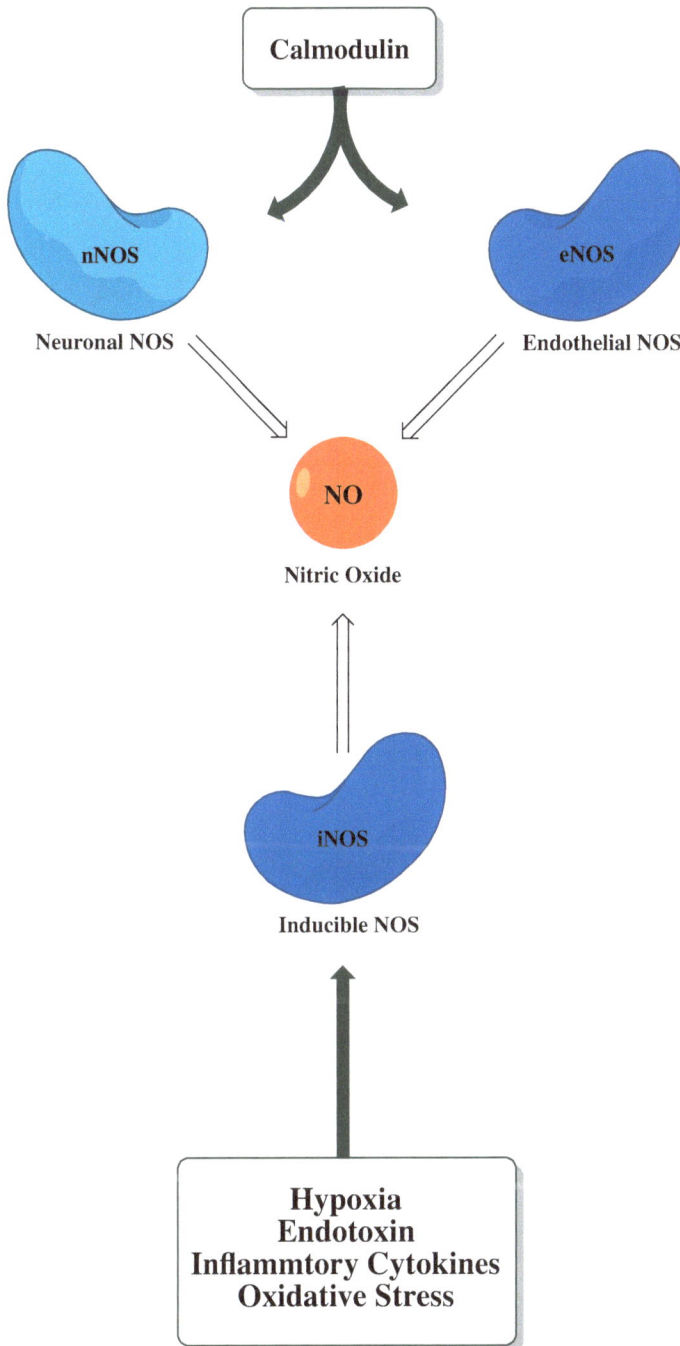

Fig. (2): NOS isoforms include two calcium-calmodulin regulated forms (upper: nNOS and eNOS) and one inducible form (lower: iNOS).

A variety of biological processes are facilitated by nitric oxide which can be grouped within two mechanistic pathways, namely cGMP-dependent or – independent. The principal route by which nitric oxide mediates physiological processes is cGMP-dependent. In this pathway, NO interacts with guanylate cyclase thereby triggering cyclic nucleotide-gated ion channels and cGMP-governed kinases as well as phosphodiesterases [15]. Activating such channels ultimately imparts such physiological outcomes as relaxation of smooth muscle, neurotransmission, inhibition of platelet aggregation, and vasodilation [15]. The mode of action for NO which is generated by eNOS and nNOS occurs by way of such cGMP-dependent mechanisms [13, 15].

The NO cGMP-independent pathways include reactivity with metals and molecular O_2. These often govern post-translational modifications including nitration and nitrosylation. For instance, S-nitrosylation of cysteines represents a common mechanism for cell signaling in the control of enzymatic functions [16]. NO produced by iNOS operates in such cGMP-independent pathways [17] whereby it maintains an essential role in the cytotoxicity of T-lymphocytes along with other immunological outcomes [18].

In recent years, NO has been the subject of increasing research related to its capacity to serve as a mediator of radio-sensitization. Numerous findings have reported the involvement of NO in the control of anticancer immunological mechanisms [19-21]. Likewise, NO interaction with superoxide anions has been correlated with the induction of cancer cell apoptosis by way of its formation of peroxynitrite and the consequent outcomes involving mitochondrial membrane permeability resulting in the release of cytochrome c oxidase [22-25]. As a result, prospective therapeutic applications for nitric oxide donors have been underscored in numerous articles and patent applications [26-29]. However, seemingly conflicting studies correlate the expression of NOS and the production of NO with tumorigenic outcomes including head and neck, pancreatic, breast, and cervical tumors [30-32]. Thus, a picture is emerging of NO where factors such as concentration and timing of release dictate its role as either a promoter or inhibitor of tumors. Further research related to the antitumor mechanisms of nitric oxide and the corresponding circumstances required to activate those mechanisms, in tandem with the analysis of nitric oxide donors with the ability to discharge NO at controlled concentrations in a temporally governed way, are necessary in the development of effective NO-based therapeutics. Here, we focus on the capacity of nitric oxide to serve as a radio-sensitizing, adjuvant therapeutic in the clinical management of malignancies.

NITRIC OXIDE AND THE ROLE OF OXYGEN IN RADIO-SENSITIZATION

The ability of radiotherapy to induce apoptosis in tumor cells is significantly enhanced by the presence of oxygen [30] due to indirect DNA damage induced by reactive species of oxygen [33]. Conversely, tumor cells exhibit greater resistance to radiotherapy under hypoxic conditions. This disparity in outcomes can be explained by the relative ability of cells to repair radio-induced DNA damage in the absence *versus* presence of oxygen. In hypoxic conditions, damaged DNA can be repaired by a mechanism involving reversal of DNA radicals by thiol-hydrogen donation. In aerobic conditions, however, oxygen interactions with damaged DNA produce peroxy DNA radicals thereby thwarting DNA repair mechanisms [34].

The cytotoxic contributions of NO in radiotherapy are two-fold. First, as previously mentioned, NO reactions with superoxide anions produce peroxynitrite resulting in mitochondrial-mediated apoptosis or necrosis. These outcomes are driven by the ability of peroxynitrite to impart peroxidation of lipids, DNA lesions, nitration of protein tyrosines, thiol oxidation, and upregulation of poly(ADP-ribose) polymerase activity [22-25, 35-37]. The second contributing cytotoxic factor of NO is its ability to impact oxygen delivery to, and depletion within, cells [4-7].

APPLICATIONS OF NO-MEDIATED RADIO-SENSITIZATION

One approach to achieving NO-mediated radio-sensitization exploits the radio-protective conditions of hypoxia. Specifically, several NO donors have been developed that are activated under hypoxic conditions. For example, RRx-001 is an NO-donor which is currently being studied for its ability to increase oxygen delivery to tumors *via* vasodilation [38]. Early research has indicated that RRx-001 is highly effective at inducing radio-sensitization. Likewise, nitrosonium ion donors are capable of producing NO in hypoxic tissues resulting in enhancement of radio-sensitization [39].

Activation of NOS has also been proven effective in radio-sensitization of tumors. For instance, ONO-4007 is a synthetically produced analog of lipid A which up-regulates activity of NOS thereby resulting in radio-sensitization [40-41]. Likewise, indirect activation of NOS *via* introduction of insulin followed by a series of electric stimulations has been shown to achieve radio-sensitization in several tumor lines [40, 42].

CONTROLLING NO DELIVERY

The function of NO in cytotoxic pathways has garnered much interest with relation to potential uses of nitric oxide donors as therapeutics in the treatment of malignancies. Variations in biological effects of NO derived from the three isoforms of NOS underscores the relevance of timing, longevity and concentration of NO at the site of the desired impacts. While processes requiring eNOS and nNOS function through the presence of moderate concentrations of NO for brief durations [43-45], to achieve cytotoxicity, the concentration of NO levels must be relatively high and long lasting. With inducible NOS, nitric oxide is produced at micromolar concentrations for durations of days or more [46-48]. The differences between concentration and duration of nitric oxide seem to differentiate cell signal processes such as those imparted by the neuronal and endothelial forms of NOS from events which affect the survival and growth of cells such as those imparted by the inducible from of NOS. Thus, the investigation of NO donors for their potential roles in cancer therapies is often conceived to identify those that most closely exhibit the NO release specifications of iNOS.

Indirect regulators of NO concentrations such as lipid A and its synthetic derivatives such as ONO-4007 have yielded promising results in their potential to induce anti-tumor immune responses [49]. However, the majority of NO-donors are deficient in several respects including directed targeting, protracted half-lives, and governance of release kinetics. Thus, NO-donating pro-drugs that are able to discharge NO in a site-specific and in a concentration-controlled way have been the subjects of increasing research. For example, JS-K (O_2-(2,4-dinitrophenyl) 1-[(4-ethoxycarbonyl) piperazin-1-yl] diazen-1-ium-1,2-diolate) represents a diazeniumdiolate-based NO-donor being investigated as a prospective cytotoxic pro-drug for use against human malignancies [50-52]. Likewise, site specific delivery of glyco-S-nitrosothiols have proven effective against prostate cancer cells [53].

CONCLUDING REMARKS

Cytotoxic resistance represents a serious impediment in the clinical management of cancer. Likewise, dose-limiting toxicity and accompanying adverse events introduce yet another hindrance in the application of traditional therapeutics. To enhance the sensitivity of tumors to radio-therapeutics, NO has been identified as a potentially robust adjuvant to existing therapies. Proven methods for radio-sensitization of tumors continue to represent a gap in the clinical management of malignancies. A thorough examination of the cytotoxic effects of nitric oxide and the corresponding conditions required to prompt those effects, in tandem with the study of prospective NO donors that have the ability to release nitric oxide at the controlled concentrations and in a temporally governed, site-specific manner will result to a robust cadre of adjuvant tumor therapeutics.

ACKNOWLEDGEMENTS

MAB thankfully acknowledges support from the National Science Foundation (1060548), the CVMBS College Council, and the Flint Animal Cancer Center.

CONFLICT OF INTEREST

The authors confirm that this chapter contents have no conflict of interest.

REFERENCES

[1]   Hughes MN. Chemistry of nitric oxide and related species. Methods in Enzymology 2008; 3-19.

[2]   Kroncke KD. Cysteine–Zn2+ complexes: Unique molecular switches for inducible nitric oxide synthase-derived NO. The FASEB Journal 2001; 15(13): 2503-7.

[3]   Osorio J, Recchia F. The role of nitric oxide in metabolism regulation: From basic sciences to the clinical setting. Intensive Care Medicine 2000; 26: 1395-8.

[4] Moncada S. Nitric oxide: Discovery and impact on clinical medicine. Journal of the Royal Society of Medicine 1999; 92: 164-9.

[5] Umansky V, Shirrmacher V. Nitric oxide-induced apoptosis in tumor cells. Advanced Cancer Research 2001; 82: 107-31.

[6] Albina J, Reichner J. Role of nitric oxide in mediation of macrophage cytotoxicity and apoptosis. Cancer Metastasis Reviews 1998; 17: 39-53.

[7] Li H, Hu J, Xin W, Zhao B. Production and interaction of oxygen and nitric oxide free radicals in PMA stimulated macrophages during the respiratory burst. Redox Report 2000; 5: 353-8.

[8] Leiro J, Iglesias R, Paramá A, Sanmartin ML, Ubeira FM, Respiratory burst responses of rat macrophages to microsporidian spores. Experimental Parasitology 2001; 98: 1-9.

[9] Gkaliagkousi E, Ferro A. Nitric oxide signaling in the regulation of cardiovascular and platelet function. Frontiers in Bioscience 2011; 16: 1873-97.

[10] Somers M, Harrison D. Reactive oxygen species and the control of vasomotor tone. Current Hypertension Reports 1999; 1: 102-8.

[11] Andrew PJ, Mayer B. Enzymatic function of nitric oxide synthases. Cardiovascular Research 1999; 43: 521-31.

[12] Lefèvre-Groboillot D, Boucher JL, Mansuy D, Stuehr DJ. Reactivity of the heme–dioxygen complex of the inducible nitric oxide synthase in the presence of alternative substrates. FEBS Journal 2006; 273: 180-91.

[13] Huerta S, Chilka S, Bonavida B. Nitric oxide donors: Novel cancer therapeutics, International Journal of Oncology 2008; 33: 909-27.

[14] Bredt D. Endogenous nitric oxide synthesis: Biological functions and pathophysiology. Free Radical Research 1999; 31: 577-96.

[15] Derbyshire ER, Marletta MA. Structure and regulation of soluble guanylate cyclase. Annual Review of Biochemistry 2012; 81: 533-59.

[16] Hess DT, Stamler JS. Regulation by s-nitrosylation of protein post-translational modification. Journal of Biological Chemistry 2012; 287: 4411-8.

[17] MacMicking J, Xie QW, Nathan C. Nitric oxide and macrophage function. Annual Review of Immunology 1997; 15: 323-50.

[18] Hirst D, Robson T. Nitrosative stress as a mediator of apoptosis: Implications for cancer therapy. Current Pharmaceutical Design 2010; 16: 45-55.

[19] Wink D, Hines H, Cheng R, *et al.* Nitric oxide and the redox mechanisms in the immune response. Journal of Leukocyte Biology 2011; 89: 873-91.

[20] Binder C, Schulz M, Hiddemann W, Oellerich M. Induction of inducible nitric oxide synthase is an essential part of tumor necrosis factor-alpha-induced apoptosis. Laboratory Investigations 1999; 79: 1703-12.

[21] Farias-Eisner R, Sherman MP, Aeberhard E, Chaudhuri G. Nitric oxide is an important mediator for tumoricidal activity *in vivo*. Proceedings of the National Academy of Sciences 1994; 91: 9407-11.

[22] Sarti P, Forte E, Mastronicola D, Giuffrè A, Arese M. Cytochrome c oxidase and nitric oxide in action: Molecular mechanisms and pathophysiological implications. Biochimica et Biophysica Acta (BBA) - Bioenergetics 2012; 1817: 610-9.

[23] Boyd CS, Cadenas E. Nitric oxide and cell signaling pathways in mitochondrial-dependent apoptosis. Biological Chemistry 2002; 411.

[24]   Oh-hashi K, Maruyama W, Yi H, Takahashi T, Naoi M, Isobe K. Mitogen-activated protein kinase pathway mediates peroxynitrite-induced apoptosis in human dopaminergic neuroblastoma SH-SY5Y cells. Biochemical and Biophysical Research Communications 1999; 263(2): 504-9.

[25]   Dairou J, Atmane N, Rodrigues-Lima F, Dupret J. Peroxynitrite irreversibly inactivates the human xenobioticmetabolizing enzyme arylamine n-acetyltransferase 1 (NAT1) in human breast cancer cells - A cellular and mechanistic study. Journal of Biological Chemistry 2004; 279(9): 7708-14.

[26]   Switzer CH, Flores-Santana W, Mancardi D, *et al.* The emergence of nitroxyl (HNO) as a pharmacological agent. Biochimica et Biophysica Acta (BBA) - Bioenergetics 2009; 1787: 835-40.

[27]   Serafim R, Primi M, Trossini G, Ferreira E. Nitric oxide: State of the art in drug design. Current Medicinal Chemistry 2012; 19: 386-405.

[28]   Burgaud J, Ongini E, Del Soldato P. Nitric oxide-releasing drugs: A novel class of effective and safe therapeutic agents. Annals of the New York Academy of Sciences 2002; 962: 360-71.

[29]   Huerta S, Chilka S, Bonavida B. Nitric oxide donors: Novel cancer therapeutics. International Journal of Oncology 2008; 33: 909-27.

[30]   Beckman JS, Koppenol WH. Nitric oxide, superoxide, and peroxynitrite: The good, the bad, and ugly. *Am J Physiol* 1996; 271: 1424-7.

[31]   Wang J, Torbenson M, Wang Q, Ro JY, Becich M. Expression of inducible nitric oxide synthase in paired neoplastic and non-neoplastic primary prostate cell cultures and prostatectomy specimen. Urol Oncol 2003; 21: 117-22.

[32]   Jadeski LC, Hum KO, Chakraborty C, Lala PK. Nitric oxide promotes murine mammary tumor growth and metastasis by stimulating tumor cell migration, invasiveness, and angiogenesis. Int J Cancer 2000; 85: 30-9.

[33]   Oronsky BT, Knox SJ, Scicinski JJ. Is nitric oxide the last word in radiosensitization? Transl Oncol 2012; 5: 66-71.

[34]   Oronsky BT, Knox SJ, Scicinski JJ. Six degrees of separation: The oxygen effect in the development of radiosensitizers. Transl Oncol 2011; 4: 189-98.

[35]   Szabo C, Ischiropoulos H, Radi R. Peroxynitrite: Biochemistry, pathophysiology and development of therapeutics. Nat Rev Drug Discov 2007; 6: 662-90.

[36]   Obrosova IG, Drel VR, Pacher P, *et al.* Oxidative-nitrosative stress and poly(ADP-ribose) polymerase (PARP) activation in experimental diabetic neuropathy: The relation is revisited. Diabetes 2005; 54: 3435-41.

[37]   Martinez GR, Di Mascio P, Bonini MG, *et al.* Peroxynitrite does not decompose to singlet oxygen andnitroxyl. Proc Natl Acad Sci USA 2000; 97: 10307-12.

[38]   Ning S, Bednarski M, Orongsky B, Scicinsky J, Saul G, Knox, S. Dinitroazetidines are a novel class of anticancer agents and hypoxia-activated radiation sensitizers developed from highly energetic materials. Proceedings of the 102nd Annual Meeting of the American Association for Cancer Research; 2011 April 2-6; Orlando, FL. American Association for Cancer Research, Philadelphia, PA, Abstract no. 676.

[39]   Janssens MY, Verovski VN, Van den Berge DL, Monsaert C, Storme GA. Radiosensitization of hypoxic tumour cells by S-nitroso-N-acetylpenicillamine implicates a bioreductive mechanism of nitric oxide generation. Br J Cancer 1999; 79: 1085-9.

[40]   De Ridder M, Verellen D, Verovski V, Storme G. Hypoxic tumor cell radiosensitizer through nitric oxide. Nitric Oxide 2008; 19: 164-9.

[41]   Wardman P. Chemical radiosensitizers for use in radiotherapy. Clin Oncol 2007; 19: 397-417.

[42]   Jordan BF, Sonveaux P, Feron O, *et al.* Nitric oxide as a radiosensitizer: Evidence for an intrinsic role in addition to it effect on oxygen delivery and consumption. Int J Cancer 2004; 109: 768-73.

[43]   Singh S, Gupta A. Nitric oxide: Role in tumour biology and iNOS/NO-based anticancer therapies. Cancer Chemotherapy and Pharmacology 2011; 67: 1211-24.

[44]   Masini E, Cianchi F, Mastroianni R, Cuzzocrea S. Nitric oxide expression in cancer. Nitric Oxide (NO) and Cancer 2010; 59-82.

[45]   Kröncke KD, Fehsel K, Kolb-Bachofen V. Nitric oxide: cytotoxicity *versus* cytoprotection - how, why, when, and where? *Nitric Oxide* 1997; 1: 107-20.

[46]   Wang Z. Protein S-nitrosylation and cancer. Cancer Letters 2012; 320: 123-9.

[47]   Rigas B. Novel agents for cancer prevention based on nitric oxide. Biochemical Society Transactions 2007; 35: 1364-8.

[48]   Hibbs Jr J, Taintor R, Vavrin Z. Macrophage cytotoxicity: Role for l-arginine deiminase and imino nitrogen oxidation to nitrite. *Science* 1987; 235: 473-6.

[49]   Matsushita K, Kuramitsu Y, Ohiro Y, Kobayashi I, Watanabe T, Kobayashi M, Hosokawa M. ONO-4007, a synthetic lipid A analog, induces Th1-type immune response in tumor eradication and restores nitric oxide production by peritoneal macrophages. Int J Oncol; 2003: 23: 489-493.

[50]   Maciag AE, Chakrapani H, Saavedra JE, *et al.* The nitric oxide prodrug JS-K is effective against non–small-cell lung cancer cells *in vitro* and *in vivo*: Involvement of reactive oxygen species. Journal of Pharmacology and Experimental Therapeutics 2011; 336: 313-20.

[51]   Kiziltepe T, Hideshima T, Ishitsuka K, *et al.* JS-K, a GST-activated nitric oxide generator, induces DNA double-strand breaks, activates DNA damage response pathways, and induces apoptosis *in vitro* and *in vivo* in human multiple myeloma cells. Blood 2007; 110: 709-18.

[52]   Reynolds MM, Witzeling SD, Damodaran VB, *et al.* Applications for nitric oxide in halting proliferation of tumor cells. Biochem Biophys Res Comm 2013; 431: 647-51.

[53]   Hou Y, Wang J, Andreana PR, *et al.* Targeting nitric oxide to cancer cells: Cytotoxicity studies of glyco-S-nitrosothiols. Bioorganic & Medicinal Chemistry Letters 1999; 9: 2255-8.

Send Orders for Reprints to reprints@benthamscience.net

Frontiers in Anti-Cancer Drug Discovery, 2014, 3, 201-232

CHAPTER 6

Molecular and Genetic Mechanisms of Various Types of Cancers

Sanath Kumar* and Mira M. Shah

Department of Radiation Oncology, Henry Ford Hospital, Detroit, MI 48202, USA

Abstract: Cancer is a multistep process in which multiple genetic changes result in the transformation of normal cells into malignant cells. These genetic alterations are a result of various environmental or endogenous DNA-damaging agents. They can be inherited through germ cells or more commonly acquired as somatic mutations. Somatic mutations include point mutations, chromosomal translocations, deletions, inversions or amplifications. These genetic changes lead to the malignant transformation of normal cells through self-sufficiency in growth signals, insensitivity to growth-inhibitory signals, evasion of apoptosis, replicative immortality, sustained angiogenesis, tissue invasion and metastasis. Characteristic genetic alterations have been identified in various types of cancers. This review focuses on the key molecular mechanisms underlying various human cancers.

Keywords: Cancer, carcinogenesis, genetics, molecular biology, pathogenesis.

INTRODUCTION

Cancer is a disease characterized by uncontrolled cell division and distant spread. According to the World Health Organization (WHO) classification, cancer is categorized by cell-type of origin, such as carcinoma (epithelial cells); lymphoma and leukemia (blood and bone marrow cells); sarcoma (mesenchymal cells); mesothelioma (mesothelial cells of peritoneal and pleural cavities); glioma (brain cell), germinoma (germ cells of the ovary or testes) and choriocarcinoma (placental cells) [1]. Multiple genetic changes underlie the process of carcinogenesis, whereby normal cells undergo malignant transformation.

MODELS OF CARCINOGENESIS

Various models of carcinogenesis have been proposed. The single gene model was one of the earliest models proposed to explain the pathogenesis of chromic

Address correspondence to Sanath Kumar: Department of Radiation Oncology, Henry Ford Hospital, Detroit, MI 48202, USA; Tel: (313) 916-1021; Fax: (313) 916-3264; E-mail: skumar4@hfhs.org

myeloid leukemia [2]. The underlying molecular mechanism was characterized by the Philadelphia chromosome, which was due to the reciprocal translocation of genetic material between chromosomes 9 and 22 [3-6]. Another well-characterized genetic model was introduced by Vogelstein to explain the causation of colorectal cancer [7]. According to this model, the tumor is thought to arise as a result of mutational activation of oncogenes and mutational inactivation of tumor suppressor genes [8].

The most widely accepted model of carcinogenesis was proposed by Hanahan and Weinberg [9, 10] (Fig. **1**). According to their model, six classical determinants are involved in the malignant transformation of a normal cell: (a) self-sufficiency in growth signals; (b) insensitivity to anti-growth signals; (c) evasion of apoptosis; (d) limitless replicative potential; (e) sustained angiogenesis; and (f) tissue invasion and metastasis [9]. In addition to these six classical characteristics, two additional features were added to this list- reprogramming of energy metabolism and evading immune destruction [10]. Multiple signal transduction pathways have been identified in each of these eight cases. The cell is believed to become cancerous by acquiring the aforementioned characteristics. Hanahan and Weinberg have also proposed two cancer enabling characteristics; tumor promoting inflammation and genome instability and mutation [10].

In addition to the classic hallmarks, malignant cells are also characterized by the loss of differentiation, loss of contact inhibition [11-14], vascular mimicry [15], vessel abnormalization [16], and loss of cell polarity [17].

FACTORS UNDERLYING CARCINOGENESIS AND CLINICAL RELEVANCE

Sustained Cell Proliferation

Normal cells maintain a tight control over the production and release of growth-promoting signals. In contrast, cancer cells are characterized by sustained growth signaling resulting in tumor formation. This is achieved by either the self-production of growth factors and ligands by cancer cells, stimulation of nearby normal cells to produce growth signals, or up-regulation of receptors on the cell membrane [18-23]. Examples include mutations affecting the genes encoding epithelial growth factor receptor (EGFR) in adenocarcinoma of lung and Her2/neu receptor in breast cancer. Identification of growth promoting receptors has led to development of targeted agents such as cetuximab and trastuzumab in the treatment of lung and breast cancer respectively (Fig. **1**).

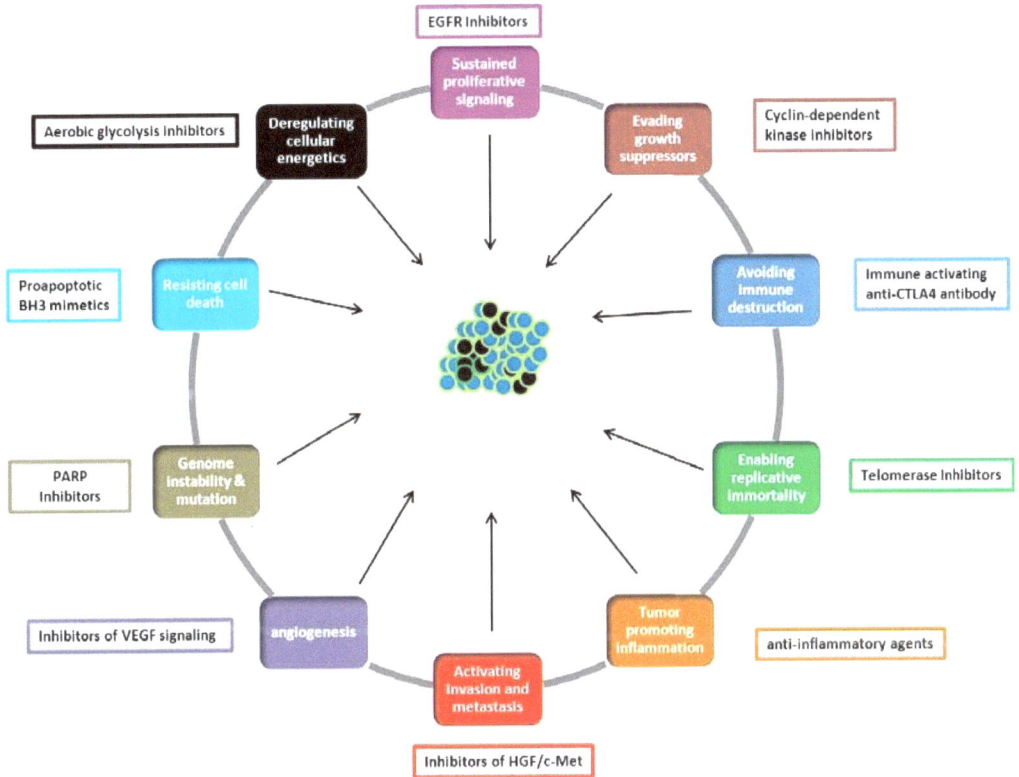

Fig. (1). Schematic of factors underlying carcinogenesis and potential therapeutic interventions.

Inactivation of Growth Suppressors

Growth and proliferation of normal cells are kept in check by the activation of tumor suppressor genes. However, mutations in these genes allow cancer cells to overcome the negative regulation. The two most important tumor suppressor genes that are known to regulate cell proliferation are the retinoblastoma gene (Rb) and TP53 gene [24]. In humans, the TP53 protein is coded by the TP53 gene located on the short arm of chromosome 17. The tumor suppressor activity is due to p21 mediated arrest of cell cycle at G1/S checkpoint allowing for DNA damage repair. Rb protein is encoded by the RB1gene located on the long arm of chromosome 13. Similar to TP53, Rb protein prevents cancer formation by regulating cell cycle at G1/S checkpoint by binding to transcription factors of the E2F family. Mutations in TP53 and Rb gene are a common finding in the majority of human cancers making them attractive targets for therapy. Therapeutic strategies include inactivation of the mutant TP53 protein or inhibition of downstream pathways such as cyclin dependent kinases (Fig. **1**).

Evasion of Apoptosis

Programmed cell death (apoptosis) is an evolutionary mechanism to prevent carcinogenesis in multi-cellular organisms [25, 26]. This process is tightly controlled by the balance between pro- (Bcl-2-associated X protein; Bax protein) and anti-apoptotic (Bcl-2 family proteins) factors. In addition to unrestricted proliferation, evading apoptosis constitutes a major mechanism in carcinogenesis. Pro-apoptotic signals are activated in damaged cells that still retain potential for DNA replication, and therefore are liable to carcinogenesis. Factors that cause loss of apoptosis following cell damage could potentially lead to tumor formation [27]. Targeted therapies aimed at increasing apoptosis in tumor cells could be developed by inhibiting the expression or activity of Bcl-2 protein [28]. One such approach is the use of BH3 mimetic that binds to Bcl-2 and promotes apoptosis in leukemia cells.

Replicative Immortality

Normal cells are unable to form visible tumors due to cellular senescence and cell death [29]. However, cancer cells acquire the capacity for infinite cell growth and are thus able to form macroscopic tumors. This is thought to be due to an increase in the activity of the telomerase, a ribonucleoprotein reverse transcriptase, which prevents cellular senescence and apoptosis [30, 31]. Unlike the cancer cells, most normal cells are telomerase negative and hence could be exploited for developing tumor directed therapy. Many clinical trials are currently underway using telomerase inhibitors in the treatment of various human cancers [32].

Angiogenesis

Essential nutrients and oxygen required for cellular growth and maintenance is supplied by blood vessels that course through the tissue. The nutritional and metabolic requirements of tumor cells are met by new blood vessels that are formed during the process of angiogenesis [33]. Activation of the vascular endothelial growth factor (VEGF) gene in tumor cells is believed to be involved in the induction of angiogenesis [34, 35]. Since the identification of its role in angiogenesis, many targeted agents have been developed that inhibit VEGF mediated angiogenesis. Bevacizumab (Avastin) is the most widely used anti-angiogenic agent. It has been used in the treatment of metastatic colon and breast cancer, ovarian cancer, and recurrent glioblastoma. Recent evidence indicates that tumor neovascularization is not solely driven by VEGF, but includes alternative pathways such as vasculogenesis, vascular mimicry, and tumor cell trans-differentiation [36].

Tissue Invasion and Metastasis

Cancer cells are characterized by their ability to invade local tissue structures and spread to distant sites. This phenomenon is believed to be secondary to the loss of the E-cadherin molecule, which maintains normal cell-to-cell adhesion [37, 38]. The loss of the E-cadherin molecule leads to local tissue invasion by cancer cells, followed by metastasis [39]. The c-Met/HGF (hepatocyte growth factor) signaling pathway is known to play an important role in epithelial--stromal interactions and tumor metastasis. Increased expression of c-Met/HGF has been noted in metastatic cancers [40]. Many c-Met/HGF inhibitors, including small molecule tyrosine kinase inhibitors and antibodies that bind to HGF or c-Met, are currently under investigation in clinical trials.

Evading Immune Surveillance

For the formation and spread of tumors to be successful, cancer cells must evade the host's immune system. Malignant cells are believed to suppress the action of cytotoxic T lymphocytes (CTL) by secreting various cytokines and immunosuppressive factors [41-43]. Use of anti-cytotoxic T lymphocyte-associated antigen 4 (CTLA-4) agents such as Ipilimumab, has been shown to improve survival in metastatic melanoma [44].

Alteration in Cellular Metabolism

Uncontrolled cell proliferation requires higher than normal energy to maintain tumor growth. Cancer cells have been observed to switch their energy metabolism to glycolysis even in the presence of oxygen [45]. The glycolytic switch is believed to divert cellular resources towards much needed biosynthetic pathways in proliferating tumor cells [46]. Drugs that inhibit glycolysis in the tumors could be a potential target for anti-cancer therapy.

Role of Inflammation and Tumor Microenvironment

Inflammatory cells are known to promote carcinogenesis by producing various cytokines, growth factors, and pro-angiogenic factors [47-50]. The interaction between inflammatory cells and tumor microenvironment enables tumor growth and progression. Cancer stem cells along with pericytes, fibroblasts, endothelial cells, cytotoxic T- lymphocytes (CTL), natural killer cells, and tumor stroma are believed to participate in a complex process that leads to tumor formation. The use of anti-inflammatory agents could potentially prevent tumor formation and further studies would be required to test this hypothesis. Observational studies have indicated a decrease in the prevalence of colorectal cancer in patients with ulcerative colitis using anti-inflammatory agents [51].

MOLECULAR AND GENETIC MECHANISMS UNDERLYING SPECIFIC CANCERS

Although carcinogenesis is a multi-step process involving multiple changes in the cell, many cancers in the human body are well characterized by molecular changes believed to underlie the process of malignant transformation. Below is a brief overview of the distinct molecular changes found in various cancers of the human body.

LUNG CANCER

Smoking is considered to be a major risk factor for lung cancer. However, 25% of lung cancers occur in non-smokers suggesting the role of other environmental and genetic factors [52]. Table **1** lists common molecular mechanisms underlying lung cancer. Mutations in the growth promoting K-ras oncogene have been reported in 30% of adenocarcinomas and, to a smaller extent in the squamous cell carcinoma subtype [53]. K-ras mutations appear to be more common in patients with history of smoking. A K-ras mutation renders ras proteins insensitive to GDP, leading to over-stimulation of downstream effectors [54]. Mutations in the EGFR, a receptor tyrosine kinase, have been observed in 40% of adenocarcinomas and in about 30% of adeno-squamous carcinoma [55, 56]. EGFR mutations are also observed in high frequency among non-smokers. EML4-ALK fusion gene is seen in about 10% of all non-small cell lung cancer (NSCLC) [57]. Anaplastic lymphoma kinase (ALK), a receptor tyrosine kinase, is fused with the N-terminal echinoderm microtubule associated protein-like 4 (EML4) resulting in constitutive activation of the kinase. Like EGFR mutations, EML4-ALK mutations are primarily seen in adenocarcinoma sub-type and non-smokers [58].

Table 1:   Common Molecular Mechanisms Underlying Lung Cancer

Molecular Characteristic	Molecular Pathway	Histological Subtype	Clinical Relevance
EGFR mutation	enhanced tyrosine kinase activity	adenocarcinoma	Treatment with anti EGFR agents (TKIs): cetuximab, gefetinib
EML4-ALK rearrangement	constitutional activation of protein tyrosine kinase	adenocarcinoma	crizotinib (ALK tyrosine kinase inhibitor)
K-ras activation	RAS/MAPK1 signaling pathway of many growth factor receptors	adenocarcinoma	Negative predictor of response to TKIs
ERCC1 expression	nucleotide excision repair	adenocarcinoma	Predicts response to platinum based chemotherapy
c-MET overexpression	c-MET	small cell carcinoma, adenocarcinoma, squamous cell carcinoma	
Bcl-2 overexpression	anti-apoptotic	small cell carcinoma	

Mutations involving TP53 are seen in a vast majority of NSCLCs and small cell lung cancers (SCLC). Tumor suppressor gene TP53 is responsible for cell cycle regulation and apoptosis [59]. Mutational inactivation of TP53 leads to loss of DNA damage repair and unrestricted cell proliferation. TP53 alterations are more commonly seen with smoking associated lung cancers, demonstrating a link between carcinogen exposure and cancer development [60].

In contrast to NSCLC, mutations involving the Rb gene occur in >70% of neuroendocrine tumors and SCLC [61]. The anti-apoptotic factor Bcl-2 is also over expressed in most of the SCLC and neuroendocrine tumors [62].

CENTRAL NERVOUS SYSTEM TUMORS

Gliomas are the most common tumors of the central nervous system. They are a histologically heterogeneous group of tumors. Current classification is based on the WHO system, which relies on histological features including cellularity, mitosis, nuclear atypia, vascularity, and necrosis [63].

Astrocytoma

TP53 mutation is the most common genetic alteration seen in adult astrocytomas [64]. Low-grade astrocytomas show overexpression of platelet-derived growth factor (PDGF) receptors, which may lead to cell proliferation [64, 65]. Additional genetic alterations include loss of heterozygosity (LOH) of 22q, gain of chromosome 7, amplification of 8q, mutation of Rb1, and the deletion of negative regulators CDKN2A /CDKN2B [64].

Oligodendroglioma

The combined loss of chromosome arms 1p and 19q is the most common genetic change observed in 50-80% of oligodendrogliomas, irrespective of the grade [66, 67]. This abnormality arises due to the unbalanced centomeric translocation between chromosomes 1p and 19q. Complete co-deletion is associated with better prognosis and survival [68]. Unlike astrocytomas, TP53 mutations and gene amplifications are rarely seen [66].

Glioblastoma (GBM)

GBMs arising *de novo* are characterized by EGFR amplification, deletion of negative regulators p14^{ARF} or p16^{INK4a}, loss of chromosome 10, and a mutation in the PTEN gene that negatively regulates PI3kinase pathway [69]. EGFR amplification is rarely seen in secondary GBM. O^{6}-methylguanine-DNA methyltransferase (MGMT) is a DNA repair enzyme that removes alkyl groups from the O^6 position of guanine in DNA following alkylation and methylation. The MGMT gene is silenced by epigenetic hyper-methylation in 45% of all GBM patients, which results in an increased response to Temozolamide and radiation therapy [70]. Point mutations involving the IDH1 gene have been identified in about 10% of GBM cases [71]. These mutations are more common in patients who are younger, have secondary GBMs, and are associated with an increase in survival. Mutations in IDH1 are believed to lead to GBM formation through the induction of the hypoxia-inducible factor 1 (HIF-1] pathway [72].

Pediatric Gliomas

Low-grade gliomas of the optic tract and hypothalamus are frequently seen in patients with Neurofibromatosis 1 (NF1). The NF1 is caused by mutations within the neurofibromin gene located on chromosome 17q [73]. It may also cause tumors by activating the mitogen-activated protein kinase (MAPK) pathway. Low-grade astrocytomas are seen in patients with Li-Fraumeni syndrome, which is triggered by a germ line mutation in TP53 [74]. Unlike adults, EGFR amplifications are uncommon in pediatric high-grade gliomas [75].

GENITOURINARY CANCERS

Prostate Cancer

Although prostate cancer is the second most common malignancy among men worldwide, the molecular biology of prostate cancer is not completely understood. Family history of prostate cancer is a significant risk factor, suggesting a genetic predisposition for the disease. Evidence suggests that the long arm of chromosome 1 carries the Hereditary Prostate Cancer 1 (HPC1) susceptibility locus in hereditary prostate cancer [76]. An increased risk of prostate cancer has also been found in carriers of the mutation for the BRCA gene, a DNA repair enzyme. The BRCA2 mutation has been associated with 3-fold risk of prostate cancer, and mutations in BRCA1 or BRCA2 are associated with aggressive disease (Table **2**) [77].

No single oncogene has been conclusively proven to initiate prostate cancer [78], however, overexpression of the insulin like growth factor receptor (IGFR) and the

EGFR leading to activation of Phosphoinositide-3Kinase (PI3K) pathway has been documented. Together with the loss of PTEN, a lipid phosphatase, this leads to constitutional activation of Akt, leading to activation of androgen receptors (AR). Activated ARs in turn lead to an increase in cell proliferation of prostate cancer cells [79]. Recently, genomic rearrangement leading to the fusion of TMPRSS2 to ERG, which encodes oncogenic transcription factor ETS has been identified to be an early event in prostate cancer [80]. Overexpression of the Myc oncogene has been identified in advanced prostate cancers [81].

Inactivation of tumor suppressor genes TP53, Rb1, and CDKN2A are frequently seen in metastatic and hormone refractory disease, but are less common in primary prostate cancer [81].

Table 2:   Common Molecular Mechanisms Underlying Prostate Cancer

Molecular Characteristic	Molecular Pathway	Clinical Relevance
TMPRSS2-ERG fusion	aberrant expression of transcription factor ETS	possibly predicts response to abiraterone acetate
BRCA-2 mutation	DNA repair	family history of prostate cancer
PTEN deletion	tumor suppressor gene	

Renal Cell Carcinoma (RCC)

The most common histological subtype accounting for >80% of RCC case is the clear cell carcinoma. Most cases are sporadic and <4% are familial. Almost all familial clear cell RCCs arise from an inherited mutation in the von Hippel-Lindau (VHL) tumor suppressor gene located on chromosome 3p [82]. The protein encoded by the VHL gene is involved in the degradation of hypoxia-inducible-factor (HIF). Inactivation of the VHL gene leads to activation of the hypoxia pathway through HIF, which in turn activates expression of genes involved in the hypoxia response, angiogenesis, and other signaling pathways involving VEGF [83]. The most common genetic alterations in sporadic cases of RCC are chromosome 3p deletion and inactivation of VHL tumor suppressor gene [83].

Bladder Cancer

The second most frequent genitourinary cancer is the bladder cancer. Carcinoma *in situ* is a precursor of invasive cancer, and is characterized by mutations affecting tumor suppressor genes TP53, Rb, and PTEN. Non-muscle invasive superficial bladder cancers arise secondary to mutations affecting oncogenes H-ras, FGFR3, and PI3K, and deletions of the long arm of chromosome 9 [84].

Testicular Cancer

Germ cell tumor of the testes (TGCT) is the most common testicular neoplasm, and is the most common tumor in men between the ages 15 and 35 years [85]. The different subtypes of TGCT include teratomas, yolk sac tumors, seminomas and non-seminomas. The most widely accepted risk factor for TGCT is cryptorchidism. The characteristic genetic abnormality in these tumors is the excess genetic material of the short arm of chromosome 12, usually in the form of isochromosome [i [12p]]. The initiating event is thought to be aberrant chromatid exchange leading to an increase in 12p number in the spermatocyte. The resulting genomic instability in the cell is believed to enable it to escape TP53 mediated apoptosis [86]. Another theory proposed suggests that the primordial germ cells undergo abnormal cell division (polyploidization) due environmental factors in utero, leading to development of intratubular germ cell neoplasia followed by TGCT [87].

BREAST CANCER

Breast cancer is the most common cancer among women worldwide. One of the risk factors for breast cancer is inheritance of a mutation in the BRCA1 or BRCA2 genes (Table **3**). It is estimated that BRCA mutations account for about 5-7% of all breast cancers. The tumor suppressor genes, BRCA1 and BRCA 2, play an important role in homologous recombination repair during DNA replication [88]. Mutations in BRCA genes are inherited in an autosomal dominant manner, and individuals are at an increased risk of developing breast and ovarian cancer [89].

Table 3:   **Common Molecular Mechanisms Underlying Breast Cancer**

Molecular Characteristic	Molecular Pathway	Clinical Relevance
HER-2 amplification	increased receptor tyrosine kinase activity	targeted therapy with trastuzumab, lapatinib
BRCA 1&2 mutation	DNA repair	family history of breast cancer; autosomal dominant
Estrogen/Progesterone receptor expression	Estrogen/progesterone stimulated growth and differentiation	favorable prognosis; endocrine therapies with tamoxifen, anastrozole
PI3KCA mutation	activated PI3K/Akt/mTOR pathway	

About 50-60% of breast cancer is luminal A type. This type is characterized by the up regulation of the estrogen (ER) transcription factor, low rate of proliferation, and low histological grade [90]. About 10-20% of breast cancer is luminal B type. This type has an increased expression of MKI67, cyclin B1, EGFR and Her2 genes, and carries a worse prognosis than luminal A tumors.

Increased cell proliferation secondary to the amplification of the Her-2/neu oncogene has been documented in 15-20% of breast cancers [91]. The Her-2 membrane receptor belongs to the human epidermal receptor (HER) family, and can activate three major signaling pathways: Ras/Raf/ MAPK, JAK/Stat and PI3K/AKT/mTOR. These pathways are involved in the growth and cell survival, along with proliferation, division, metabolism, apoptosis and migration capabilities. Also, mutations involving these signal transduction pathways could lead to sustained cell proliferation and aggressive disease [92]. The activation of the PI3K pathway has been documented in estrogen receptor positive breast cancer [93]. The role of VEGF in promoting angiogenesis and subsequent tumor development in breast cancer is a matter of debate in the oncology community [94].

GYNECOLOGICAL CANCERS

Common gynecological malignancies include cancers of the endometrium, cervix, and ovary. Genetic alterations have been documented in all of the major types of gynecological cancers.

Cervical Cancer

Cervical cancer is the second most common cancer among women worldwide. The Human papilloma virus (HPV) infection is one of the major risk factor for cervical cancer. More than 90% of cervical cancers contain HPV DNA [95]. HPV 16 and 18 are considered high-risk oncogenic types that are known to cause high-grade intraepithelial neoplasia and cervical cancer [96]. The E6 protein associated with HPV binds to and degrades TP53. The E7 protein binds to the Rb gene, causing decreased cell cycle arrest and malignant transformation of cervical cells (Table **4**). Mutations in K-ras and myc oncogenes have also been found in a small number of cervical cancers [97].

Table 4:   **Molecular Mechanisms Underlying Cervical Cancer**

Molecular Characteristic	Molecular Pathway
E6 protein	Binds p53 causing cell proliferation (*via* p53 degradation) and by preventing/targeting activation or expression of pro-apoptotic genes
E7 protein	Binds pRb causing cell proliferation (*via* pRb degradation); Mediates structural changes in the genomic structure of epithelial cells

Endometrial Cancer

Mutations involving PTEN, a tumor suppressor gene, is the most common genetic alteration in endometrioid adenocarcinoma (type I) [98]. Microsatellite instability (MSI), where short segments of repetitive DNA bases are found predominantly throughout noncoding DNA, is seen in about 20% of all endometrioid carcinoma cases [99]. Thus, patients with familial hereditary non-polyposis colorectal carcinoma (HNPCC) are at increased risk of endometrioid carcinoma. Other genetic alterations in endometrioid adenocarcinoma include mutations in K-ras and β-catenin genes [100]. Mutations involving TP53 are the most common genetic alteration in type II endometrial carcinoma (serous carcinoma). Inactivation of P16 and overexpression of Her-2/neu is also seen in about 50% of type II endometrial carcinoma (Table **5**) [100].

Ovarian Cancer

Ovarian cancer is the leading cause of death among in women with gynecological cancers. Germline mutations in BRCA1 and BRCA2 genes have been implicated in hereditary ovarian cancer [101]. Patients have an estimated 20-30% lifetime risk of ovarian carcinoma. Heritable mutations in DNA mismatch repair genes, such as hMLH1 and hMSH2, underlie ovarian cancer associated with Lynch syndrome (Table **6**). TP53 mutations appear to be the initiating event in high-grade epithelial ovarian tumors [102]. Mutations in K-ras, Braf, β -catenin or PTEN genes are more commonly found in borderline or low-grade tumors. In contrast to primary tumors, metastatic ovarian cancers overexpress stromal factors and metastatic genes, such as metalloproteinase, VEGF, endothelin, fibroblast growth factor, thrombospondins, integrins, and chemokines.

Table 5:   Common Molecular Mechanisms Underlying Endometrial Cancer

Genetic Alteration	Molecular Pathway	Clinical Relevance
PTEN mutation/loss of function	Loss of tyrosine kinase and tumor suppressor function → uncontrolled/ aberrant cell growth and decreased cell death; involved pathways: (PI3K-AKT-mTOR)	Investigation of targeted therapy with m-TOR inhibitors (temsirolimus, ridaforolimus, everolimus) and PARP inhibitors
Microsatellite instability	mismatch repair deficiency leading to genomic instability	
K-ras mutation	oncogene	
B-catenin mutation	cell differentiation, normal tissue architecture, signal transduction, accumulation of B-catenin protein	
p53 mutation	uncontrolled cell division	
p16 inactivation	uncontrolled cell division	
HER-2/neu overexpression	Increased receptor tyrosine kinase activity	combination therapy with trastuzumab under investigation

Table 6:   Molecular Mechanisms Underlying Ovarian Cancer

Molecular Characteristic	Molecular Pathway	Clinical Relevance
hMLH1, hMSH2 mutation	Mismatch repair genes	Hereditary ovarian cancer
BRCA 1&2 mutation	DNA repair	hereditary ovarian cancer
K-ras, Braf mutation	oncogenes	
PTEN, TP53 mutation	tumor suppressor gene	
PGR, ESR1, CYP3A4, CYP19A1, SRD5A2 mutation	steroid hormone regulation	

GASTROINTESTINAL TUMORS

Esophageal Cancer

The two most common histological subtypes of esophageal cancer are adenocarcinoma and squamous cell carcinoma, each with different risk factors and distinct pathways of oncogenesis. Known risk factors of esophageal adenocarcinoma include obesity and gastroesophageal reflux; chronic acid refluxes linked to Barrett's esophagus. Patients with Barrett's esophagus have a 30-150 fold higher risk of developing esophageal adenocarcinoma compared to those without this abnormality. The homeobox gene CDX-2 – a transcription factor that drives intestinal differentiation, is markedly up-regulated in the intestinal cells of Barrett's esophagus (Table 7) [103]. Alterations in EGFR and Her2/Neu expression are also seen in esophageal adenocarcinomas [104]. Smoking and alcohol consumption are risk factors in the development of squamous cell carcinoma. Alcohol is known to induce cancer by the production of acetaldehyde in the mucosa which induces genetic mutations, by the generation of reactive oxygen species and by the inhibition of DNA methylation which leads to oncogene overexpression [104]. While a direct causal link has not been defined in esophageal cancer, cigarette smoke contains polycyclic aromatic hydrocarbons and N-nitrosamines, both carcinogens that create DNA adducts, alter gene methylation and induce mutations [104]. A number of gene mutations have also been identified in squamous cell esophageal cancers – p53, p21, p16, cyclin D, EGFR, COX-2, E-cadherin, and BRCA1. Use of erlotinib, an EGFR tyrosine kinase inhibitor, is being studied in advanced squamous cell carcinoma of the esophagus.

Table 7:   **Common Molecular Mechanisms Underlying Esophageal Cancer**

Molecular Characteristic	Molecular Pathway	Clinical Relevance
CDX-2 transcription factor	Upregulated in Barrett esophagus cells, induces intestinal differentiation	Underlying factor in adenocarcinomas
EGFR mutation	Oncogene, upregulated in Barrett and esophageal adenocarcinoma	increased expression correlates with high tumor stages and worse overall survival, investigation of cetuximab and pantitumab in esophageal adenocarcinoma
Her2/Neu receptor	"gene amplification" in 17-34% of esophageal adenocarcinomas	Investigation of trastuzumab in esophageal adenocarcinoma

Gastric Cancer

Helicobacter pylori (*H. Pylori*) *infection* is known to be a significant risk factor for the development of gastric cancer, however the definite mechanisms of carcinogenesis from infection are not clear [105]. *H. pylori* infection induces increased levels of Bcl-2, an anti-apoptotic protein, leading to decreased apoptosis in gastric epithelial cells [106]. Other risk factors include high intake of smoked, salted and nitrated foods [107]. Multiple molecular abnormalities have been identified in gastric cancers including microsatellite instability, inactivation of tumor suppressor genes (p53, p16, APC, DCC (decreased in colon cancer), FHIT (fragile histidine triad) and TTF-1), overexpression of oncogenes (such as HER-2/neu), and telomerase reactivation (Table **8**) [107].

Pancreatic Cancer

Pancreatic cancer is one of the most lethal cancers of the gastrointestinal tract. Mutational activation of K-ras is the most commonly observed change in pancreatic cancer (Table **9**) [108]. p16 tumor suppressor gene is inactivated in more 90% of pancreatic cancer. Other mutations seen include overexpression of Braf and EGFR, and SMAD4/DPC4 deletion. Familial pancreatic cancer is seen in patients with mutations in BRCA2 and LKB1 genes. LKB1 gene acts as a tumor suppressor gene and is associated with Peutz-Jeghers syndrome.

Table 8:   Common Molecular Mechanisms Underlying Gastric Cancer

Molecular Characteristic	Molecular Pathway	Clinical Relevance
Microsatellite instability	Mismatch repair deficiency leading to genomic instability	One of the earliest changes in carcinogenesis, associated with antral tumors, intestinal-type differentiation, better prognosis, marker for screening of genetic instability
p53 (loss of heterozygosity)	Tumor suppressor gene	p53 alteration reported in up to 80% gastric cancer cases, assist in diagnosis
p16 (loss of hetereozygosity)	Tumor suppressor genes, hypermethylation of p16 promoter	
APC	Tumor suppressor genes, altered interaction with B-catenin	Assist in diagnosis
HER-2/neu	Tyrosine kinase receptor overexpression	Her-2/neu overexpression implicated as a marker of poor prognosis

Liver Cancer

Hepatocellular carcinoma (HCC) is the most common type of liver cancer and a leading cause of cancer death. Risk factors include chronic hepatitis B (HBV) and

C (HCV) viral infections, genetic disorders such as hemochromatosis, dietary aflotoxin B1 intake, smoking, and heavy alcohol consumption. Cirrhosis is an independent risk factor for the development of HCC. Somatic mutations in TP53 and genomic instability are believed to be major mechanisms leading to HCC [109, 110]. HBV and HCV act as oncoviruses in the development of HCC. HBV is believed to cause an inactivation of TP53 through HBx, a protein required for the transcription of viral genome. HCV is known to cause chronic infection and higher propensity for causing cirrhosis. Along with TP53 inactivation, chronic inflammation and evasion of the host immune system has been implicated to cause HCC by HCV [110]. Alcohol-induced HCC is associated with the induction of inflammation, oxidative stress, and cirrhosis [110].

Table 9:   Common Molecular Mechanisms Underlying Pancreatic Cancer

Molecular Characteristic	Molecular Pathway	Clinical Relevance
BRCA-2 mutation	DNA repair	Hereditary pancreatic cancer
P16/CDKN2A	Tumor suppressor gene	Hereditary pancreatic cancer
K-ras	Oncogene	Most common mutation
TP53 mutation	Tumor suppressor gene	
SMAD4 mutation	Tumor suppressor gene	

Table 10:   Common Molecular Mechanisms Underlying Colon Cancer

Molecular Characteristic	Molecular Pathway	Clinical Relevance
hMLH1, hMSH2 mutation	Mismatch repair; microsatellite instability	Lynch syndrome
APC mutation	Tumor suppressor gene	Familial adenomatous polyposis, sporadic colorectal cancer
LKB1 mutation	Tumor suppressor gene	Peutz-Jeghers syndrome.
TP53 mutation	Tumor suppressor gene	Sporadic colorectal cancer
CpG island methylation	Inactivation of promoter sites of tumor suppressor genes	Aggressive tumors; Kras/Braf mutation
Kras mutation	Oncogene	Predicts poor response to anti- EGFR therapy
SMAD4 mutation	Tumor suppressor gene	

Colorectal Cancer

Colorectal cancer (CRC) is a major cause of morbidity and mortality in the western world. Most CRCs are believed to arise from adenomatous polyps over a period of years or even decades. CRCs result from the cumulative accumulation of multiple sequential genetic alterations (Table **10**). These alterations can either be acquired, as it happens in the sporadic forms, or inherited, as in genetic cancer predisposition syndromes. About 15-30% of CRCs are believed to be inherited secondary to germ line mutations [111]. Various hereditary syndromes have been documented where the individual is predisposed to develop colorectal cancer. Familial adenomatous polyposis (FAP) is an autosomal dominant syndrome caused by germ line mutations in the APC, a tumor suppressor gene [112]. Similarly, Gardner and Turcot's syndromes, caused by mutations in APC gene, are associated with colorectal cancer and extra colonic malignancy. Lynch syndrome, also known as HNPCC, is an autosomal dominant disorder caused by mutations in the DNA mismatch repair genes hMLH1 and hMSH2 [112]. Mutations that involve LKB1 tumor suppressor gene are associated with development of Peutz-Jeghers syndrome. In case of sporadic CRCs, tumor formation is secondary to chromosomal instability, which is characterized by multiple allelic loss of tumor-suppressor genes and mutations of the oncogene. Alternatively, mutations in mismatch repair genes, lead to a micro-satellite instability phenotype as in the Lynch syndrome, can also lead to sporadic CRCs. TP53 mutations have been found in approximately 70% of CRCs [7, 8]. TP53 protein functions as a key transcriptional regulator of genes that encodes proteins with functions in the cell-cycle checkpoints G1/S and G2/M phase and also in promoting apoptosis. Deletions of the APC gene on chromosome 5q lead to the disruption of *wnt* signaling pathway, which has been observed in up to 50% of cases [8]. Alterations in chromosome 18q are observed in approximately 70% of CRCs. As a result, the two tumor suppressor genes, SMAD2 and SMAD4, that encode proteins functioning downstream of the TGF-β receptor complex are mutated [113]. Mutational activation of K-ras oncogene has been reported in 40% of CRCs [113]. Along with alterations in tumor suppressor genes and oncogenes, DNA methylation changes that include hypermethylation at CpG sites of promoters that lead to transcriptional silencing have been documented in CRCs

[113]. Tumors carrying CpG island methylation exhibit distinct genetic and clinical features [114]. These tumors are located more proximally, have a high rate of mutations in Kras or Braf, and wild type TP53, occur in older patients and females. These tumors carry worse prognosis than other subtypes of colon cancers.

Anal Cancer

The majority of anal cancers are induced by an infection with HPV types 16 and 18. As in cervical cancer, an HPV infection causes decreased apoptosis from inactivation of tumor suppressor genes which leads to uninhibited cell proliferation and tumor formation.

HEAD AND NECK CANCERS

Head and neck cancers arise in the oral cavity, oropharynx, larynx or hypopharynx. Squamous cell carcinoma (SCC) is the most common type of head and neck cancer. Risk factors include smoking, alcohol consumption, and viral infections with HPV and Epstein Barr virus (EBV). About 20% of oral tongue and oropharyngeal cancers arise secondary to HPV infection. HPV contains two oncogenes, E6 and E7, whereby the expression inactivates TP53 and Rb respectively, and causing unregulated cell cycle in the infected cells leading to tumor formation [95]. Characteristics common to HPV positive tumors include younger patients, the absence of TP53 mutations, and favorable prognosis after treatment [115]. Overexpression of the EGFR oncogene has been implicated in the pathogenesis of head and neck SCC [116]. The role of the PI3K–PTEN–Akt pathway in SCC of the head and neck has been investigated. Mutational activation of PIK3 causes activation of Akt, resulting in evasion of apoptosis [115]. EBV virus has been implicated in the pathogenesis of nasopharyngeal carcinoma. EBV induced carcinogenesis is thought to be secondary to DNA methylation of promoter regions, regulation of host gene expressions and signal pathways due to viral proteins, viral small RNAs that target host genes, altered expression of microRNAs, and epigenetic alterations [117].

LYMPHOMA

Cancer arising from lymphatic tissue is broadly classified into Hodgkin's lymphoma (HL) and non-Hodgkin lymphoma (NHL), which arise from either the B-cell or the T-cell.

Hodgkin's Lymphoma

In classical HL, cells lose the expression of the B-cell typical genes and acquire expression of multiple genes that are typical for other cell types of the immune system. Classical HL is characterized by the presence of pathognomonic Reed-Sternberg cells, and lymphocytic and histiocytic (L&H) cells in nodular lymphocyte predominant HL (NLPHL). It is believed that Reed-Sternberg cells are derived from B-cells of the germinal center that acquired immunoglobulin variable chain gene mutations. L&H cells of NLPHL appear to derive from the antigen-selected germinal center B-cells. Few cases of classical HL are believed to originate from T-cells [118]. EBV infection has been implicated in the pathogenesis of classic HL [119]. The transforming events involved in the generation of RS probably involve the nuclear factor-κB or Jak–Stat signaling pathway. The RS cells attract many cells into the local tissue, resulting in an inflammatory microenvironment, which promotes the survival of RS cells, and helps them to evade cytotoxic T-cells or natural killer cells [118].

Non-Hodgkin Lymphoma (NHL)

The majority of NHL are B-cell lymphomas, and are characterized by reciprocal chromosomal translocations involving one of the immunoglobulin loci and a proto-oncogene (Table **11**). As a result, the oncogene is controlled by the active immunoglobulin locus (Ig), causing deregulated, and constitutive expression of the translocated gene [120]. About 15 different types of B-cell lymphomas are distinguished in the current WHO lymphoma classification. Diffuse large B-cell lymphoma is the most common NHL. The various molecular changes include reciprocal translocations between oncogenes Bcl-6, Bcl-2, Myc and Ig [120]. Mutations in the tumor suppressor genes TP53, ATM and CQ95 have also been identified. Follicular lymphoma is seen in about 20% of the patients, and of the most cases is associated with Bcl- 2–IgH rearrangement secondary to t [14; 18]. Mantle cell lymphoma is seen in about 5% of the patients, and arises from cells that populate the mantle zone of follicles. The cells are CD5+, show aberration in cyclin-D1 expression, and are associated with CCND1–IgH rearrangement due to t [11; 14]. MALT lymphoma arises from marginal zone cells in acquired lymphatic tissues, such as the mucosa of GI tract. Underlying translocations include API2–MALT1 [t[11;18]], Bcl10–IgH [t[1;14]], MALT1–IgH [t[14;18]], and FOXP1–IgH [t[3;14]]. *H. Pylori* infection has been implicated in the pathogenesis of MALT lymphoma [121]. Burkitt's lymphoma is a high grade B-cell lymphoma endemic in certain parts of Africa. The endemic variant is strongly associated with EBV [119]. Virtually all cases are associated with Myc–IgH [t [8; 14]] or Myc–IgL [[8;22]] translocations.

Table 11:　Common Molecular Mechanisms Underlying Non-Hodgkin Lymphoma

Molecular Characteristic	Molecular Pathway	Clinical Relevance
t [14: 18]	Bcl-2 rearrangement, decreased apoptosis	Follicular lymphoma
t [11;14]	Aberrant cyclin-D1 expression	Mantle cell lymphoma
t [14: 18]	Bcl-2 rearrangement, decreased apoptosis	Diffuse large B-cell lymphoma
t [8: 14]	C-myc oncogene	Burkitt's lymphoma
t [11: 18]	Fusion protein activates NFκB pathway	MALT lymphoma

Cutaneous T-Cell Lymphomas (CTCL)

These cancers are derived from CD4+ T-cells in the skin. The most common subtypes include Mycosis fungoides (MF) and Sezary syndrome (SS) [23]. The exact mechanism underlying MF pathogenesis is unclear. Current evidence points towards the role of cancer immunosurviellance in the pathogenesis of CTCL [122]. The disease manifestation is secondary to margination and extravasation of T-cells in the cutaneous microvasculature, followed by migration into the epidermis. This process is secondary to the expression of a cutaneous lymphocyte antigen, which is a ligand for E-selectin. Additional adhesion molecules and chemokines, such as CCR4, CCR10, and their respective ligands CCL17/TARC and CCL27/CTACK, are known to play a role in attracting T-cells to the skin [123].

Multiple Myeloma (MM)

MM is characterized by an abnormal clonal plasma cell (a terminally differentiated B-cell) that infiltrates into the bone marrow. Central to the pathogenesis of MM are the myeloma propagating cells (MPCs) [124]. Environmental factors, inherited traits, or normal physiological process of generating antibody diversity, leads to genetic changes like the loss of heterozygosity, gene amplification, or mutations with the end result being immortalization of MPCs. This results in clonal proliferation of cells in the bone marrow resulting in clinical signs and symptoms of MM. Progression of the disease results in extramedullary plasmacytoma and plasma cell leukemia. Hyperdiploidy as a primary genetic event is seen in about 50% of the cases. Other genetic events underlying initiation and progression of MM include chromosomal translocations [15%], deletions [45%], and gain of function [40%].

LEUKEMIA

T- Cell Acute Lymphoblastic Leukemia (ALL)

ALL comprises 15% of pediatric and 25% of adult acute lymphoblastic leukemia cases. Radiation exposure is a well-known risk factor in the development of ALL. Chromosomal aberrations are seen in about 50% of the patients [125]. The aberrations include rearrangements of proto-oncogenes to T-cell receptor (TCR) genes leading to overexpression of the proto-oncogene, rearrangements of two transcription factor coding genes resulting in the production of an aberrant fusion transcription factor protein, and rearrangements in the ALL1 (MLL) gene. Mutations involving NOTCH1, FBXW7, FLT3, BCL11B, PTPN2, PHF6, WT1, NRAS, CDKN2A and IL7R genes have also been implicated in ALL pathogenesis [125]. CpG island methylation and Ig/TCR rearrangements may also play a role in ALL development.

Myeloid Leukemia

Myeloid malignancies are clonal diseases of the hematopoietic progenitor cells. They result from genetic alterations that disrupt cellular processes like self-renewal, proliferation and differentiation. Acute stages of the disease include acute myeloid leukemia (AML), which originates *de novo* or less commonly following a chronic stage (secondary AML). Chronic stages of the disease include myeloproliferative neoplasms like chronic myeloid leukemia (CML), myelodysplastic syndromes (MDS) and chronic myelomonocytic leukemia (CMML). Mutations responsible for myeloid leukemia occur in several genes encoding proteins belonging to five classes: signaling pathways [CBL, FLT3, JAK2, RAS], transcription factors [CEBPA, ETV6, RUNX1], epigenetic regulators [ASXL1, DNMT3A, EZH2, IDH1, IDH2, SUZ12, TET2, UTX], tumor suppressors [TP53], and spliceosome [SF3B1, SRSF2] [126].

Acute promyelocytic leukemia (APL) variant of AML is characterized by the translocation involving the retinoic acid receptor-alpha (RARa) locus on chromosome 17 [127]. RARa is a member of a family of retinoid-binding transcription factors that regulate gene expression. The vast majority of these cases contain t [15; 17], although several variant translocations involving RARa have been identified, including t [11; 17] and t [5; 17].

CML is caused by a somatic mutation involving reciprocal translocation between chromosomes 9 and 22 [t [9; 22] [q34; q11]] which results in the Philadelphia chromosome, an abnormally short chromosome 22. The translocation juxtaposes the *abl* gene on chromosome 9 with the *bcr* gene on chromosome 22, generating the chimeric *bcr-abl* mRNA [128]. The *bcr-abl* protein is a constitutively activated form of the *abl* tyrosine kinase which is believed cause CML.

MELANOMA

Melanoma arises from the malignant transformation of melanocytes. Both environmental and genetic factors contribute to the development of melanoma. Familial melanomas represent 10% of the cases, and is due inheritance of defective tumor suppressor genes, CDKN2A and CDK4 [130]. Activation of the MAPK pathway, which regulates cellular proliferation, has been implicated in more than 90% sporadic cutaneous melanoma [129]. Mutations in Braf proto-oncogene has been documented in 70% malignant melanoma, and a significant proportion of both benign and dysplastic melanocytic nevi [129]. Mutations in the c-KIT proto-oncogene are also believed to underlie significant cases of melanoma [130].

SARCOMA

Sarcomas are malignancies arising from mesenchymal cell. Many sarcomas arise due to a single genetic abnormality. The genetic alterations underlying sarcomas include genetic rearrangements leading to aberrant fusion proteins, somatic mutations in signaling pathways, and karyotype abnormalities [131]. Gastrointestinal Stromal Tumors (GISTs) are believed to be due to the somatic mutations in c-KIT and PDGFR oncogenes [132]. HHV-8, a gamma herpes virus, has been implicated in the causation of Kaposi's sarcoma [133]. Partial or complete loss of the hSNF5/INI1 gene on chromosome 22q has been implicated in the pathogenesis of rhabdoid tumors, malignant peripheral nerve sheath tumor, and epithelioid sarcomas. hSNF5/INI1 gene is a core member of the SWI/SNF chromatin remodeling complex, and its deletion leads to cell cycle progression. Amplification of the murine double minute gene (MDM2) and CDK4 are seen in many cases of lipsarcomas (LPS). Various reciprocal translocations have been implicated in the pathogenesis of sarcomas. More than 85% of all patients with Ewing sarcoma have translocation between the EWSR1 gene on chromosome 22q12 and the FLI1 gene (Friend leukemia virus integration 1) on chromosome 11q24. The fusion gene encodes an aberrant transcription factor which alters cell signaling pathways affecting proliferation and apoptosis [134]. Fusion genes including [t[X; 22] [p11.23; q11]] and [t [2; 23] [q35; q14]] have been documented in synovial sarcoma and alveolar rhabdomyosarcoma respectively [135].

THYROID CANCER

Benign tumors of the thyroid gland care more common with malignant neoplasms representing <1% of all thyroid cancers. The most common histology is the papillary thyroid carcinoma, followed by follicular thyroid carcinoma. Radiation exposure is a well-known risk factor in the pathogenesis of thyroid malignancy. About 5% of all the thyroid cancers are inherited as a part of familial syndromes like familial polyposis of colon, Cowden's disease, Sipple syndrome (MEN 2 syndrome) and Carney complex. The most common genetic alterations seen in thyroid cancers include the activation of oncogenes Baf, Ras, RET, and NTRK1 and the silencing of tumor suppressor genes PTEN and TP53 [136]. Mutations in Braf appear to indicate an aggressive clinical course.

CONCLUSION AND FUTURE DIRECTIONS

Recent advances in molecular biology have led to an increased understanding of the genetic and molecular factors underlying various types of human cancers. There has been a coordinated effort in the recent years to catalogue the genetic mutations underlying various human cancers. The Cancer Genome Atlas project (CGAP) has set out to investigate genomic changes in 20 different cancer types, and so far have published results on three cancers- GBM, ovarian cancer, and colorectal cancer [137-139]. The findings from CGAP have greatly helped in increasing our knowledge of the molecular basis of cancer. This could potentially help in developing novel therapeutic strategies for human cancers in future.

ACKNOWLEDGEMENTS

Authors thank Dr. Stephen L. Brown for reading the manuscript and providing with valuable suggestions.

CONFLICT OF INTEREST

The authors confirm that this chapter contents have no conflict of interest.

REFERENCES

[1]   International Classification of Diseases for Oncology, 3rd Edition (ICD-O-3).
[2]   Nowell PC, Hungerford DA (1960). A minute chromosome in chronic granulocytic leukemia. Science; 132: 1497.
[3]   Rowley JD (1973): A new consistent chromosomal abnormality in chronic myelogenous leukaemia identified by quinacrine fluorescence and Giemsa staining. Nature; 243: 290-293.
[4]   De Klein A, Guerts van Kessel A, Grosveld G, Bertram CR, Hagemeijer A, Bootsma D, *et al.* (1982) A cellular oncogene is translocated to the Philadelphia chromosome in chronic myelocytic leukaemia. Nature; 300: 765-767.
[5]   Groffen J, Stephenson JR, Heisterkamp N, de Klein A, Bertram CR, Grosveld G (1984): Philadelphia chromosomal breakpoints are clustered within a limited region, bcr, on chromosome 22. Cell; 36: 93-99.

[6]   Heisterkamp N, Stem K, Groffen J, de Klein A, Grosveld G (1985): Structural organization of the bcr gene and its role in the Ph' translocation. Nature; 315: 758-761.

[7]   Fearon ER, Vogelstein B (1990). A genetic model for colorectal tumorigenesis. Cell; 61: 759-67.

[8]   Vogelstein B, Fearon ER, Hamilton SR, Kern SE, Preisinger AC, Leppert M, *et al.* (1988). Genetic alterations during colorectal-tumor development. N. Engl. J. Med. 319: 525-532.

[9]   Hanahan D, Weinberg RA (2000). The hallmarks of cancer. Cell ; 100: 57-70.

[10]   Hanahan D, Weinberg RA (2011). Hallmarks of cancer: the next generation. Cell 4; 144: 646-74.

[11]   Delys L, Detours V, Franc B, Thomas G, Bogdanova T, Tronko M, *et al.* (2007) Gene expression and the biological phenotype of papillary thyroid carcinomas. Oncogene; 26: 7894-7903.

[12]   Tomás G, Tarabichi M, Gacquer D, Hébrant A, Dom G, Dumont JE, *et al.* (2012). A general method to derive robust organ-specific gene expression-based differentiation indices: application to thyroid cancer diagnostic. Oncogene; 31: 4490-4498.

[13]   Floor SL, Dumont JE, Maenhaut C, Raspe E (2012). Hallmarks of cancer: of all cancer cells, all the time? Trends Mol Med. 18: 509-515.

[14]   Küppers M, Faust D, Linz B, Dietrich C (2011). Regulation of ERK1/2 activity upon contact inhibition in fibroblasts. Biochem. Biophys. Res. Commun. 406: 483- 487.

[15]   Hendrix MJ, Seftor EA, Hess AR, Seftor RE (2003) Vasculogenic mimicry and tumour-cell plasticity: lessons from melanoma. Nat. Rev. Cancer; 3: 411-421.

[16]   De Bock K, Cauwenberghs S, Carmeliet P (2011). Vessel abnormalization: another hallmark of cancer? Molecular mechanisms and therapeutic implications. Curr. Opin. Genet. Dev. 21: 73-79.

[17]   Royer, C. and Lu, X. (2011). Epithelial cell polarity: a major gatekeeper against cancer? Cell Death Differ. 18: 1470-1477.

[18]   Witsch, E., Sela, M., and Yarden, Y. (2010). Roles for growth factors in cancer progression. Physiology (Bethesda); 25: 85-101.

[19]   Lemmon, MA and Schlessinger, J. (2010). Cell signaling by receptor tyrosine kinases. Cell; 141: 1117-1134.

[20]   Hynes NE and MacDonald G (2009). ErbB receptors and signaling pathways in cancer. Curr. Opin. Cell Biol. 21; 177-184.

[21]   Perona, R. (2006). Cell signaling: growth factors and tyrosine kinase receptors. Clin. Transl. Oncol. 8: 77-82.

[22]   Cheng N, Chytil A, Shyr Y, Joly A, Moses HL. (2008). Transforming growth factor-beta signaling-deficient fibroblasts enhance hepatocyte growth factor signaling in mammary carcinoma cells to promote scattering and invasion. Mol. Cancer Res. 6: 1521-1533.

[23]   Bhowmick NA, Neilson EG, Moses HL (2004). Stromal fibroblasts in cancer initiation and progression. Nature; 432: 332-337.

[24]   Sherr CJ and McCormick F (2002). The RB and p53 pathways in cancer. Cancer Cell; 2: 103-112.

[25]   Evan G and Littlewood T (1998). A matter of life and cell death. Science; 281: 1317-1322.

[26]   Lowe SW, Cepero E, Evan G (2004). Intrinsic tumor suppression. Nature; 432 : 307-315.

[27]   Adams JM, and Cory S (2007). The Bcl-2 apoptotic switch in cancer development and therapy. Oncogene; 26: 1324-1337.

[28]   Azmi AS, Wang Z, Philip PA, Mohammad RM, Sarkar FH (2011). Emerging Bcl-2 inhibitors for the treatment of cancer. Expert Opin Emerg Drugs; 16: 59-70.

[29]   Hayflick L (1997). Mortality and immortality at the cellular level. Biochemistry; 62: 1180-1190.

[30]   Blasco MA (2005). Telomeres and human disease: ageing, cancer and beyond. Nat. Rev. Genet. 6: 611-622.

[31]   Wright WE, Pereira-Smith OM, Shay JW (1989). Reversible cellular senescence: implications for immortalization of normal human diploid fibroblasts. Mol. Cell. Biol. 9: 3088-3092.

[32]   Buseman CM, Wright WE, Shay JW (2012). Is telomerase a viable target in cancer? Mutat Res. 2012 ; 730: 90-7.

[33]   Hanahan D and Folkman J (1996). Patterns and emerging mechanisms of the angiogenic switch during tumorigenesis. Cell; 86: 353-364.

[34]   Ferrara N (2009). Vascular endothelial growth factor. Arterioscler. Thromb. Vasc. Biol. 29: 789-791.

[35]   Carmeliet P (2005). VEGF as a key mediator of angiogenesis in cancer. Oncology; 69 (Suppl 3); 4-10.

[36]   Weis SM, Cheresh DA (2011). Tumor angiogenesis: molecular pathways and therapeutic targets. Nat Med. ; 17 (11): 1359-70.

[37]   Berx G and van Roy F (2009). Involvement of members of the cadherin superfamily in cancer. Cold Spring Harb. Perspect. Biol. 1: a003129.

[38]   Cavallaro U and Christofori G (2004). Cell adhesion and signalling by cadherins and Ig CAMs in cancer. Nat. Rev. Cancer; 4: 118-132.

[39]   Talmadge JE and Fidler IJ (2010). AACR centennial series: the biology of cancer metastasis: historical perspective. Cancer Res. 70: 5649-5669.

[40]   Cecchi F, Rabe DC, Bottaro DP (2012). Targeting the HGF/Met signaling pathway in cancer therapy. Expert Opin Ther Targets.; 16: 553-72.

[41]   Shields JD, Kourtis IC, Tomei AA, Roberts JM, Swartz MA (2010). Induction of lymphoidlike stroma and immune escape by tumors that express the chemokine CCL21. Science; 328: 749-752.

[42]   Yang L, Pang Y, Moses HL (2010). TGF-beta and immune cells: an important regulatory axis in the tumor microenvironment and progression. Trends Immunol. 31: 220-227.

[43]   Mougiakakos D, Choudhury A, Lladser A, Kiessling R, Johansson CC (2010). Regulatory T cells in cancer. Adv. Cancer Res. 107: 57-117.

[44]   Hodi FS, O'Day SJ, McDermott DF, Weber RW, *et al.* (2010). Improved survival with ipilimumab in patients with metastatic melanoma. N Engl J Med.; 363: 711-23.

[45]   Warburg O (1956). On respiratory impairment in cancer cells. Science; 124: 269-270.

[46]   Vander Heiden MG, Cantley LC, Thompson CB (2009). Understanding the Warburg effect: the metabolic requirements of cell proliferation. Science; 324: 1029-1033.

[47]   Qian BZ and Pollard JW (2010). Macrophage diversity enhances tumor progression and metastasis. Cell; 141: 39-51.

[48]   Karnoub AE, Dash AB, Vo AP, Sullivan A, Brooks MW, Bell GW, *et al.* (2007). Mesenchymal stem cells within tumour stroma promote breast cancer metastasis. Nature; 449: 557-563.

[49]   DeNardo DG, Andreu P, Coussens LM (2010). Interactions between lymphocytes and myeloid cells regulate pro- *versus* anti-tumor immunity. Cancer Metastasis Rev. 29: 309-316.

[50]   Grivennikov SI Greten FR and Karin M (2010). Immunity, inflammation, and cancer. Cell 140: 883-899.

[51]   Velayos FS, Terdiman JP, Walsh JM (2005). Effect of 5-aminosalicylate use on colorectal cancer and dysplasia risk: a systematic review and metaanalysis of observational studies. Am J Gastroenterol; 100 (6): 1345-53.

[52]   Sun S, Schiller JH, Gazdar AF (2007). Lung cancer in never smokers—a different disease. Nature Reviews Cancer; 7: 778-790.

[53]   Mao C, Qiu LX, Liao RY, Du FB, Ding H, Yang WC, Li J, Chen Q (2010). KRAS mutations and resistance to EGFR-TKIs treatment in patients with nonsmall cell lung cancer: a meta-analysis of 22 studies. Lung Cancer; 69: 272-278.

[54]   Santos E, Martin-Zanca D, Reddy EP, Pierotti MA, Della Porta G, Barbacid M (1984). Malignant activation of a Kras oncogene in lung carcinoma but not in normal tissue of the same patient. Science; 223: 661-664.

[55]   Pao W, Miller V, Zakowski M, Doherty J, Politi K, Sarkaria I, *et al.* (2004). EGF receptor gene mutations are common in lung cancers from "never smokers" and are associated with sensitivity of tumors to gefitinib and erlotinib. Proceedings of the National Academy of Sciences; 101: 13306-13311.

[56]   Marchetti A, Martella C, Felicioni L, Barassi F, Salvatore S, Chella A, *et al.* (2005). EGFR mutations in non-small-cell lung cancer: analysis of a large series of cases and development of a rapid and sensitive method for diagnostic screening with potential implications on pharmacologic treatment. Journal of Clinical Oncology; 23: 857-865.

[57]   Soda M, Choi YL, Enomoto M, Takada S, Yamashita Y, Ishikawa S, *et al.* (2007). Identification of the transforming EML4-ALK fusion gene in non-small-cell lung cancer. Nature; 448: 561-566.

[58]   Horn L and Pao W (2009). EML4-ALK: honing in on a new target in non-small-cell lung cancer. Journal of Clinical Oncology; 27: 4232-4235.

[59]   Mao L (2001). Molecular abnormalities in lung carcinogenesis and their potential clinical implications. Lung Cancer; 34: S27-S34.

[60]   Hainaut P and Pfeifer GP (2001). Patterns of p53→T transversions in lung cancers reflect the primary mutagenic signature of DNA-damage by tobacco smoke. Carcinogenesis; 22: 367-374.

[61]   Brambilla E and Gazdar A. (2009). Pathogenesis of lung cancer signaling pathways: roadmap for therapies. Eur Respir J.33: 1485-1497.

[62]   Brambilla E, Negoescu A, Gazzeri S, Lantuejoul S, Moro D, Brambilla C, *et al.* (1996). Apoptosis-related factors p53, Bcl2, and Bax in neuroendocrine lung tumors. Am J Pathol ; 149: 1941-1952.

[63]   Kleihues P, Louis DN, Wiestler OD, Burger PC, Scheithauer BW (2007). WHO grading of tumours of the central nervous system. WHO Classification of tumors of the central nervous system. Lyon, France: IARC Press : 10-11.

[64]   Reifenberger G, Collins VP (2004). Pathology and molecular genetics of astrocytic gliomas. J Mol Med ; 82: 656-670.

[65]   Hermanson M, Funa K, Koopmann J, Maintz D, Waha A, Westermark B, *et al.* (1996). Association of loss of heterozygosity on chromosome 17p with high platelet-derived

growth factor alpha receptor expression in human malignant gliomas. Cancer Res; 56: 164-171.

[66]   Reifenberger G, Louis DN. Oligodendroglioma (2003). Toward molecular definitions in diagnostic neuro-oncology. J Neuropathol Exp Neurol; 62: 111-126.

[67]   Hartmann C, Mueller W, von Deimling A (2004). Pathology and molecular genetics of oligodendroglial tumors. J Mol Med; 82: 638-655.

[68]   Smith JS, Perry A, Borell TJ, Lee HK, O'Fallon J, Hosek SM, *et al.* (2000). Alterations of chromosome arms 1p and 19q as predictors of survival in oligodendrogliomas, astrocytomas, and mixed oligoastrocytomas. J Clin Oncol ; 18: 636-645.

[69]   Ohgaki H (2005). Genetic pathways to glioblastomas. Neuropathology; 25: 1-7.

[70]   Hegi ME, Diserens AC, Gorlia T, Hamou MF, de Tribolet N, Weller M, *et al.* (2005). MGMT gene silencing and benefit from temozolomide in glioblastoma. N Engl J Med ; 352: 997-1003.

[71]   Parsons DW, Jones S, Zhang X, Lin JC, Leary RJ, Angenendt P, *et al.* (2008). An integrated genomic analysis of human glioblastoma multiforme. Science; 321: 1807-1812.

[72]   Zhao S, Lin Y, XuW, Jiang W, Zha Z, Wang P, *et al.* (2009). Glioma derived mutations in IDH1 dominantly inhibit IDH1 catalytic activity and induce HIF-1alpha. Science ; 324: 261-265.

[73]   Vinchon M, Soto-Ares G, Ruchoux MM, Dhellemmes P (2000). Cerebellar gliomas in children with NF1: pathology and surgery. Childs Nerv Syst ; 16: 417-420.

[74]   Nakamura M, Shimada K, Ishida E, Higuchi T, Nakase H, Sakaki T, *et al.* (2007). Molecular pathogenesis of pediatric astrocytic tumors. Neuro Oncol ; 9: 113-123.

[75]   Bredel M, Pollack IF, Hamilton RL, James CD (1999). Epidermal growth factor receptor expression and gene amplification in high-grade non-brainstem gliomas of childhood. Clin Cancer Res; 5: 1786-1792.

[76]   Smith JR, Freije D, Carpten JD, Grönberg H, Xu J, Isaacs SD, *et al.* (1996). Major susceptibility locus for prostate cancer on chromosome 1 suggested by a genome-wide search. Science; 274: 1571-1574.

[77]   Gallagher DJ, Gaudet MM, Pal P, Kirchhoff T, Balistreri L, Vora K, *et al.* (2010). Germline BRCA mutations denote a clinicopathologic subset of prostate cancer. Clin Cancer Res. ; 16: 2115-2121.

[78]   Dasgupta S, Srinidhi S, Vishwanatha JK. (2012). Oncogenic activation in prostate cancer progression and metastasis. Molecular insights and future challenges. J Carcinog.11: 4.

[79]   Mosquera JM, Perner S, Genega EM, Sanda M, Hofer MD, Mertz KD, *et al.* (2008). Characterization of TMPRSS2-ERG fusion high-grade prostatic intraepithelial neoplasia and potential clinical implications. Clin Cancer Res; 14: 3380-3385.

[80]   Van Den Berg C, Guan XY, Von Hoff D, Jenkins R, Bittner, Griffin C, *et al.* (1995). DNA sequence amplification in human prostate cancer identified by chromosome micro dissection: potential prognostic implications. Clin Cancer Res. 1: 11-8.

[81]   Bookstein R (2005). Tumor suppressor genes in prostate cancer. In: Totowa NJ, ed. Prostate cancer: biology genetics and the new therapeutics. Humana Press: 61-95.

[82]   Gnarra JR, Tory K, Weng Y, Schmidt L, Wei MH, Li H, *et al.* (1994). Mutations of the VHL tumour suppressor gene in renal carcinoma. Nat Genet. 7: 85-90.

[83]   Kaelin WG Jr (2007). The von Hippel-Lindau tumor suppressor protein and clear cell renal carcinoma. Clin Cancer Res. 13: 680-684.

[84]   Castillo-Martin M, Domingo-Domenech J, Karni-Schmidt O, Matos T, Cordon-Cardo C (2010). Molecular pathways of urothelial development and bladder tumorigenesis. Urol Oncol.28: 401-408.

[85]   Bosl GJ and Motzer RJ (1997). Testicular germ-cell cancer. N Engl J Med. 337: 242-253.

[86]   Chaganti RS, Houldsworth J (2000). Genetics and biology of adult human male germ cell tumors. Cancer Res. 60: 1475-1482.

[87]   Grigor KM, Skakkebaek NE (1993). Pathogenesis and cell biology of germ cell neoplasia: general discussion. Eur Urol. 23: 46-53.

[88]   Roy R, Chun J, Powell SN (2011). BRCA1 and BRCA2: different roles in a common pathway of genome protection. Nat Rev Cancer. 12: 68-78.

[89]   Foulkes WD (2008). Molecular origins of cancer: inherited susceptibility to common cancers. N. Engl. J. Med. 359: 2143-2153.

[90]   Sorlie T, Perou CM, Tibshirani R, Aas T, Geisler S, Johnsen H, *et al.* (2001). Gene expression patterns of breast carcinomas distinguish tumor subclasses with clinical implications. Proc Natl Acad Sci ; 98: 10869-10874.

[91]   Slamon DJ, Clark GM, Wong SG, Levin WJ, Ullrich A, McGuire WL (1987). Human breast cancer: correlation of relapse and survival with amplification of the HER-2/neu oncogene. Science; 235: 177-182.

[92]   Eroles P, Bosch A, Pérez-Fidalgo JA, Lluch A (2012). Molecular biology in breast cancer: intrinsic subtypes and signaling pathways. Cancer Treat Rev. 38: 698-707.

[93]   Baselga J (2011). Targeting the phosphoinositide-3 (PI3) kinase pathway in breast cancer. Oncologist ; 16: 12-19.

[94]   O'Shaughnessy J, Miles D, Gray RJ, *et al.* (2010). A meta-analysis of overall survival data from three randomized trials of bevacizumab (BV) and first-line chemotherapy as treatment for patients with metastatic breast cancer (MBC). J Clin Oncol ; 28: 12-14. abstract

[95]   zur Hausen H (1991). Viruses in human cancers. Science; 254: 1167-1173.

[96]   Ibeanu OA (2011). Molecular pathogenesis of cervical cancer. Caner Biol Ther; 11: 295-306.

[97]   Spandidos DA, Dokianakis DN, Kallergi G, Aggelakis E (2000). Molecular basis of gynecological cancer. Ann N Y Acad Sci ; 900: 56-64.

[98]   Mutter GL, Lin MC, Fitzgerald JT, Kum JB, Baak JP, Lees JA, *et al.* (2000). Altered PTEN expression as a diagnostic marker for the earliest endometrial precancers. J Natl Cancer Inst.92: 924-930.

[99]   Basil JB, Goodfellow PJ, Rader JS, Mutch DG, Herzog TJ (2000). Clinical significance of micro - satellite instability in endometrial carcinoma. Cancer; 89: 1758-1764.

[100]   Bansal N, Yendluri V, Wenham RM (2009). The Molecular Biology of Endometrial Cancers and the Implications for Pathogenesis, Classification, and Targeted Therapies. Cancer Control; 16: 8-13.

[101]   Norquist BM, Garcia RL, Allison KH, Jokinen CH, Kernochan LE, Pizzi CC, *et al.* (2010). The molecular pathogenesis of hereditary ovarian carcinoma: alterations in the tubal epithelium of women with BRCA1 and BRCA2 mutations. Cancer; 116: 5261-5271.

[102]   Chien JR, Aletti G, Bell DA, Keeney GL, Shridhar V, Hartmann LC (2007). Molecular pathogenesis and therapeutic targets in epithelial ovarian cancer. J Cell Biochem.102: 1117-1129.

[103] Groisman GM, Amar M, Meir A (2004). Expression of the intestinal marker Cdx2 in the columnar-lined esophagus with and without intestinal (Barrett's) metaplasia. Mod Pathol ; 17: 1282-1288.

[104] Denlinger CE, Thompson RK (2012). Molecular basis of esophageal cancer development and progression. Surg Clin North Am. 92: 1089-1103.

[105] Uemura N, Okamoto S, Yamamoto S, Matsumura N, Yamaguchi S, *et al.* (2001) Helicobacter pylori infection and the development of gastric cancer. N Engl J Med 345: 784-789.

[106] Lauwers GY, Scott GV, Hendricks J (1994). Immunohistochemical evidence of aberrant bcl-2 protein expression in gastric epithelial dysplasia. Cancer ; 73: 2900.

[107] Zheng L, Wang L, Ajani J, Xie K (2004). Molecular basis of gastric cancer development and progression. Gastric Cancer.7: 61-77.

[108] Hruban RH, Maitra A, Schulick R, Laheru D, Herman J, Kern SE, *et al.* (2008). Emerging molecular biology of pancreatic cancer. Gastrointest Cancer Res.2: S10-5.

[109] Hussain SP, Schwank J, Staib F, Wang XW, Harris CC (2007). TP53 mutations and hepatocellular carcinoma: insights into the etiology and pathogenesis of liver cancer. Oncogene 26: 2166-2176.

[110] Farazi PA, DePinho RA (2006). Hepatocellular carcinoma pathogenesis: from genes to environment. Nat Rev Cancer. 6: 674-687.

[111] Taylor DP, Burt RW, Williams MS, Haug PJ, Cannon-Albright LA (2010). Population-based family history-specific risks for colorectal cancer: a constellation approach. Gastroenterology; 138: 877-885.

[112] Rustgi AK (2007). The genetics of hereditary colon cancer. Genes Dev. 21: 2525-2538.

[113] Fearon ER (2011). Molecular genetics of colorectal cancer. Annu Rev Pathol. 6: 479-507.

[114] Issa JP. CpG island methylator phenotype in cancer. Nat Rev Cancer 2004; 4: 988 -993.

[115] Leemans CR, Braakhuis BJ, Brakenhoff RH (2011). The molecular biology of head and neck cancer. Nat Rev Cancer; 11: 9-22.

[116] Hama T, Yuza Y, Saito Y, O-uchi J, Kondo S, Okabe M, *et al.* (2009). Prognostic significance of epidermal growth factor receptor phosphorylation and mutation in head and neck squamous cell carcinoma. Oncologist; 14: 900-908.

[117] Kaneda A, Matsusaka K, Aburatani H, Fukayama M (2012). Epstein-Barr virus infection as an epigenetic driver of tumorigenesis. Cancer Res. 15; 72: 3445-3450.

[118] Kuppers R (2009). The biology of Hodgkin's lymphoma. Nat Rev Cancer. 9: 15-27.

[119] Rickinson AB and Kieff E (2001). Epstein-Barr virus. in Fields Virology. Lippincott-Raven, Philadelphia, 2575-2627.

[120] Kuppers R (2005). Mechanisms of B-cell lymphoma pathogenesis. Nat Rev Cancer ; 5: 251-262.

[121] Hussell T, Isaacson PG, Crabtree JE, Spencer J (1996). Helicobacter pylori-specific tumour-infiltrating T cells provide contact dependent help for the growth of malignant B cells in low-grade gastric lymphoma of mucosa-associated lymphoid tissue. J. Pathol. 178: 122-127.

[122] Wong HK, Mishra A, Hake T, Porcu P (2011). Evolving insights in the pathogenesis and therapy of cutaneous T-cell lymphoma (mycosis fungoides and Sezary syndrome). Br J Haematol. 155: 150-166.

[123] Kallinich T, Muche JM, Qin S, Sterry W, Audring H, Kroczek RA (2003) Chemokine receptor expression on neoplastic and reactive T cells in the skin at different stages of mycosis fungoides. Journal of Investigative Dermatology; 121: 1045-1052.

[124] Morgan GJ, Walker BA, Davies FE (2012). The genetic architecture of multiple myeloma. Nat Rev Cancer. 12: 335-348.

[125] Kraszewska MD, Dawidowska M, Szczepański T, Witt M (2012). T-cell acute lymphoblastic leukaemia: recent molecular biology findings. Br J Haematol.156: 303-315.

[126] Murati A, Brecqueville M, Devillier R, Mozziconacci MJ, Gelsi-Boyer V, Birnbaum D (2012). Myeloid malignancies: mutations, models and management. BMC Cancer; 12: 304.

[127] de Thé H, Chomienne C, Lanotte M, Degos L, Dejean A (1990). The t (15; 17) translocation of acute promyelocytic leukaemia fuses the retinoic acid receptor alpha gene to a novel transcribed locus. Nature; 347: 558.

[128] de Klein A, van Kessel AG, Grosveld G, Bartram CR, Hagemeijer A, Bootsma D, *et al.* (1982). A cellular oncogene is translocated to the Philadelphia chromosome in chronic myelocytic leukaemia. Nature; 300: 765-7.

[129] Ibrahim N and Haluska FG (2009). Molecular pathogenesis of cutaneous melanocytic neoplasms. Annual Review of Pathology; 4: 551-579.

[130] Beadling C, Jacobson-Dunlop E, Hodi FS, Le C, Warrick A, Patterson J, *et al.* (2008). KIT gene mutations and copy number in melanoma subtypes. Clinical Cancer Research; 14: 6821 -6828.

[131] Taylor BS, Barretina J, Maki RG, Antonescu CR, Singer S, Ladanyi M (2011). Advances in sarcoma genomics and new therapeutic targets. Nat Rev Cancer.11: 541-557.

[132] Hirota S, Isozaki K, Moriyama Y, Hashimoto K, Nishida T, Ishiguro S, *et al.* (1998). Gain-of-function mutations of c-KIT in human gastrointestinal stromal tumors, Science; 279: 577-580.

[133] P. S. Moore and Y. Chang (1995), Detection of herpesvirus-like dna sequences in Kaposi's sarcoma in patients with and those without HIV infection,"New England Journal of Medicine; 332: 1181-1185,

[134] Le Deley MC, Delattre O, Schaefer KL, Burchill SA, Koehler G, Hogendoorn PC, *et al.* (2010). Impact of EWS-ETS fusion type on disease progression in ewing's sarcoma/peripheral primitive neuroectodermal tumor: prospective results from the cooperative Euro- E.W.I.N.G. 99 trial. Journal of Clinical Oncology; 28: 1982-1988.

[135] Quesada J and Amato R (2012). The molecular biology of soft-tissue sarcomas and current trends in therapy. Sarcoma; 2012: 849456.

[136] Giusti F, Falchetti A, Franceschelli F, Marini F, Tanini A, Brandi ML (2010). Thyroid cancer: current molecular perspectives. J Oncol. 2010: 351679.

[137] The Cancer Genome Atlas Research Network (2008). Comprehensive genomic characterization defines human glioblastoma genes and core pathways. Nature 455, 1061-1068.

[138] The Cancer Genome Atlas Research Network (2011). Integrated genomic analyses of ovarian carcinoma. Nature 474, 609-615.

[139] The Cancer Genome Atlas Research Network (2012). Comprehensive molecular characterization of human colon and rectal cancer. Nature.; 487: 330-7.

Frontiers in Anti-Cancer Drug Discovery, 2014, 3, 233-261   233

CHAPTER 7

Novel Strategies in the Drug Delivery Development of Anticancer Drugs: The Nanoparticulate Formulations

Deepak Yadav[*,1], Mohammad F. Anwar[2], Suruchi Suri[2], Hemant Kardum[3], Manju Belwal[4], Sunanda Singh[5], Veena Garg[5] and Mohd Asif[1]

[1]Department of Ilmul-Advia (Pharmacology), Faculty of Medicine, Jamia Hamdard, New Delhi-110062, India; [2]Department of Chemistry, Faculty of Science, Jamia Hamdard, New Delhi-110062, India; [3]Department of Botany, Faculty of Science, Jamia Hamdard, New Delhi-110062, India; [4]Department of Pharmaceutics, B. S. Anangpuria Institute of Pharmacy, Faridabad, India; [5]Department of Biotechnology, Banasthali University, Banasthali, Rajasthan, India

Abstract: Cytotoxic drugs are a diverse class of compounds that treat cancer primarily by killing cancerous cells that are rapidly growing and dividing along with cells that are meant for normal tissue function. A novel and suitable delivery system delivers the chemotherapeutic agents to cancerous tissues without harming healthy tissues and also retains these chemotherapeutic agents in the tumor area for a longer period of time that gives a boost to the therapy. Smaller size increases the surface area of the nanoparticles that enhances drug absorption or encapsulation and carries the drug into the blood in a shorter time period. In comparison with already existing delivery systems, nano sized delivery systems can penetrate much deeper into tumor tissue, generally taken up more efficiently by cells and reduce the toxicity of cancerous drug to healthy tissues. However, nanoparticulate systems are being researched throughout the world to increase the drug efficacy and to reduce toxicity. Thus, generally nanoparticulate systems work on passive targeting as well as on active targeting of the drug to the tumors. However, the research is still at a nascent stage and there is a need to understand the role of nano carriers in cancer treatment. This article summarizes various drug delivery technologies for chemotherapeutic agents, which are gaining more attention for better therapeutic response.

Keywords: Active targeting, dendrimers, micelles, nanoparticles, passive targeting, polymeric and solid lipid nanoparticles.

***Address correspondence to Deepak Yadav:** Department of Ilmul-Advia (Pharmacology), Faculty of Medicine, Jamia Hamdard, New Delhi-110062, India; Tel: +911126059688; Fax: +911126059689; E-mail: deepaknano@gmail.com

INTRODUCTION

Nanotechnology uses techniques, processes and materials at the supramolecular level, at 1 - 100 nanometers (nm) scale when some defining up to 1 μ (micron), in order to create new properties and to stimulate particular desired functionalities. Nanoengineering has now been evidenced as an innovatory journey to develop control, measure and manipulate matter to change the properties and functions of materials on anatomic scale level [1]. Three applications of nanotechnology are particularly suited to biomedicine: diagnostic techniques, drugs, prostheses and implants. It is an interdisciplinary field for potential regions of various fields as molecular biology, biotechnology, physics, advanced chemistry *etc*. Nanoparticles are being used in different ways in health and medicine system as biocatalysts [2], photocatalysts, biosensors [3] and ferrofluids. Nanoparticulate systems have been recognized for their material properties for application to optical, electronic, and magnetic devices. Such formulations of different types of metals, polymers and lipids *etc*. are being utilized in imaging and regulated drug delivery system for the treatment and diagnosis of several fatal diseases such as arthritis, filarial, cancer, leishmaniasis, diabetes, viral infections *etc*. [4]. There are many drugs being used for nano preparation such as cisplatin, carboplatin, bleomycin, 5-fluorouracil, doxorubicin, dactinomycin, 6-mercaptopurine, paclitaxel, topotecan, vinblastin, etoposide *etc*.

NANOCARRIERS

Cancer can be defined as the anomalous growth of cells at a particular tissue. Treatments available involve a lot of patient incompliance. This draws interest of scientists to develop alternative treatments other than invasive and deadly painful chemotherapies. Conventional methods available for the treatment include surgery of the tumor bearing tissue followed by residual cell killing by radiations and so called chemotherapeutic molecules to prevent the recurrence. The effectiveness of cancer therapy in solid tumors depends on adequate delivery of the therapeutic agent to tumor cells to prevent the relapse through few left behind neoplastic cells. Except for a few cancer types (*e.g.* breast cancer), for which hormonal therapy or immunotherapy is used, cytotoxic drugs remain the major form of chemotherapy for cancer. Cancerous cells rapidly grow and divide along with cells that are meant for normal tissue function.

Despite the long history of their use, and the development of numerous new multiple drug regimens for improved clinical success, treatment failure is still frequently encountered. Existing conventional therapies have much extreme toxicity to the healthy cells. However, chemotherapeutics needs a scientific approach to deliver the chemotherapeutic agents in a sustained and targeted manner to increase patient compliance and reduce dose adverse effects. This can be achieved by designing novel nano drug delivery systems for chemotherapeutic agents as depicted in Fig. (**1**). Nano drug delivery systems do not only reduce the repeated administration to overcome non-compliance, but also help to increase the therapeutic efficacy by reducing toxicity. As recently described, PLGA nanoparticles were developed for curcumin (CUR) to enhance its oral bioavailability, to have higher release rate in the intestinal juice, inhibition of P-glycoprotein (P-gp)-mediated efflux, and increased residence time in the intestinal cavity [5, 6]. Pharmaceutical scientists have been working on the novel drug delivery systems development for chemotherapeutic agents in more triggered manner. However, modern chemo-pharmaceutical research has revealed many novel delivery systems, which paves the way for developing novel formulations such as nanoparticles, microemulsions, solid dispersions, liposomes, solid lipid nanoparticles *etc*. By enhanced permeability and retention (EPR) effect, nanoparticulate systems accumulate in tumor, release the drug at the site of action and increase the chemotherapeutic agents' bio efficacy [7]. Though in cancer treatment, existing marketed chemotherapeutic agents have limited toxicity to healthy tissues and also short half-life period, and poor aqueous solubility which put barrier in their therapeutic potential [8]. Nanoparticulate drug delivery systems exhibit passive targeting and active targeting. Nanoparticles extravasate through the leaky vasculature and accumulate through the enhanced permeability and retention (EPR) effect. Nanoparticle drug carriers deliver the drug in the extracellular environment and diffuse into tissue by passive targeting. In active targeting, ligand conjugated nanoparticles are prepared which interact with the receptors present on the cell surface and result in endocytosis. Researchers have formulated many formulations to overcome these problems such as liposomes, microparticles, nanoparticles, micelles, vesicles, nanotubes *etc.* so that the drugs can be delivered at specific site by entrapping in these novel formulations to eliminate the toxicity and enhance the efficacy [1, 9].

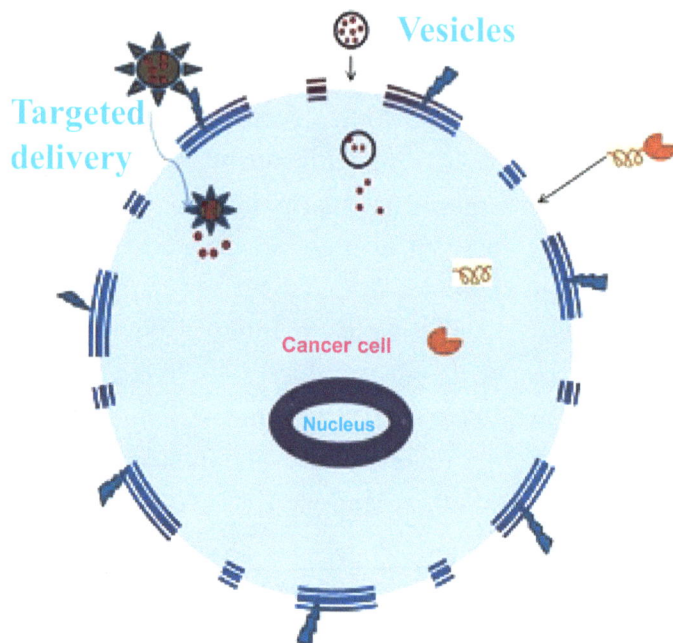

Fig. (1): Nano drug delivery systems for chemotherapeutic agents.

Polymeric micelles having core-shell architecture, the new class of polymeric nanoparticles, are an emerging field in drug delivery development to deliver hydrophobic, aqueous insoluble drugs to tumor site [10, 11]. The human beings possess homeostatic mechanisms to adjust a variety of physiological parameters within an assured range like temperature, pH and salt content and the body maintains homeostasis for appropriate conditions for enzyme reactions and metabolism [12, 13]. Various formulations have been developed by scientists to deliver the anticancer chemical drugs and molecular drugs like paclitaxel, docetaxel, several proteins, hormones and enzymes [14]. Polyethylene glycol (PEG) is a polymer having different molecular weights contributing in drugs safeguard within the body atmosphere by pegylation of drugs which escapes drug contact with plasma components and enhances the half-life period of the drug and also avoids uptake by the reticulo-endothelial system and phagocytosis [15]. At present, anticancer drugs development is in demand because of the controlled release after their administration in the body to a better treatment and patient compliance. Stimuli reactive biodegradable polymeric nanoparticles have become the keen interest of scientists in recent years due to their fascinated delivery of the drugs in a controlled manner [16]. These stimuli reactive polymeric systems have established precise advantages in the treatment of world's life threatening diseases and also in the release of vaccines [17, 18]. Novel nanoparticulate delivery systems have advantages over conventional drug delivery systems such as regulated release manner, sustained release of drugs, direct act on site of action, and the ability to extravasate into the tumor [19, 20]. Moreover, the nanoparticles have more advantages as early detection of disease and bypassing the mononuclear phagocyte system [21].

Particles indistinguishable to the body defense system, which can avoid clearance from the blood system, are called theft or extensive circulating particles, which can be realized by attaining tremendously small particle size as well as applying proper matrix material and surface engineering [22, 23]. Researchers have proved that dissolution of drug is indirectly proportional to particle size as particle size decreases, rate of dissolution increases. Decreasing the particle size of these drugs, which causes increase in surface area, improves their rate of dissolution [24]. There are different techniques to minimize the particle size which stimulates the drug absorption as described by the scientists such as the wet grinding technique which is more beneficial than dry milling techniques [25]. Smart polymers are polymers which react to external environmental factor such as temperature, pH, ions, and solvent *etc.* and have straightforward injectable formulation preparation [26]. This category of polymer solution is injected into a target site as the polymer gels, and diffuses the drug from the solid gel which allows for sustained-release formulations such as a protein bovine serum albumin (BSA) from temperature-responsive chitosan grafted with PEG (PEG-g-chitosan) [27]. These delivery systems acquire, prolonged drug delivery periods, localized drug delivery for a site-specific achievement, reduce body drug dosage with concurrent diminution in possible objectionable effects which are common to most forms of systemic drug delivery, the nontoxic degradability, and better patient compliance and relief [28].

Scientists are developing better suitable delivery systems than the existing ones. The nano carriers should be strong and biocompatible. Much work is going on in understanding the ways to develop more compatible and biodegradable delivery systems that can trigger drug release.

Various Drug Delivery Systems

The goal in the nanomedicine is to develop nanometer-sized drugs. However, gold nanoparticles, carbon buckyballs and nanotubes are being used as imaging and as drug delivery vehicles because of their nanometer size which enables them to move easily inside the body various polymeric nanoparticles, solid lipid nanoparticles and liposomes have also their use. The active compound might be encapsulated into delivery carriers or bonded to a particle's surface so that the drug delivery system may be used to enhance cancer therapeutics by reducing drug side effects. Nanophase Technologies Corporation produces nanocrystalline materials such as zinc oxide, titanium oxide for use in sunscreens and other products. Recent efforts towards drug delivery systems in cancer research have been designed as the prodrugs, various polymeric drug carriers and specially designed triggered release systems *etc.*

Prodrugs

Prodrugs are the compounds that need to be transformed before exhibiting their pharmacological action. Their main advantages include:

a)   Increased bioavailability hence, improved pharmacokinetics of the antitumor agents.

b)   Local delivery of the antitumor agents.

Limited bioavailability is the result of low chemical stability, limited oral absorption and rapid *in vivo* breakdown due to first pass metabolism [2]. An ideal prodrug is designed into chemotherapeutic drug that slowly activates in blood (*i.e.* activated from prodrug) and acts in order to have higher bioavailability. But a major limitation is that slower drug release also affects the neighboring non-tumor tissues due to the reactivity of most antitumor drugs. Moreover, slower drug release can also result in the conversion of the other competing enzymes into inactive metabolites [3]. In another approach, prodrugs are designed to achieve a high local concentration of antitumor agents in order to decrease unwanted side effects [29]. Hypoxic environment of the tumor tissue can also be exploited for the bioreductive activation of the prodrug. Prodrugs remove toxins that undergo biotransformation and superoxide radical outcome of this route is detoxified by superoxide dismutase, confirming bioreductive agents' reveled negligible toxicity to normal tissues [30-32]. No new agents have been approved for clinical use. But several reductively activated prodrugs are in various stages of clinical trial as nitro (hetero) cyclic compounds, aromatic and aliphatic N-oxides, and metal complexes *etc*. [33]. Antigens expressed on tumor cells are used to target enzymes with the help of antibodies to the tumor site prior to the prodrug administration as cytochrome P450 isozymes [34].

Liposomes as the Drug Carriers

Liposomes are bilayered membrane vesicles made of natural or synthetic amphiphilic lipid molecules with aqueous core shown in Fig. (**2**) and reveal several exclusive properties such as long systemic circulation half-life, ease of surface modifications and safety profiles for both hydrophilic and lipophilic drugs [35]. Liposomes are below 100 nm but might be of different sizes in the range of 10 nm - 100 μm depending upon their various architecture types [36]. Liposome drug delivery for doxorubicin (DOXIL®) was the first nano-therapeutics to get FDA approval for clinical use followed by several other nano-therapeutics [37, 38]. A cationic lipid-based liposome system Allovectin-7 delivers the plasmid DNA in the treatment of cancer [39].

Ligand-conjugated liposomes also exhibit promising therapeutic efficacy of drugs through targeted delivery. In a research study, an N -glutarylphosphatidyl ethanolamine (NGPE) liposome which is conjugated to the human transferrin (Tf) was developed to deliver oxaliplatin to cancerous cells [40]. In another study, scientists conjugated mAb 2C5 to DOXIL liposomes to enhance the drug efficacy and signify cell targeting. The monoclonal antibody 2C5 recognizes nucleosomes by binding to the surface of liver tumor cell [41]. However, liposomes have a major flaw not to be able to show sustain release for drugs these liposomes show several unique properties such as safety profiles, long systemic circulation half-life *etc.* [42]. Most of the liposomes are now PEG coated because pegylated liposomes decrease the monocyte system uptake, prolong circulation time and reduce immune recognition [43]. Anticancer drugs have several drawbacks in the treatment such as low aqueous solubility, lack of stability, rapid metabolism and other adverse consequences such as dose-limitation *etc.* Liposome encapsulated drugs have been developed to overcome the above mentioned drawbacks and many biological, biophysical, and biomedical barriers and reduce the toxic effects of anticancer drugs [44]. Scientists from all over the world have presented several methodologies for liposomes drug delivery such as hyperthermia, enzymatic and pH based delivery approaches for cancer treatment [45-47].

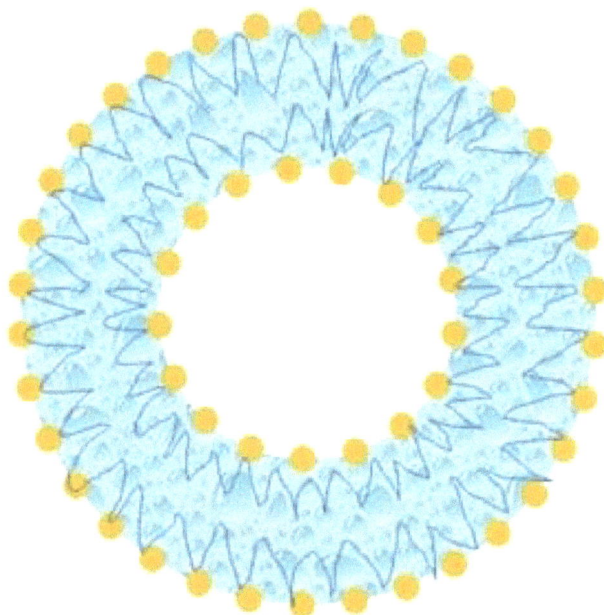

Fig. (2): Liposome.

Polymersomes as Drug Carriers

Polymersomes are self-assembled polymeric vesicles with bi-layered membrane structures that are analogs of liposomes, which comprise of amphiphilic block copolymers as depicted in Fig. (**3**). They are formed from a diverse array of synthetic amphiphilic block copolymers [48]. They differ from liposomes in the way that they have improved storage stability [49] and prolonged circulation time. While the hydrophilic aqueous core houses water-soluble drugs, the thick hydrophobic outer membrane accommodates the hydrophobic drugs [50].

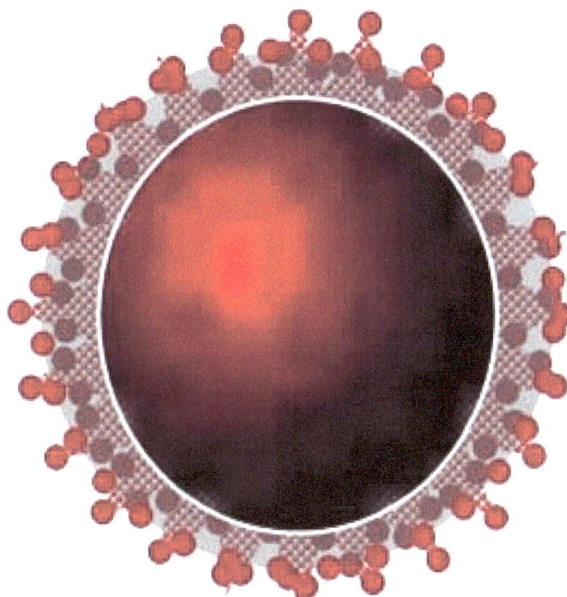

Fig. (3): Polymersome.

In addition, multifunctional polymersomes can be designed from functional block copolymers [51]. Poly (ethylene glycol) (PEG) is generally used as a hydrophilic outer shell, and provides a stealth-like character to the drug, which increases circulation time and biocompatibility [52]. The ratio of the hydrophilic-to-hydrophobic volume fraction is the key in determining the mesoscopic formulations among micelles (spherical or oblate) or polymersomes in aqueous solution [53-55]. Conceptually, when a proportion of hydrophilic block-to-total polymer ranges from 25 to 45%, it favors polymersomes formation. Whereas, block copolymers that have proportions greater than 45%, favor micelle formation [56]. Hydrophobic blocks that are used for polymersomes fabrication include inert polyethylethylene, polybutadiene, polystyrene, polydimethylsiloxane, degradable poly(lactic acid) (PLA), and poly(e-caprolactone) (PCL). Hydrophilic blocks include negatively charged poly (acrylic acid) and cross-linkable polymethyloxazoline. Neutral PEG is more common for bio applications.

Polymeric Nanoparticles as Drug Carriers

Polymeric drug carriers are of various types including conjugates, dendrimers, micelles, nanoparticles, nanogels and polymerosomes. Drug molecules that are covalently linked to a polymer backbone as side groups or end groups are referred to as polymer-drug conjugates [57]. Drug conjugate system has at least three components: a water-soluble polymer, bioactive anticancer agents, and a biodegradable spacer between the polymer and the drug [58]. The system is customized by selecting the appropriate polymer, and drug molecules, changing the polymer's molecular weight, altering number of drug molecules that are conjugated per polymer chain and /or by introducing bio-responsive elements and moieties for specific targets. The conjugates so obtained are regarded as new chemical entities (NCEs) [59]. In PG-TXL, paclitaxel is conjugated to a synthetic polyamino acid, poly (L-glutamic acid) (PG) through its 2'-hydroxyl group *via* an ester linkage. The conjugate is highly water soluble (>20 mg/kg) and has significantly higher antitumor efficacy and improved safety as compared to paclitaxel in preclinical studies [60]. Studies with paclitaxel resistant tumors (NMP-1 and HEY ovarian tumor) were also found to be successful with significant improvement in survival [61]. Over the last one decade, nearly a dozen polymer-drug conjugates have entered clinical studies besides PG-TXL.

Another form of polymeric carriers that are gaining popularity is micelles. Polymeric micelles were pioneered by Bader *et al.*, in 1984 and are well defined core-shell structures formed by the assembly of amphiphilic block copolymers in an aqueous environment [62]. The hydrophobic core can incorporate water insoluble drugs through chemical, physical, or electrostatic interactions. In the past two decades, many groups have reported on the development and optimization of polymeric micelles for the delivery of anti-cancer drugs. Presently, several doxorubicin- (*i.e.*, NK911, SP1049C) and paclitaxel-loaded (*i.e.*, Genexol-PM, NK105) micelle formulations have entered into clinical trials. Doxorubicin has been successfully loaded into micelles formed from PEG-b-poly(3-caprolactone) (PEG-b-PCL), PEG-b-poly(D,L-lactide-co-glycolide) (PEG-b-PLGA) [63], and PEG-b-poly(propylene oxide)-b-PEG (PEG-b-PPO-b-PEG; Pluronic) [64, 65]. Currently, two doxorubicin-loaded micelle formulations, NK911 and SP1049C have entered into clinical trials. NK911 is a doxorubicin-loaded PEG-b-PAsp copolymer micelle formulation that entered into phase I trial in 2001 and the results revealed it to exhibit longer circulation half-life, larger area under curve (AUC), and reduced toxicities in comparison to the conventional formulation. It is a micelle formed from the assembly of two different types of pluronic copolymers, L61 and F127 in 1: 8 w/w ratios [66]. Paclitaxel has been successfully loaded into PEG-b-poly(D,L-lactide) (PEG-b-PDLLA) [67-70], poly(N-vinyl-pyrrolidone)-b-PDLLA (PVP-b-PDLLA) [71], PEG-b-PCL, and PEG-b-poly(d-valerolactone) (PEG-b-PVL) [72]. Genexol-PM (*i.e.*, PEG-b-PDLLA) and NK105 (*i.e.*, PEG-b-PAsp) are two paclitaxel-loaded polymeric micelle formulations that have entered into clinical trials. In 2004, results from a phase II clinical trial evaluated Genexol-PM and cisplatin for treatment of patients with advanced gastric cancer [73]. Firstly, liquid-like core of PDLLA acts as a solubilization site for paclitaxel and secondly, decrease in AUC and Cmax occurs as a result of the shift in the drug accumulation to the tumor tissues that was evidenced in preclinical biodistribution studies [74].

There has been substantial interest in developing biodegradable nanoparticles (NPs) for drug delivery due to their exclusive size that ranges from 10 to 1000 nm, stability and controlled release properties [75]. Depending upon their fabrication method, they can be classified into two categories: nanospheres and nanocapsules. Nanospheres are matrix systems in which the drug molecules are dissolved or dispersed while nanocapsules are the vesicular systems in which the drug is enclosed into a polymer cavity as shown below in Fig. (**4**).

Typical biodegradable polymers that are used for NPs include poly(D, Lactide), poly(D, L-glycolide), poly(lactide-co-glycolide) (PLGA), polyanhydride, and poly(alkyl cyanoacrylate). PLGA/PLA nanoparticles and their modification have enticed the attention of number of researchers for the delivery of anti-cancer and other therapeutic agents [76]. Recently, research has been done on the transferrin conjugated PLGA nanoparticles with the loading of paclitaxel, both in *In vitro* and in an animal model of prostate carcinoma [77]. Cegnar *et al.*, developed the cystatin-loaded PLGA nanoparticles with the tactic of inhibiting the tumor-associated activity of intracellular cysteine proteases. *In vitro* studies of the same cystatin-loaded PLGA nanoparticles demonstrated 160-fold greater cytotoxic effect in MCF-10A neoT cells when compared to free cystatin ones [78].

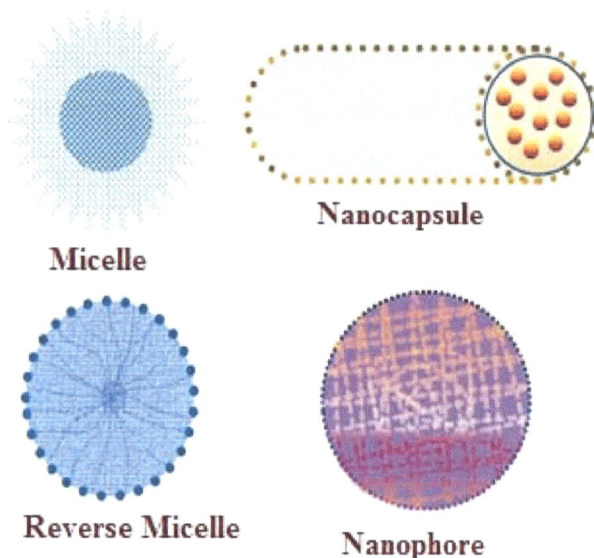

Fig. (4): Different types of polymeric nanoparticles.

Dendrimers as Drug Carriers

Another type of carrier systems includes dendrimers that are highly branched macromolecular architecture synthesized by polymers shown in Fig. (**5**). Paleos *et al.* reported first time the concept of branching growth in 2010 by constructing low molecular weight dendrimers [79]. Dendrimers with molecular weights ranging from several hundreds to over 1 million Daltons were prepared in high yields. Their characteristic features include a controlled size (15 nm in diameter), multivalency, and the surface charge of ionizable dendron terminal groups, which can vary in the generation number which further determines the drug content of the dendrimers.

The linkages between the drug and the dendrimer control the release of the drug [80]. Duncan *et al.*, 2005, studied the conjugates of a polyamidoamine (PAMAM) dendrimer with cisplatin [81]. This dendrimer-drug conjugate showed increased drug solubility, decreased systemic toxicity of the drug, and selective accumulation in solid tumors. The results using dendrimer-cisplastin conjugate showed increased efficacy when compared with free cisplatin in the treatment of subcutaneous B16F10 melanoma. Similar studies were carried out with fluorouracil by Zhuo *et al.*, 1999 where 5- Fluorouracil was attached to the periphery of a cyclic tetra-amine core [82]. Dendrimers are being used extensively in diagnostics and treatments of cancer at the nanoscale. These dendritic macromolecules have been synthesized for target delivery through wide functionality and specificity. Recently, dendrimers are utilized in the delivery of antineoplastic and contrast agents, neutron capture therapy, photodynamic therapy, and most-recently, photothermal therapy. Dendrimers are nearly mono disperse, globular macromolecules with a large number of peripheral groups and are formulated either as grown outwards from a central core by Tomalia and Newkome [83-85], or from the periphery inwards, terminating at the core by Frechet's convergent method [86]. Dendrimers have been known as perfect delivery carriers for the properties of less cytotoxicity, more internalization, enhanced blood plasma retention time, and filtration due to polymer size, charge, and composition.

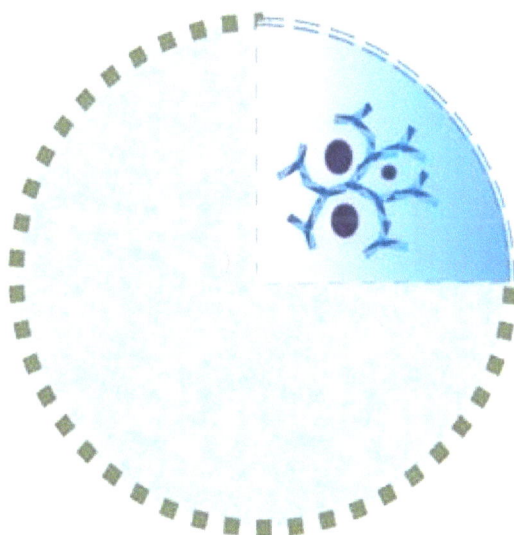

Fig. (5): Dendrimer.

Nanogels as Drug Carriers

When talking of delivery systems of nanorange, nanogels cannot be overlooked. These can be described as nanosized hydrogels made of physically or chemically cross linked polymers that are water-soluble. These are generally made up of polymers that may change volume depending on the external environment [87]. A nanogel of poly (ethylene glycol)-cl-polyethyleneimine using a modified emulsification-solvent evaporation method was prepared by Vinogradov *et al.*, 2005 [87]. Bae recently studied a virus-mimetic (VM) nanogel that consisted of a hydrophobic core comprising of poly (histidine-co-phenylalanine) (poly (Hisco-Phe) [88] and two layers of hydrophilic shells [PEG and bovine serum albumin (BSA)] [89]. A significant amount of DOX being released at endosomal pHs (6.4) has closely been linked to the reduction of DOX release rate at cytosolic or extracellular pHs (*e.g.*, pH 6.8-7.4). Therefore, VM nanogels and the anticancer drug that is enclosed get transferred from the endosomes to the cytosol. They shrink to their original size as a result of the more neutral local pH, thereby reducing the drug release rate. Release of the drug as triggered by endosomal pH would be in the cytosol. Lastly, the drug diffuses into the nucleus, which is the target site and hence, nanogels have been observed to show effect in drug resistant tumor cells as well.

Triggered Release Systems

Triggered Release Systems are of various types and used in imaging as well as in the treatment of cancer, some of them are summarized in Fig. (**6**).

Macromolecular water soluble carriers have been most commonly used for the release of the drug on the basis of the pH. At a particular pH, the carriers would release the free drug or may sometimes elicit changes in the physicochemical properties of the drug in the presence of the acidic environment of the tumor [90]. For instance, the novel pH- sensitive polymeric micelles for delivery of doxorubicin (DOX) have been formulated which self-assemble in aqueous solutions due to amphiphilic diblock copolymers comprising of poly(ethylene oxide) blocks and a hydrophobic block in which DOX was incorporated by covalent bonding to the core. DOX hydrazine bonding was pH sensitive which led to free drug release at 37°C and pH 5 which is close to the pH of the tumor [91]. A similar formulation as exemplified above was made using poly (ethylene oxide) (PEO)-modified poly (β-amino ester) (PbAE) and its biodistribution profiles were described. It was compared with non pH sensitive PEO-PCL (PEO-modified poly

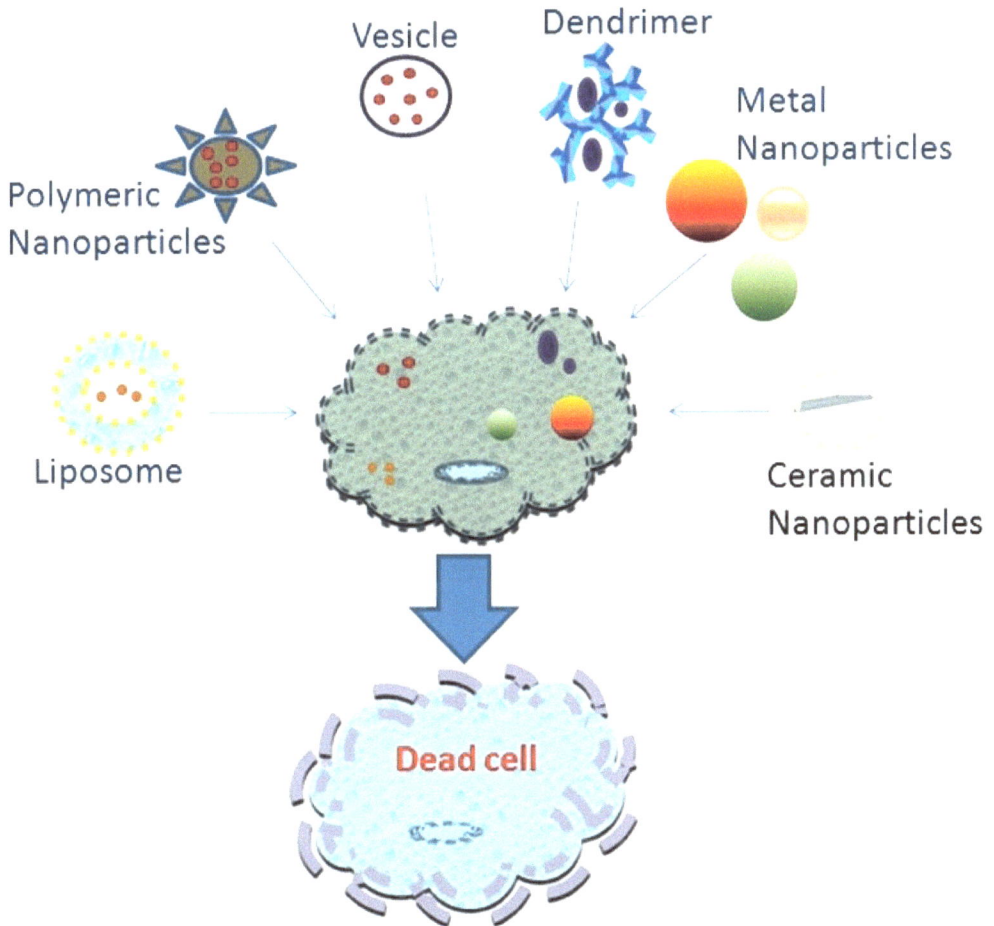

Fig. (6): Various triggered release systems.

(epsilon-caprolactone)) which was chosen as a control [92]. The method chosen for the loading of drug was by continuous solvent displacement and formulation was given to human ovarian adenocarcinoma cell line previously injected in athymic (Nu/Nu) model with predetermined dose of 20 mg/kg. Additionally low toxicity of the drug was observed with PEO modified formulation as compared to the aqueous formulation [93]. While talking of di-block copolymers, the NIPAAM copolymers cannot be overlooked. Many NIPAAM based pH sensitive polymers have also been investigated. The polymer was fabricated from the block copolymers of polyHis/PEG-folate and PLLA/PEG-folate and then folate tagged polymer was loaded with DOX and administered to the DOX resistant MCF-7 cell lines. The formulation showed more than 90% of cytotoxicity. This allowed the carrier system to bypass the Pgp efflux pump and accumulation of the DOX in the acidic environment which was up to 20 times more than the free DOX to the MCF-7 xenograft model. Thereby, it can be concluded that pH sensitivity as well as folate designing of the polymer made the formulation better [94]. Another recent work demonstrated that pH sensitive formulations can even prevent metastasis as demonstrated on 4T1 murine cancer model described by Gao *et al.*, 2011 [95]. Other than those discussed above, many more pH sensitive anticancer formulations are being developed which use pH as an internal stimuli for the drug release.

Temperature sensitivity acts as an external stimulus to induce apoptosis at initial exposure and to inhibit it at another consecutive exposure [96]. The same can be used as an internal stimulus as cancer region tends to have higher temperature due to increased blood circulation in that area. Higher temperature of a selective region can be utilized in a way that formulation can be developed which is particularly functional at elevated temperature of the tumor and is less or nonfunctional at the normal body temperatures. Such property of the formulation avoids the chemotherapeutic drugs to act at the normal sites thus drastically reducing the developmental side effects. Such formulations are known as thermo responsive drug delivery systems. Core-shell polymeric micelles of block copolymers of NIPAAm have been suitably employed for the purpose. Poly (N-isopropylacrylamide) (PNIPAAm) is one such thermosensitive polymer which exhibits lower critical solution temperature (LCST) of about 30-34°C [97, 98]. Below this temperature range, the polymer remains soluble whereas above this temperature it precipitates out or rather becomes insoluble. This makes the formulation to act in a controlled and targeted manner. Core shell structure is composed of both hydrophobic and hydrophilic portions which arrange themselves in an aqueous solution to form micelles. Micelles remain in their native state only at a critical temperature, above which the structure is deformed due to change in the equilibrium of the core shell structure, making them insoluble. This property is exploited in a way that if the LCST of the polymer is above 37°C, drug will remain intact inside the polymer but as soon as it reaches the tumor site, the polymer will be deformed, exposing the drug to the site of its action. Conversely, the thermoresponsive behavior of materials with LCST lower than normal body temperature can be exploited for delivery of drugs to regions of low temperature such as hypoxic tissue [96]. One such example of thermo responsive drug delivery is polymeric micelle that has been prepared from amphiphilic block copolymers consisting of *N*-isopropylacrylamide (NIPAAm) as outer shell and styrene (St) as hydrophobic core. Their transition temperature was about 32°C, above which the outer shell chains got dehydrated and collapsed, allowing aggregation between micelles and also supporting them in binding to the cell membrane surface. Such changes were reversible. Added advantage was that due to their unique size, they had longer circulation times and lower RES uptake. Hydrophobic drug molecules were integrated with the inner hydrophobic core of the thermo-responsive micelles and therefore, these were found to be of great use for site-specific delivery of drugs making use of changes in temperature as a trigger [96]. As described above, the heat can be utilized as an internal stimuli while targeting the hyperthermia of the tumor environment and can also be employed externally to trigger the thermosensitive polymers. Often a combination of both can offer better and effective drug delivery.

Temperature Reactive Polymeric Nanoparticles

The recent concern and keen interests of scientists are to develop and build up thermo-reactive delivery systems and devices so that clinically promoted modified delivery transporters can release the drug in a temperature dependent manner as discussed in Fig. (**7**). Researchers have developed various approaches to alter the temperature of carriers such as heating pads, exothermic chemical reactions and light *etc.* [99]. Stimuli reactive delivery systems show the exact potency of the release profiles of these transporters as required by the diseases the patients. Polymeric nanoparticles have not only been reported for stimuli regulated drug release, but also to reduce the adverse effects of the drugs, for providing protection from inactivation before releasing the anticancer agent at the particular site of action and in increment of the intracellular penetration and the pharmacological activities [100].

Several polymers have the properties to change the solubility depending upon different physical factors like temperature [101, 102]. As the discovery and

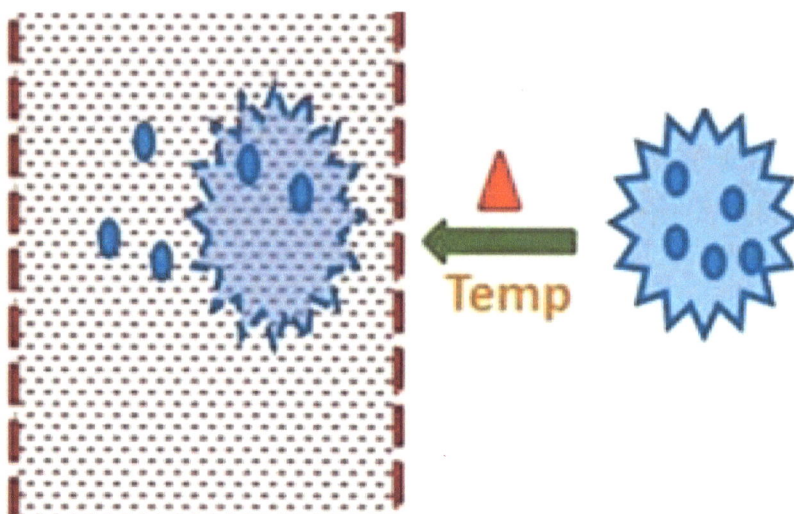

Fig. (7): Temperature dependent releases of nanoparticles.

evaluation of scientists report, there are several polymers and co-polymers which show the temperature sensitive behavior such as poly (*N*-isopropylacrylamide) (PNIPAAm), poly(lactic-co-glycolic) acid, poly(ethylene oxide) - poly(propylene oxide)-poly(ethylene oxide) triblock copolymers (PEO-PPO-PEO), poly(ethylene glycol)-poly(lactic acid)-poly(ethylene glycol) triblocks (PEG-PLA-PEG) poly (ethylene oxide) *etc.* [103]. Polymeric nanoparticulate system releases the drug when temperature reaches to a lower critical solution temperature (LCST) and above LCST polymeric configuration breaks and undergoes a reversible phase transition, resulting in drug release in thermosensitive manner [104]. A triblock co-polymeric particles formulation MarcoMed, ReGel®, was developed having hydrophobic and hydrophilic blocks, containing poly (lactide-co-glycolide) and poly (ethylene glycol) as (PLGA-PEG-PLGA) and applied to deliver paclitaxel and protein *e.g.* insulin. Paclitaxel, OncoGel®, formulation showed sustain release of the drug on cancer site [105, 106]. Though NIPAAm is a good temperature stimulant having LCST 30°C, scientists formulated NIPAAm copolymeric nanoparticles (NIPAAM/VP/AA), (NIPAAM/MMA/AA) *etc.* to enhance the LCST to 45-50°C. LCST may be increased by adding vinyl derivatives like vinylpyrrolidone (VP) and methyl methacrylate (MMA) [107]. Nanoparticulate carriers should possess the LCST above ~37°C body temperature to get better drug release, stability of nanoparticles in blood and no side effects and stimuli reactive controlled delivery. NIPAAm co-polymeric nanoparticulate system is used extensively for various synthetic chemotherapeutic agents as paclitaxel, vinblastine, rapamycin and natural agents as curcumin *etc.* for the treatment of cancer [108-110].

In another study, poly N-isopropylacrylamide and acrylamide hydrogels were formulated and these NIPAAm-co-AAm hydrogels showed 50°C temperature for temperature activities in 0-60 min in buffer. NIPAAm has hydrophobia core and acrylamide hydrophilic outer thin surface to make the release of the anticancer drug more precise and specific after bursting the polymer. As LCST of NIPAAm-co-AAm was found between 30-65°C depending upon the amount added of acrylamide to the formulation [111, 112].

pH Reactive Polymeric Nanoparticles

The pH reactive nanoparticulate systems for anticancer drugs have become novel and an emerging trend to the researchers for controlled delivery within time. Many novel and innovative requests are building utilization of the unique pH-sensitive polymeric nanoparticles. The pH reactive nanoparticulate delivery systems release the drug in an acidic atmosphere of the cancerous tissue which becomes acidic due to inflammation and other pathological and biochemical changes. Here, through the pH reactive delivery, various macromolecules can be delivered instead of synthetic drugs such as DNA, RNA, interleukins proteins and antibody as shown in Fig. (**8**). The two classes of anticancer drug used by the scientists to deliver into the cytoplasm polymer are polyanions and polycations [113]. Drugs such as adramycine, doxorubicine *etc.* have been delivered through the pH reactive polymeric micelles.

All solid tumors exhibit distinctive extracellular pH 5.7 to 7.8 and are mounted around the healthy tissue of the body. Recently, researchers have built the poly (L-histidine)-poly(ethylene glycol) micelles to release the drug in response to pH [114]. Various polymers are being evaluated for their pH reactive response and are being used in the formulation so that formulation can be converted into triggered carrier systems. Some of them include esters, anhydrides, amides, ureas, ethers, acrylates *etc.* [115, 116]. These polymers have basic and acidic groups by

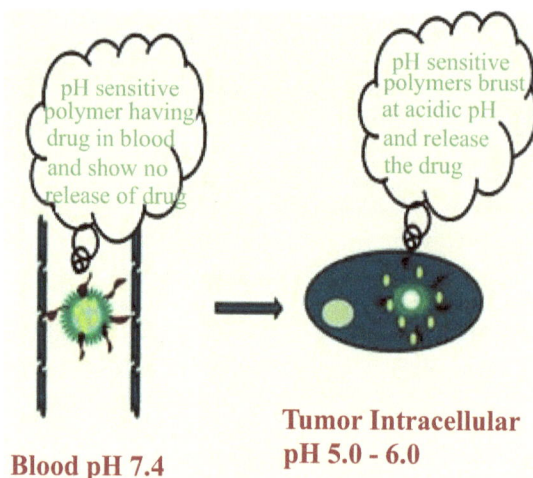

Fig. (8): Delivery of the drug through pH sensitive nanoparticles.

which these become a donor or acceptor of protons from the external environment and make pH reactive class. Polyacrylic acid is being used in many pH reactive nanoparticulate carriers formulation such as Carbopol® and methacrylic acid. Some amino acids such as L-lysine *etc.* are also very helpful in the formulation of pH reactive nanoparticles to deliver the anticancer drugs [117]. In the era of nanotechnology, many colloids of polymers have been built by addition of conductive additives. Researchers have built up polypyrrole that exteriorly has a colloidal nature of acid [118].

There exist a number of polymeric formulations built up by the smart polymers to deliver the drug in more than one stimuli factor and can be much better carrier than other particles which respond to only single stimuli factor and can be helpful in enhancing controlled release profile of the drugs. In a recent research, hydrogels were studied for their thermosensitivity and pH reactive properties and showed regulated drug release [119]. Studies by Bae *et al.*, 2005 reported chitosan which reacts to pH factor and releases drug and is found to be non-toxic having polysaccharide that is soft tissue compatible [88].

Photosensitive Nanoparticles as Carriers

Besides the photodynamic therapy, a number of other photosensitive nanoparticulate drug delivery systems have been investigated. Various photosensitive nanoformulations such as nanofibers, nanotubes, dendrimers *etc.* have been investigated for the delivery of the drug on stimulation with the light of the particular wavelength. The gold nanoparticles were conjugated to 5-Fluorouracil through a photocleavable *o*-nitrobenzyl linkage [89]. The US patent US 2009/0028946A1 has designated the cross linking of physiologically compatible matrix with the photosensitive matrix with suitable crosslinkers [120] which can be used for encapsulating chemotherapeutic drugs. These formulations are synthesized from photoisomerizable and photochromic substances *e.g.* dipalmitoyl-l-α-phosphatidyl choline (DPPC) which isomerizes on exposure to near-UV light. Bisby *et al.*, in 2000 made a formulation of doxorubicin using polymers and cholesterol. Such photoinduced release of chemotherapeutic drugs from sensitized liposomes might provide a useful adjunct photodynamic therapy [121]. Comurin implanted silica nanoparticles were designated for controlled anticancer drug release [122-124]. Photosensitizer DNA-crosslinked hydrogels exhibit the molecular approach to photoregulated by two wavelengths with a reversible sol-gel conversion [125].

CONCLUSIONS

The most common observation of this review is that nano drug delivery systems deliver the drugs at the site of the tumor rather than to other tissues in the body. These characteristics however can be utilized for targeting as well as for controlled or timely release of the anticancer drug at that particular site. As adverse effects of all anticancer formulations have been well known for centuries, they have a cytotoxic effect at the tumor site and they also invariably kill other cells of the body and thus make the therapy very harsh and painful. If any such method can be deigned that will cause the formulation when administered intravenously to release the drug only at the tumor site, then definitely it will though not vanish but decrease number of side effects and will also increase the efficacy of the drug. For reasons of patient convenience, controlled release formulations seem a valuable addition to standard formulations. In addition, controlled release formulations are of benefit in therapies that require prolonged exposure by means of a protracted treatment course. The positive perspectives of the patient, the oncologist and the pharmaceutical industry on the use of novel nano drug delivery dependent controlled and timed release formulations are being focused. Sustained release for the longer period of time will also reduce the number of in-patient and out-patient hospital visits with their associated medical and nursing administrative costs. In cancer, most of the times it is seen that patient does not die of the cancer itself but with the side effects of the chemotherapy. So, it is the need of the hour that the therapies must be made gentler to the patient and at the same time harsher to the tumor. The well-known hyperthermia therapies in such cases can be used as the adjuvant and are expected to be highly effective and highly target specific as compared to the ones which are used alone with the chemotherapeutic agents. Hence, nanocarriers release therapies will increase the revenues for cancer treatment.

ACKNOWLEDGEMENTS

Declared none.

CONFLICT OF INTEREST

The authors confirm that this chapter contents have no conflict of interest.

REFERENCES

[1]   Torchilin VP. Structure and design of polymeric surfactant-based drug delivery systems. J Control Rel 2001; 73(2-3): 137-172.
[2]   Connors T. Prodrugs in cancer chemotherapy. Xenobio 1986; 16: 975-988.
[3]   Boddy A, Yule S. Metabolism and pharmacokinetics of Oxazaphosphorines. Clin Pharmaco 2000; 38: 291-304.
[4]   Deepak, Suri S, Sikender M, Garg V, Samim M. Entrapment of seed extract *Nigella sativa* into thermosensitive (NIPAAm-co-VP) copolymeric micelles and its antibacterial activity. Int J Pharmaceu Sci Drug Res 2011; 3(3): 246-252.
[5]   Xie X, Tao Q, Zou Y, Zhang F, Guo M, Wang Y, Wang H, Zhou Q, Yu S. PLGA nanoparticles improve the oral bioavailability of curcumin in rats: characterizations and mechanisms. J Agric Food Chem 2011; 59(17): 9280-9.
[6]   Yadav D, Suri S, Choudhary AA, Sikender M, Hemant, Beg NM, Garg V, Ahmad A, Asif M. Novel approach: Herbal remedies and natural products in pharmaceutical science as nano drug delivery systems. Int J Pharm Tech 2011; 3: 3092-116.
[7]   Maeda H. The enhanced permeability and retention (EPR) effect in tumour vasculature: the key role of tumour-selective macromolecular drug targeting. Adv Enzyme Reg 2001; 41: 189-207.

[8]   Hoshino A, Fujioka K, Oku T. Physicochemical properties and cellular toxicity of nanocrystal quantum dots depend on their surface modification. *Nano Lett* 2004; 4(11): 2163-2169.

[9]   Connor EE, Mwamuka J, Gole A, Murphy CJ, Wyatt MD. Gold nanoparticles are taken up by human cells but do not cause acute cytotoxicity. *Small* 2005; 1(3): 325-327.

[10]   Wu XY, Lee PI. Preparation and characterization of thermal and pH sensitive nanospheres. Pharmaceu Res1993; 10(10): 1544-1547.

[11]   Huang M, Khor E, Lim LY. Uptake and cytotoxicity of chitosan molecules and nanoparticles: effects of molecular weight and degree of deacetylation. *Pharmaceu Res* 2004; 21: 344-353.

[12]   Kabanov AV, Alakhov VY. Pluronic block copolymers in drug delivery: From micellarnanocontainers to biological response modifiers. *Cri Rev Ther Drug Carr Sys* 2002; 19(1): 1-72.

[13]   Chavanpatil MD, Patil Y, Panyam J. Susceptibility of nanoparticle-encapsulated paclitaxel to p-glycoprotein-mediated drug efflux. *Int J Pharmaceu* 2006; 320: 150-156.

[14]   Pettit DK, Gombotz WR. The development of site-specific drug-delivery systems for protein and peptide biopharmaceuticals. Trends Biotech 1998; 16(8): 343-349.

[15]   Bellocq NC, Pun SH, Jensen GS, Davis ME. Transferrin-containing, cyclodextrin polymer-based particles for tumor-targeted gene delivery. Biocon Chem 2003; 14(6): 1122-1132.

[16]   Feng SS. Nanoparticles of biodegradable polymers for new-concept chemotherapy. Exp Rev Med Dev 2004; 1(1): 115-125.

[17]   Qiao W, Wang B, Wang Y, Yang L, Zhang Y, Shao P. Cancer Therapy Based on Nanomaterials and Nanocarrier Systems. J Nanomater 2010; DOI: 10.1155/2010/796303.

[18]   Sona PS. Nanoparticulate Drug Delivery Systems for the Treatment of Diabetes. Digest J Nanomater Biostruc 2010; 5(2): 411-418.

[19]   Vlerken LEV, Amiji MM. Multi-functional polymeric nanoparticles for tumor-targeted drug delivery. Exp Opi Drug Del 2006; 3(2): 205-16.

[20]   Avgoustakis K. Pegylated poly(lactide) and poly(lactide-co-glycolide) nanoparticles: preparation, properties and possible application in drug delivery. Curr Drug Del 2004; 1(4): 321-333.

[21]   Yam F, Wu XY, Zhang Q. A novel composite membrane for temperature and pH responsive permeation. In: Controlled Drug Delivery: Designing Technology for the Future. Ed K. Park. Washington, DC: ACS2000; pp. 263-272.

[22]   Senior J, Gregoriadis G. Is half-life of circulating small unilamellar liposomes determined by changes in their permeability? *Feder Eur Biochem Soc Lett* 1982; *145(1)*: 109-114.

[23]   Shenoy D, Fu W, Li J, Crasto C, Jones G, Dimarzio C. Surface fictionalization of gold nanoparticles using hetero-bifunctional poly (ethylene glycol) spacer for intracellular tracking and delivery. *Int J Nanomed* 2006; 1(1): 51-57.

[24]   Savjani KT, Gajjar AK, Savjani JK. Drug Solubility: Importance and Enhancement Techniques ISRN Pharm 2012; 2012: 195727.

[25]   Pathak P, Katiyar VK. Multi-functional nanoparticles and their role in cancer drug delivery - A Review. J Nanotech 2007; 3: 1-17.

[26]   Yin H, Lee ES, Kim D, Lee KH, Oh KT, Bae YH. Physicochemical characteristics of pH-sensitive poly (L-Histidine)-b-poly (ethylene glycol)/ poly (L-lactic acid)-b-poly (ethylene glycol) mixed micelles. *J Control Rel* 2008; 126(2): 130-138.

[27]   Bhattarai N, Ramay HR, Gunn J, Matsen FA, Zhang M. PEG-grafted chitosan as an injectable thermosensitive hydrogel for sustained protein release. J Control Rel 2005; 103(3): 609-24.

[28]   Yoshida R, Kaneko Y, Sakai K, Okano T, Sakurai Y, Bae YH, Positive thermosensitive pulsatile drug release using negative thermosensitive hydrogels. J Control Rel 1994; 32(1): 97-102.

[29]   Lowenthal R, Eaton K. Toxicity of chemotherapy. Hemato/OncolClini North Am 1996; 10: 967-990.

[30]   Dubowchik G, Walker M. Receptor-mediated and enzyme-dependent targeting of cytotoxic anticancer drugs. Pharmaco Ther 1999; 83: 67-123.

[31]   Lin J, Lu A. Interindividual variability in inhibition and induction of cytochrome P450 enzymes. An Rev Pharmaco Toxico 2001; 41: 535-567.

[32]   Begleiter A. Clinical applications of quinone-containing alkylating agents. Front Biosci 2000; 5: E153-E171.

[33]   Denny W. Hypoxia-activated prodrugs in cancer therapy: progress to the clinic. Future Oncol 2010; 6: 419-428.

[34]   Philpott G, Shearer W, Bower R, Parker C. Selective cytotoxicity of hapten-substituted cells with an antibody-enzyme conjugate. J Immuno 1973; 111: 921-929.

[35]   Antimisiaris SG, Kallinteri P, Fatouros DG. Liposomes and drug delivery. New York: Wiley 2007; pp. 443-533.

[36]   Brigger I, Dubernet C, Couvreur P. Nanoparticles in cancer therapy and diagnosis. Adv Drug Deliv Rev 2002; 54(5): 631-651.

[37]   Zhang L, Gu FX, Chan JM, Wang AZ, Langer AS, Farikhzad OC. Nanoparticles in medicine: therapeutic applications and developments. Clin Pharmacol Ther 2007; 83(5): 761-769.

[38]   Kale AA, Torchilin VP. Environment-responsive multifunctional liposomes. Methods Mol Biol 2010; 605: 213-242.

[39]   Chowdhery R, Gonzalez R. Immunologic therapy targeting metastatic melanoma: Allovectin-7. Immunother 2011; 3(1): 17-21.

[40]   Sankhala KK, Mita AC, Adinin R, Wood L, Beeram M, Bullock S. A phase I pharmacokinetic (PK) study of MBP-426, a novel liposome encapsulated oxaliplatin. J Clin Oncol 2009; 27(15S): 25-35.

[41]   Lukyanov AN, Elbayoumi TA, Chakilam AR, Torchilin VP. Tumor-targeted liposomes: doxorubicin-loaded long-circulating liposomes modified with anti-cancer antibody. J Control Rel 2004; 100(1): 135-144.

[42]   Torchilin VP. Recent advances with liposomes as pharmaceutical carriers. Nat Rev Drug Discov 2005; 4(2): 145-160.

[43]   Sahoo SK, Sawa T, Fang J, Tanaka S, Miyamoto Y, Akaike T. Pegylated zinc protoporphyrin: a water soluble hemeoxygenase inhibitor with tumour targeting capacity. Biocon Chem 2002; 13: 1031-38.

[44]   Ratner BD, Hoffman S, Schoen FJ, Lemons JE. Biomaterials Science: An Introduction to Materials in Medicine. San Diego. Academic Press: 1996.

[45]   Cohen S, Yoshioka T, Lucarelli M, Hwang LH, Langer R. Controlled delivery systems for proteins based on poly(lactic/glycolic acid) microspheres. Pharm Res 1991; 8: 713-20.

[46]   Ravivarapu HB, Lee H, DeLuca PP. Enhancing initial release of peptide from poly(D,L-lactide-co-glycolide) (PLGA) microspheres by addition of a porosigen and increasing drug load. Pharm Dev Technol 2000; 5: 287-96.

[47]   Husmann M, Schenderlein S, Luck M, Lindner H, Kleinebudde P. Polymer erosion in PLGA microparticles produced by phase separation method. Int J Pharm 2002; 242: 277-80.

[48]   Dischera DE, Ortiz V, Srinivas G, Klein ML, Kim Y, Christian D. Emerging applications of polymersomes in delivery: From molecular dynamics to shrinkage of tumors. Prog Polymer Sci 2007; 32: 838-857.

[49]   Meng F, Engbers GHM, Feijen J. Biodegradable polymersomes as a basis for artificial cells: encapsulation, release and targeting. J Control Rel 2005; 101: 187-198.

[50]   Ghoroghchian PP, Frail PR, Su-sumu K, Blessington D, Brannan AK, Bates FS. Near-infrared-emissive polymersomes: Self-assembled soft matter for *in vivo* optical imaging. Polymer Nat Aca Sci 2005; 102: 2922-2927.

[51]   Levine DH, Ghoroghchian PP, Freudenberg J, Zhang G, Therien MJ, Greene MI Polymersomes: A new multi-functional tool for cancer diagnosis and therapy. Methods 2008; 46: 25-32.

[52]   Lee JCM, Bermu-dez H, Discher BM, Sheehan MA, Won YY, Bates FS. Preparation, stability, and *In vitro* performance of vesicles made with diblock copolymers. Biotech Bioeng2001; 73: 135-145.

[53]   Antonietti M, Forster S. Vesicles and liposomes: A self-assembly principle beyond lipids. Adv Mater 2003; 15: 1323-1333.

[54]   Zu-pancich JA, Bates FS, Hillmyer MA. Design and synthesis of a low band gap conjugated macroinitiator: Toward rod-coil donor-acceptor block copolymers. Macromol 2006; 39: 4286-4288.

[55]   Hillmyer MA, Bates FS. Synthesis and characterization of model polyalkane-poly(ethylene oxide) block copolymers. Macromol 1996; 29: 6994-7002.

[56]   Discher DE, Ahmed F. Polymersomes. An Rev Biomed Eng 2006; 8: 323-341.

[57]   Peer D, Karp JM, Hong S, Farokhzad OC, Margalit R, Langer R. Nanocarriers as an emerging platform for cancer therapy. Nat Nanotech 2007; 2: 751-760.

[58]   Allen TM, Cullis PR. Drug delivery systems: Entering the mainstream. Sci 2004; 303: 1818-1822.

[59]   Minko T. Soluble polymer conjugates for drug delivery. Drug Discov Today 2005; 2: 15-20.

[60]   Soppimath KS, Aminabhavi TM, Kulkarni AR, Rudzinski WE. Biodegradable polymeric nanoparticles as drug delivery devices. J Control Rel 2001; 70: 1-20.

[61]   Lee ES, Gao Z, Bae YH. Recent progress in tumor pH targeting nanotechnology. J Control Rel 2008; 132: 164-170.

[62]   Bader H, Ringsdorf H, Schmidt B. Water soluble polymers in medicine. Angew Makromolku Chem1984; 123/124: 457-485.

[63]   Yoo HS, Park TG. Biodegradable polymeric micelles composed of doxorubicin conjugated PLGA-PEG block copolymer. J Control Rel 2001; 70: 63-70.

[64]   Rapoport N, Pitt WG, Sun H, Nelson JL. Drug delivery in polymeric micelles: From *In vitro* to *In vivo*. J Control Rel 2003; 91: 85-95.

[65]   Matsumura Y, Hamaguchi T, Ura T, Muro K, Yamada Y, Shimada Y. Phase I clinical trial and pharmacokinetic evaluation of NK911, a micelle-encapsulated doxorubicin. Bri J Cancer 2004; 91: 1775-1781.

[66]   Alakhov V, Klinski E, Li SM, Pietrzynski G, Venne A, Batrakova E. Block copolymer-based formulation of doxorubicin from cell screen to clinical trials. Coll Surf B: Biointerf 1999; 16: 113-134.

[67]   Burt HM, Zhang XC, Toleikis P, Embree L, Hunter WL. Development of copolymers of poly(D,L-lactide) and methoxypolyethylene glycol as micellar carriers of paclitaxel. Coll Surf B: Biointerf 1999; 16: 161-171.

[68]   Zhang XC, Jackson JK, Burt HM. Development of amphiphilic diblock copolymers as micellar carriers of taxol. Int J Pharmaceu 1996; 132: 195-206.

[69]   Kim D, Bae YH, Khandare J, Minko T. Polymer - drug conjugates: Progress in polymeric prodrugs. Polymer Sci 2006; 31: 359-397.

[70]   Liggins RT, Burt HM. Polyether-polyester diblock copolymers for the preparation of paclitaxel loaded polymeric micelle formulations. Adv Drug Del Rev 2002; 54: 191-202.

[71]   Kang N, Leroux JC. Triblock and star-block copolymers of N-(2-hydroxypropyl) methacrylamide or N-vinyl-2-pyrrolidone and D,L-lactide: Synthesis and self-assembling properties in water. Polymer 2004; 45: 8967-8980.

[72]   Park EK, Lee SB, Lee YM. Preparation and characterization of methoxypoly(ethylene glycol)/poly(epsilon-caprolactone) amphiphilic block copolymeric nanospheres for tumor-specific folate-mediated targeting of anticancer drugs. Biomater 2005; 26: 1053-1061.

[73]   Park SR, Oh DY, Kim DW, Kim TY, Heo DS, Bang YJ. A multi-center, late phase II clinical trial of genexol (paclitaxel) and cisplatin for patients with advanced gastric cancer. Oncol Reports 2004; 12: 1059-1064.

[74]   Kim SY, Lee YM. Taxol-loaded block copolymer nanospheres composed of methoxypoly(ethylene glycol) and poly(epsilon-caprolactone) as novel anticancer drug carriers. Biomater 2001; 22: 1697-1704.

[75]   Ho KS, Shoichet MS. Design considerations of polymeric nanoparticle micelles for chemotherapeutic delivery. Curr Opin Chem Eng 2013; 2(1): 53-59.

[76]   Panyam J, Labhasetwar V. Biodegradable nanoparticles for drug and gene delivery to cells and tissue. Adv Drug Del Rev 2003; 55: 329-347.

[77]   Sahoo SK, Ma W, Labhasetwar V. Efficacy of transferrin-conjugated paclitaxel-loaded nanoparticles in a murine model of prostate cancer. Int J Cancer 2004; 112: 335-340.

[78]   Cegnar M, Premzl A, Zavasnik-Bergant V, Kristl J, Kos J. Poly(lactide-co-glycolide) nanoparticles as a carrier system for delivering cysteine protease inhibitor cystatin into tumor cells. Exp Cell Res 2004; 301: 223-231.

[79]   Paleos CM, Tsiourvas D, Sideratou Z, Tziveleka LA. Drug delivery using multifunctional dendrimers and hyperbranched polymers. Expert Opin Drug Del 2010; 7(12): 1387-1398.

[80]   Duncan R. The dawning era of polymer therapeutics. Nat Rev Drug Discov 2003; 2: 347-360.

[81]   Duncan R, Vicent MJ, Greco F, Nicholson RI. Polymer-drug conjugates: Towards a novel approach for the treatment of endrocine-related cancer. Endocr Relat Cancer 2005; 12: S189-S199.

[82]   Zhuo RX, Du B, Lu ZR. *In vitro* release of 5-fluorouracil with cyclic core dendritic polymer. J Control Rel 1999; 57: 249-257.

[83]   Tomalia DA, Baker H, Dewald J, Hall M, Kallos G, Martin S. Dendritic macromolecules: synthesis of starburst dendrimers. Macromol 1986; 19: 2466-2468.

[84]   Tomalia DA, Baker H, Dewald J, Hall M, Kallos G, Martin S. A new class of polymers: starburst-dendritic macromolecules. Polymer J 1985; 17: 117-132.

[85]   Newkome GR, Yao Z, Baker GR, Gupta YK. Cascade molecules: a new approach to micelles. Arb J Org Chem2003; 50: 367-379.

[86]   Hawker CJ, Frechet JM. Preparation of polymers with controlled molecular architecture. A new convergent approach to dendritic macromolecules. J Am Chem Soc 1990; 112: 7638-7647.

[87]   Vinogradov SV, Bronich TK, Kabanov AV. Nanosized cationic hydrogels for drug delivery: Preparation, properties and interactions with cells. Adv Drug Del Rev 2002; 54: 135-147.

[88]   Kamaly N, Xiao Z, Valencia PM, Rodovic-Moreno AF, Rarokhzad OC. Targated polymeric therapeutic nanoparticles; design, development and clinical translation. Chem Soc Rev 2012; 41(7): 2971-3010.

[89]   Chan JM, Rhee JW, Drum CL, Bronson RT, Golomb G, Langer R. *In vivo* prevention of arterial restenosis with paclitaxel-encapsulated targeted lipid-polymeric nanoparticles. *Proc Nat Acad Sci USA*2011; *108(48): 19347-19352.*

[90]   Dufresne H, Garrec DL, Sant V, Leroux JC, Ranger M. Preparation and characterization of water-soluble pH-sensitive nanocarriers for drug delivery. Int J Pharmaceu 2004; 277: 81-90.

[91]   Ulbrich K, Subr V. Polymeric anticancer drugs with pH-controlled activation. Adv Drug Del Rev 2004; 56(7): 1023-1050.

[92]   Shenoy D, Little S, Langer R, Amiji M. Poly(Ethylene Oxide)-Modified Poly(β-Amino Ester) Nanoparticles as a pH-Sensitive System for Tumor-Targeted Delivery of Hydrophobic Drugs: Part 2. *In Vivo* Distribution and Tumor Localization Studies. Pharmaceu Res2005; 22: 2107-2114.

[93]   Devalapally H, Shenoy D, LittleS, Langer R, Amiji M. Poly(ethylene oxide)-modified poly(beta-amino ester) nanoparticles as a pH-sensitive system for tumor targeted delivery of hydrophobic drugs: part 3. Therapeutic efficacy and safety studies in ovarian cancer xenograft model. Cancer Chemother Pharmaco 2007; 59: 477-484.

[94]   Lee ES, Na K, Bae YH. Doxorubicin loaded pH-sensitive polymeric micelles for reversal of resistant MCF-7 tumor. J Control Rel2005; 103: 405-418.

[95]   Gao ZGjavascript: popRef('end-a2'), Lee DHjavascript: popRef('end-a3'), Kim DI, Bae YH. javascript: popRef('end-a1')javascript: popRef('cn1')Doxorubicin loaded pH-sensitive micelle targeting acidic extracellular pH of human ovarian A2780 tumor in mice. J Drug Target 2005; 13: 391-397.

[96]   Cammas S, Suzuki K, Sone C, Sakurai Y, Kataoka K, Okano T. Thermo-responsive polymer nanoparticles with a core-shell micelle structure as site-specific drug carriers. J Control Rel 1997; 48: 157-164.

[97]   Patton JN, Palmer AF. Engineering Temperature-Sensitive Hydrogel Nanoparticles Entrapping Hemoglobin as a Novel Type of Oxygen Carrier. Biomacromol 2005; 6: 2204-2212.

[98]   Lee CF, Lin ML, Wang YC, Chiu WY. Synthesis and characteristics of poly(N-isopropylacrylamide-*co*-methacrylic acid)/Fe_3O_4 thermosensitive magnetic composite hollow latex particles. Polymer Sci J: Part A 2012; DOI: 10.1002/pola.26036.

[99]   Chang JS, Chang KLB, Hwang DF, Kong ZL. *In vitro* cytotoxicity of silica nanoparticles at high concentrations strongly depends on the metabolic activity type of the cell line. *Environ Sci Tech* 2007; 6: 2064-2068.

[100]   Vilos C, Morales FA, Solar PA, Herrera NS, Gonzalez-Nilo FD, Aguayo DA. Paclitaxel-PHBV nanoparticles and their toxicity to endometrial and primary ovarian cancer cells. Biometer 2013; 34(16): 4098-108.

[101]   Wu W, Zheng Y, Wang R, Huang W, Liu L, Hu X. Antitumor activity of folate-targated, paclitaxel-loaded polymeric micelles on a human esophageal EC9706 cancer cell line. Int J Nanomed 2012; DOI: 10.1016/j.lfs.2012.10.024.

[102]   Rapoport N. Physical stimuli-responsive polymeric micelles for anti-cancer drug delivery. Progress in Polymer Sci 2007; 32(8-9): 962-990.

[103]   Hatefi A, Amsden B. Biodegradable inject able in situforming drug delivery systems. J Control Rel 2002; 80(1-3): 9-28.

[104]   Ichikawa H, Fukumori Y. A novel positively thermosensitive controlled release microcapsule with membrane of nano-sized poly (N-isopropylacrylamide) gel spaced in ethylcellulose matrix. J Control Rel 2000; 63(1-2): 107-119.

[105]   Mitra S, Gaur U, Ghosh PC, Maitra AN. Tumour Targeted Delivery of Encapsulated Dextran-Doxorubicin Conjugate Using Chitosan Nanoparticles as Carrier. J Control Rel 2001; 74(1-6): 317-323.

[106]   Liu R, Khullar OV, Griset AP. Paclitaxel-Loaded Expansile Nanoparticles Delay Local Recurrence in a Heterotopic Murine Non-Small Cell Lung Cancer Model. Annal Thor Surg 2011; 91: 1077-84.

[107]   Singer JW, Baker B, De Vries P, Kumar A, Shaffer S, Vawter E. Poly-(L)-glutamic acid-paclitaxel (CT-2103) [XYOTAX (TM)], a biodegradable polymeric drug conjugate— Characterization, preclinical pharmacology, and preliminary clinical data. Adv Exp Med Bio 2003; 519: 81-99.

[108]   Zhao M, Zabelina Y, Rudek MA, Wolff AC, Baker SD. A rapid and sensitive method for determination of dimethyl benzoylphenyl urea in human plasma by using LC/MS/MS. J Pharmaceu Biomed Anal 2003; 33(4): 725-733.

[109]   Sung YK, Kim SW. Advances in biodegradable polymers for drug delivery systems. Korea Polymer J 2000; 8(5): 199-208.

[110]   Na K, Lee KH, Lee DH, Bae YH. Biodegradable thermo-sensitive nanoparticles from poly(L-lactic acid)/poly(ethylene glycol) alternating multi-block copolymer for potential anti-cancer drug carrier. *Euro J Pharmaceu Sci* 2006; 27(2-3): 115-122.

[111]   Rieux DA, Fievez V, Garinot M, Schneider YJ, Preat V. Nanoparticles as potential oral delivery systems of proteins and vaccines: a mechanistic approach. J Control Rel 2006; 116(1): 1-27.

[112]   Ko J, Park K, Kim YS, Kim MS, Han JK, Kim K. Tumoral acidic extracellular pH targeting of pH-responsive MPEG-poly (beta-amino ester) block copolymer micelles for cancer therapy. *J Control Rel* 2007; 123(2): 109-115.

[113]   Gelderblom H, Verweij J, Nooter K, Sparreboom A. Cremophor EL: The drawbacks and advantages of vehicle selection for drug formulation. Eur J Cancer 2001; 37: 1590-1598.

[114]   Araki T, Kono Y, Ogawara K, Watanabe T, Ono T, Kimura T. Formulation and evaluation of paclitaxel-loaded polymeric nanoparticles composed of polyethylene glycol and polylactic acid block copolymer. Bio Pharmaceu Bull 2012; 35(8): 1306-1313.

[115] Kim JJ, Park K. Modulated insulin delivery from glucose-sensitive hydrogel dosage forms. J Control Rel 2001; 77(1-2): 39-47.

[116] Deepa G, Ashwanikumar N, Pillai JJ, Kumar GS. Polymer nanoparticles--a novel strategy for administration of Paclitaxel in cancer chemotherapy. Curr Med Chem 2012; 19(36): 6207-13.

[117] Zhang S, Zou J, Elsabahy M, Karwa AK, Li A, Moore DA. Poly(ethylene oxide)-block-polyphosphester-based paclitaxel conjugates as a platform for ultra-high paclitaxel-loaded multifunctional nanoparticles. Chem Sci 2013; 4: 2122-2126.

[118] Ohya Y, Oue H, Nagatomi K, Ouchi T. Design of Macromolecular Prodrug of Cisplatin Using Dextran with Branched Galactose Units as Targeting Moieties to Hepatoma Cells. Biomacromol 2001; 2(3): 927-933.

[119] Heffernan MJ, Murthy N. Polyketal nanoparticles: A new pH-sensitive biodegradable drug delivery vehicle. Bioconju Chem 2005; 16(6): 1340-1342.

[120] Kukreja N, Onuma Y, Daemen J, Surreys PW. The future of drug-eluting stents. Pharmacol Res 2008; 57: 171-180.

[121] Bisby RH, Mead C, Morgan CG. Active uptake of Drugs into Photosensitive Liposomes and Rapid Release on UV Photolysis. Photochem Photobio 2000; 72: 57-61.

[122] Lin Q, Huang Q, Li C, Bao C, Liu Z, Li F. Anticancer Drug Release from a Mesoporous Silica Based Nanophotocage Regulated by Either a One- or Two-Photon Process. J Am Chem Soc 2010; *132:* 10645-10647.

[123] Xiao L, Isner AB, Hilt JZ, Bhattacharyy D. Temperature responsive hydrogel with reactive nanoparticles. Appl Polymer 2012; DOI: 10.1002/app.38335.

[124] Yadav D, Suri S, Chaudhary AA, Hemant, Beg MN, Garg V. Stimuli responsive polymeric nanoparticles in regulated drug delivery for cancer. Pol J Chem Tech 2012; 14(1): 57-64.

[125] Kang H, Liu H, Zhang X, Yan J, Zhu Z, Peng L. Photoresponsive DNA-cross-linked hydrogels for controllable release and cancer therapy. Langmu 2011; 271: 399-408.

CHAPTER 8

Theranostic Metallic Nanomedicine in Oncology: New Insights and Concerns

Sohail Akhter[*,1,3], Farshad Ramazani[1], Mohammad Zaki Ahmad[2], Javed Ahmad[3], Iqbal Ahmad[3], Ziyaur Rahman[4], Saima Amin[3] and Farhan Jalees Ahmad[3]

[1]Department of Pharmaceutics, Department of Pharmaceutical Sciences, Utrecht University, Universiteitsweg 99, 3584 CG, Utrecht, The Netherlands; [2]Department of Pharmaceutics, College of Pharmacy, Najran University, Kingdom of Saudi Arabia; [3]Nanomedicine Research Lab, Department of Pharmaceutics, Faculty of Pharmacy, Jamia Hamdard, New Delhi 110062, India; [4]Irma Lerma Rangel College of Pharmacy, Texas A&M Health Science Center, Kingsville, Texas, USA

Abstract: Cancer is a leading cause of mortality at global level, with recent advancements in research of anticancer drug therapy and diagnosis resulting in modest impacts on cancer therapy. Multifunctional or theranostic metallic nanoparticles gained attention in recent years as promising therapeutic paradigms, which provide attractive vehicles for diagnosis, and therapeutic delivery of diagnostic/active agents to tumor specific cells. Here, we discuss the cancer patho-physiology that acts as barrier in conventional chemotherapy and multidimensional aspects of metallic nanoparticles for effective cancer therapy, with particular focus on clinical stages. Keeping in mind the growing research in clinical application of metallic nanomedicines, toxicity and regulatory concerns related with these nanometric systems are also addressed in this review.

Keywords: Active targeting, cancer therapy, EPR, metallic nanoparticles, passive targeting, regulatory, theranostic nanoparticles, toxicity.

INTRODUCTION

In general, intracellular transport of therapeutically active substance, particularly in cancer, appears as one of the key problems with the drug delivery system. Conventionally, first line treatment of solid tumor is surgical removal followed by

---

*Address correspondence to Sohail Akhter: Department of Pharmaceutics, Department of Pharmaceutical Sciences, Utrecht University, Universiteitsweg 99, 3584 CG, Utrecht, The Netherlands; Tel: +31649517651; E-mails: sohailakhtermph@gmail.com, S.Akhtar@uu.nl

Atta-ur-Rahman & M. Iqbal Choudhary (Eds)

regimen of chemotherapy and or radiation treatment. Unfortunately, these strategies often fail and patient must discontinue the chemotherapy before the complete eradication of tumor due to severe side effects [1, 2]. At present, various anticancer agents are available that belong to different categories like plant origin, hormones, enzymes, biological, semi synthetic and synthetic molecules. However, they have certain therapeutics and toxicological limitations [3]. Distribution of drug within the cellular and tissue structure essentially depends upon its physiochemical properties, pKa, hydrophilicity, polarity and electrostatic charges, but these criteria do not necessarily fit in the characteristic of tumor cell because concentration of drug can be distributed towards healthy tissue rather than targeted ones, and this is the main limiting factor for conventional chemotherapy and imaging [4]. Furthermore, most of the anticancer drugs are not soluble in water or physiological solution, this limiting factor necessitates the use of pharmaceutical solvent for the administration of drugs that may cause life threatening effects [1, 5]. Consequently, conventional anticancer therapy by systemic delivery of chemotherapeutic agents often fails or inadequately delivers the drug to target cell/tissue and has a tremendous impact on reducing the quality and expectancy of life. Other associated disadvantages with current conventional anticancer therapy imaging technology include - inefficient cell entry, uptake by the immune system and mononuclear phagocyte system, accumulation of drugs in non-targeted organs and tissues, non-selectivity with high toxicity against normal tissues [6].

The effectiveness of a cancer therapeutic device is measured by its ability to reduce and eliminate tumors without damaging healthy tissues. The ultimate goal of anticancer therapy should include increased survival time and improved quality of life of the patient. Therefore, the utmost need for the treatment of tumor is the designing of drug delivery systems that can selectively deliver anti-cancer agents to the target tissue with high localized bioavailability thereby achieving therapeutic efficacy while minimizing toxic side effects. Therefore, new cancer therapy must deliver theranostic therapeutics agents that are capable of destroying the heterogeneous population of tumor cell. Drug delivery systems, such as nanometer-sized carriers have been shown to improve the treatment of cancer with reduced dosing frequency and lesser side effects [7-12]. Advancement in nanotechnology based drug delivery and imaging techniques allow more specific mapping of tumor cell, increase therapeutic index of drugs through site specificity, their ability to escape from multi-drug resistance, and the controlled delivery of therapeutic agent [2, 13].

The usefulness of metallic nanoparticles in cancer therapy is mainly derived from their potential to carry a large dose of drug which results into high concentration of anticancer drugs at desired site, thus avoiding toxicity arising due to high concentration of drug in other body tissues. In recent years, metallic nanoparticles showed potential application in field of magnetic resonance imaging (MRI) and colloidal mediators for cancer magnetic hyperthermia [14]. Advantages with the use of metallic nanoparticles based probe system in cancer therapeutics include: 1) it contains tumor targeting ligands that bind to particular tumor cells and are capable of sequestering anticancer drugs exclusively within tumor; therefore, 2) reduces the accumulation of the drugs in healthy organs; 3) has large surface area to a volume ratio, that provides a surface for chemical modification that improves cell entry; 4) protects the therapeutic agent from the biological milieu; and 5) improves bioavailability of the anticancer agent [15-20]. Furthermore, theranostic nanoparticles can detect and attack the heterogeneous crowd of tumor cell. The theranostic nature of metallic nanoparticles is briefly represented in Fig. (**1**). Despite all these advantages, metallic nanoparticles are still at early stages of development. So far, some of the great achievements have been attained in this area but many challenges still remain. However, their multidirectional rapid development with improved practical potential of metallic nanoparticles highlights their potency as novel tools for future cancer therapeutics modalities. The advance techniques in cancer therapeutics are progressing very quickly both, in terms of newly discovered anticancer agents and the ways of delivering both new and old anticancer agents. The application of metallic nanoparticles in cancer therapeutics probably is the largest public health contribution of Nano science. In this review, we are going to address the background, recent development and patent, application and overview of the risk assessment in the area of metallic nanoparticles as a probe and novel drug delivery carrier in cancer therapeutics.

THERANOSTIC METALLIC NANOPARTICLES

Most important characteristics of nanoparticles are their size, encapsulation efficiency, zeta potential (surface charge), and release characteristics. Since theranostic metallic nanoparticles can combine a specific targeting and therapeutic agent, they have been designed for simultaneous imaging, and targeting of cytotoxic agents. A simple proposed diagrammatic presentation of multiple functional metallic nanoparticles is given here in Fig. (**1**).

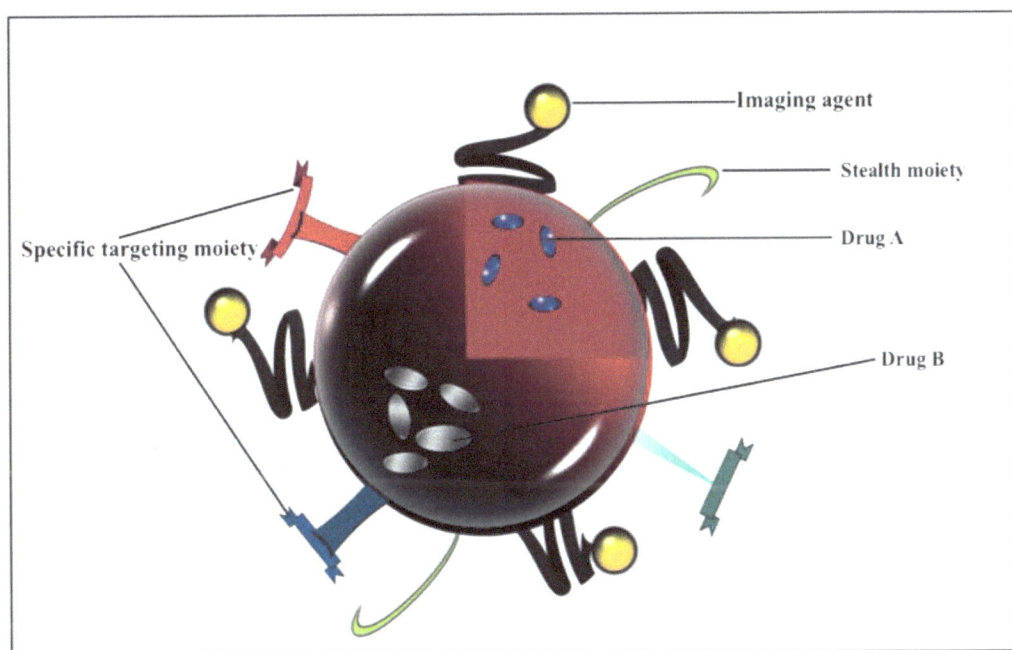

Fig. (1): Theranostic metallic nanoparticle with specific targeting and therapeutic agent.

Theranostic metallic nanoparticles can detect the early stage of cancer and deliver therapeutic agents to target tissue/organ to enhance therapeutics efficacy. They have been designed to simultaneously carry a drug, a ligand responsible for targeted delivery (for example, antibodies) and or any contrast agent. This type of theranostic character can be used to identify tumor cell, release specific antitumor drug and to monitor the treatment efficacy in time limit. Theranostic nanoparticles can also help overcome multiple drug resistance by delivering antitumor drug to tumor cell without launching the glycoprotein pump [21-33].

Site Specific Delivery and Biological Consideration

Conventionally, anticancer drugs are designed with relatively low molecular weight and have an agreement between hydrophilic and liphophilic balance (HLB), hence allowing partition across the lipid membrane very easily. Therefore, drug within systemic circulation rapidly gets distributed throughout the body, reaching non-targeted tissue/organ, and also rapidly metabolized by liver and or rapidly excreted by kidney [22-25]. For effective drug targeting, it is essential that a drug-targeting system should not be eliminated quickly. Ideally, drug carrier should provide a pharmacokinetic profile that will allow the drug to interact with its target [6, 34]. During the designing of metallic nanoparticles, the painstaking lesson learned from the polymer based and liposomal drug delivery system must be taken into consideration. Since, upon intravenous injection, the unprotected liposomal and polymer based drugs are rapidly cleared from blood by Reticuloendothelial System and accumulate in liver conditioning their rapid first pass metabolism from the systemic circulation followed by metabolic degradation and excretion. This consideration is very beneficial while designing metallic nanoparticles intended for cancer therapeutics located close by the mononuclear phagocyte system [35-39].

The performance of nanoparticles inside the vascular compartment is controlled by a complex array of factors such as shape, density nanoparticles size distribution and surface characteristics. All these factors control the flow properties of nanoparticle, bifurcation in vascular compartment as well as modulation of circulation time, and mode of entry into cell [34, 40-45].

Escaping Clearance by the Reticuloendothelial System

A major barrier that drug delivery system must be able to avoid in the systemic circulation is the removal of delivery system or drug by phagocytic cells of Mononuclear Phagocytes System (MPS). Since nanoparticles are usually taken up by the liver, spleen and other parts of the RES depending on their surface characteristics and undergo opsonization in the blood and clearance by RES [18, 46-50], the MPS presents a significant barrier to effective drug targeting, because it has the ability to filter out and destroy a drug delivery system unless appropriate formulation approaches are used to avoid the same. Therefore the nanoparticles should be designed to avoid these interactions and possible clearance from the vascular compartment, particularly opsonization process must be avoided. Opsonization is a process in which surface of the foreign particle such as bacteria and particulate drug carrier is coated with blood protein, known as opsins. The phagocytosis of these tagged particles is enhanced, because surface receptors present on phagocytes bind to opsonins and the foreign particle is engulfed and untimely digested by various lysosomes [40, 50-53]. For example, when unprotected colloidal gold nanoparticles were intravenously injected into mouse, it was observed that 95% of gold nanoparticles were cleared from vascular compartment within 10 minutes [26]. Therefore, suppression of opsonization, avoiding MPS recognition and receptor mediated phagocytosis are primary concerns while designing metallic nanoparticles.

A more practical approach to avoid RES uptake and clearance of nanoparticles is the modification of nanoparticles surface. For example, by increasing surface hydrophilicity *i.e.* adding a hydrophilic polymer coat to the metallic nanoparticles carrier makes them invisible to the RES and thus reduces opsonization and suppresses macrophage recognition. This coating is referred to as stealth moiety. Most commonly used stealth agents include polyethylene glycol (PEG) and block copolymer [54, 55]. Fig. (**1**) representing the stealth moiety on nanoparticles surface. It has been proposed that PEG has high local concentration of hydrated group which sterically inhibits the interaction with blood-born opsins [34]. Intravenous injection of sterically stabilized nanoparticles results in prolonged circulation time, and their accumulation in tumor [56-63].

Other factors affecting the opsin binding are physicochemical properties of nanoparticles *i.e.* surface characteristics such as size, surface charge in the characteristics bio-distribution and residence times of these particles *in vivo* [39, 64-70]. Neutral systems tend to remain longer in blood circulation but their charged counterparts are cleared by RES readily [2, 39]. Similarly particle size of around 1-2 micron undergoes phagocytosis and higher size *i.e.* around 6 micron is trapped in lungs capillaries [34]. Therefore, to avoid clearance by RES, metallic nanoparticles should be formulated not more than 100 nm in size and should have sterically stabilized neutral surface.

Passive Targeting of Tumor Cells by Metallic Nanoparticles

In passive targeting, the biodistribution of nanoparticles is mediated by MPS physiological condition. In passive targeting, we take the advantage of pathological condition of tumor to allow the accumulation of drug carrier at the target site [71]. For example, the pH or specific enzymes present within tumor cell can be used to facilitate the release of drugs from nanoparticles. Enzymes such as alkaline phosphatases and plasmids are present at higher level at tumor site. When the volume of tumor becomes 2 cubic millimeter, it becomes diffusion limited, and this diffusion limitation is overcome by angiogenesis (growth of new capillary in cell/ tissue) [72]. In tumor cell, one of the characteristic features of angiogenesis is that it has aberrant tortuosity and abnormalities in basement membrane [73]. Since tumor cell generally lacks the well defined lymphatic system, interstitial pressure becomes maximum at center of tumor. This incomplete vasculature of tumor results in leaky blood vessels (capillary). This hyper permeability of tumor vasculature is a key feature in passive targeting of drug carrier [74-77]. Due to leaky vasculature and poor lymphatic drainage drug carriers which are trapped in the tumor vasculature and release their loaded drug, this is called Enhanced Permeation and Retention (EPR) effect [62, 78, 79]. Fig. (**2**) represents the capillary with Enhanced Permeability at tumor sites. However, the problem associated with EPR is the accumulation of nanoparticles in blood capillaries near the healthy cells which can be recognized by MPS [80].

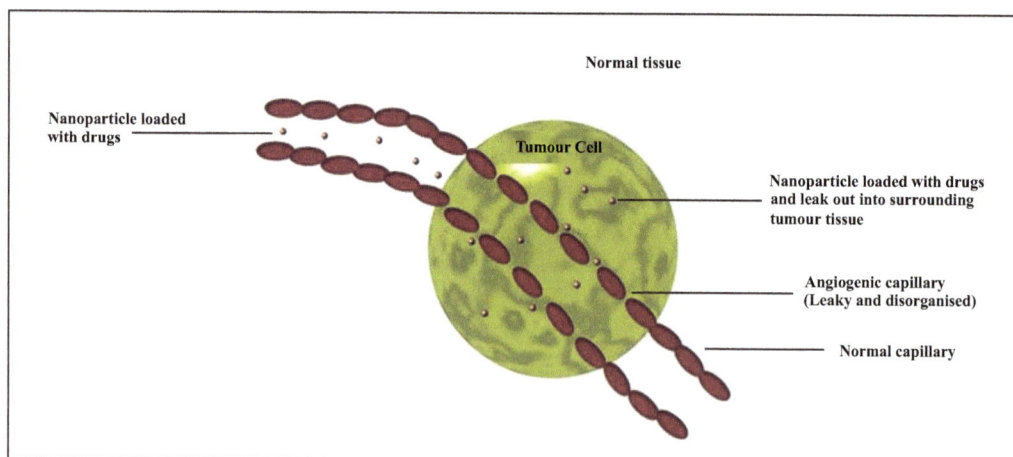

Fig. (2): Figure shows the capillary with Enhanced Permeability at tumor sites which facilitates the escape of drug loaded nanoparticles from the circulation and enhances the EPR.

Active Tumor Targeting with Metallic Nanoparticles

Since passive targeting does not necessarily assure the internalization of nanoparticles by targeted cell, therefore nanoparticles are modified with molecular targeting ligands for active targeting of tumor. Active targeting of metallic nanoparticles involves the interaction between peripherally conjugated targeting moiety and a corresponding receptor to facilitate the targeting of a carrier to specific malignant cell [81-83]. Various molecules are used to facilitate the active targeting of nanoparticles, such as aptamers [84, 85], proteins and antibodies [86-89]. The bioconjugation of ligands, such as monoclonal antibodies, proteins, or peptides to the nanocarrier surface, has been exploited on many nanoparticles for the purpose of concentrating therapeutic action to specific tumor cell [2, 7, 19, 36, 89-92].

Recent Patents on Metallic Nanoparticles Technology

There are lots of research being carried out on possible cancer therapeutics and cancer imaging techniques. Metallic nanoparticle devices are being developed for the early detection of tumor cell, imaging of cancer cell and targeted drug delivery to the cancer cell. Recently, a number of patents were generated in this area. The aim of this review is to discuss these patents and their claims. Patent number 6,165440 assigned to the Board of Regents, The University of Texas System describes interaction of electromagnetic pulse and ultrasonic radiation with nanoparticles for enhancement of drug delivery in solid tumor [93]. They claimed that nanoparticles can be attached to the antibodies targeted against antigens on the surface of tumor cells. Cavitation induced by ultrasonic wave results in perforation of cancer cell membrane, and therefore, provides enhanced delivery of therapeutic agents from blood into cancer cells. Patent number 6,689,338, assigned to the Board of Regents for Oklahoma State University describes the diagnosis and treatment of cancer by bioconjugates of nanoparticles as radiopharmaceuticals for use in connections with radioimmuno-therapy and radioimmunodetection [94]. Their claim reports that nanoparticle is covalently linked to a biological vector due to radioactive metal ion (metal sulfide or metal oxide). This biological vector may be monoclonal antibody or fragment of antibody. This bioconjugate has utility as an effective radiopharmaceutical to deliver a radiolabel in cancer treatment. Patent number 1651957 deals with process of preparing nanoparticles comprising a magnetic particle coated with a phosphor fluoride [95]. These nanoparticles can be used as both solid phase carrier which can be manipulated by a magnet and fluorescent labels for various types of immunoassay, DNA/RNA hybridization, affinity purification, cell separation and other industrial, medical and diagnostic applications. Patent number 2277548 describes the fabrication and evaluation of nanoparticles having a core comprising a magnetic material of gold, platinum or silver atoms which are covalently linked to a plurality of ligands and their composition is used in the treatment of a cancer by applying a high frequency magnetic field to kill cancer cells [96]. The present invention relates particularly to magnetic nanoparticles having immobilized ligands and their use in treating the conditions involving carbohydrate mediated interactions, potentially overcoming the difficulty in modulating the polyvalent interactions. Patent number 1746610 invention falls within nanotechnology applications. Applications are likewise in biomedicine, as tools for biomolecule recognition, in nuclear magnetic resonance imaging, drug-release control or hyperthermia treatments [97]. The nanoparticles of the present invention can be employed instead of radioactive materials used as tracers for the release of drugs and in a method of hyperthermia treatment. An external AC magnetic field is applied for locally heating a region such as tumor zone, in which the magnetic nanoparticles have been deposited or accumulated and have favored site specific accumulation of the nanoparticles. Patent number 3177868 describes the composition and methods for the treatment of cancer using a bioconjugated nanoparticle comprising a biocompatible quantum dot conjugated to a target moiety [98]. It claimed that the quantum dot, upon excitation by soft X-rays emits electromagnetic radiation of ultraviolet region, thereby allowing the disruption of the DNA found in cancer cell. Patent number 2010152 describes the use of a biocompatible nanoparticle in combination with an external non-oscillating magnetic field, for the manufacturing of a pharmaceutical composition to prevent or treat a cancer [99]. Biocompatible nanoparticle in the form of an oxide or a hydroxide of iron, nickel, cobalt and the biocompatible shell is made of a material consisting of silica, gold, alumina, sugar, PEG and dextran. Patent No.6767635 assigned to Biomedical Apherse system Gabh (Jena: DE) invention relates to magnetic nanoparticles, their production and use [100]. The object of the invention is to provide nanoparticles capable of specifically forming bonds to intracellular biomacromolecules even in the intracellular region of cells, so that separation is possible by exposure to an exterior magnetic field. This is accomplished by means of magnetic nanoparticles having biochemical activity, consisting of a magnetic core particle and an envelope layer fixed to the core particle (see Table **1**).

Table 1: **Different Patents Illustrating the Application of Theranostic Metallic Nanoparticles in Cancer**

Patent Number	Patent Title	Invention Relates to	Year	Refs.
US 6165440	Radiation and nanoparticles for enhancement of drug delivery in solid tumors	Interaction of electromagnetic pulse and ultrasonic radiation with nanoparticles for enhancement of drug delivery in solid tumors	2000	[93]
US 6689338	Bioconjugates of nanoparticles as radiopharmaceuticals	Bioconjugates of the titanium oxide nanoparticles having utility as an effective radiopharmaceutical to deliver a radiolabel in tumor treatment	2004	[94]
EP 1651957	Fluorescent magnetic nanoparticles and process of preparation	Magnetic particles coated with a phosphor fluoride can be used as both solid phase carrier which can be manipulated by a magnet and fluorescent labels for various types of medical and diagnostic applications	2011	[95]
EP 2277548	Magnetic nanoparticles linked to a ligand	Nanoparticles having a core comprising a magnetic material are covalently linked to a plurality of ligands and their use in the treating conditions involving carbohydrate mediated interactions	2013	[96]
EP 1746610	Magnetic nanoparticles of noble metals	Application of magnetic nanoparticles as tools for biomolecule recognition, in nuclear magnetic resonance imaging, drug-release control or hyperthermia treatments	2012	[97]
US3177868	Bioconjugated nanoparticles	Biocompatible quantum dot conjugated to a target moiety which emits ultraviolet radiation to disrupt DNA in cancer cells	2008	[98]
EP 2010152	Magnetic nanoparticles compositions and uses thereof	Use of biocompatible nanoparticles in combination with an external non-oscillating magnetic field to prevent or treat a cancer	2011	[99]
US 6767635	Magnetic nanoparticles having biochemical activity, method for the production thereof and their use	Magnetic nanoparticles capable of specifically binding to a binding domain of an intracellular biomacromolecule	2004	[100]

RECENT DEVELOPMENT AND FUTURE PROSPECTIVE

There is a long historical support for the application of metallic nanoparticles in biological system for the diagnostic and therapeutic rationales [26]. However, use of metallic nanoparticles in cancer therapeutics has recently been reported [92,

101, 102]. Metallic nanoparticles have the ability to treat as well as diagnose the disease and can be termed as theranostics [103]. For example, light activated theranostic nanoparticles have been reported for imaging and treatment of brain tumor [104].

Iron nanoparticles have been used as theranostic agents with specific application as contrasting agents for Magnetic Resonance Imaging (MRI) and magnetically targeted drug delivery to the tumor cells [105-110]. Mainly two types of iron oxide nanoparticles have been reported as imaging agents [105, 111], superparamagnetic iron oxides (SPIOs) and ultra-small superparamagnetic iron oxides (USPIOs). Major advantages associated with SPIOs are biocompatible and biodegradable properties of iron, which can be recycled *via* normal biochemical pathway for iron metabolism [112]. Hepatic imaging was the first application of these magnetic nanoparticles, which was possible because normal liver cell absorbed SPIOs, which resulted in darkening of image, however cancerous cells were not able to take up the SPIOs, thus resulting in bright spot in tumor cell [113-116].

There are many reports in which SPIOs have been used in combination with monoclonal antibodies to detect a variety of cancers [117-120]. Transferrin and pancreatic receptors are over expressed in some tumors [121, 122]. SPIOs have been conjugated with peptide to target these receptors and imaging of the cancer cell. Zhao reported that when SPIOs were linked with peptide synaptotagmin, they enabled the imaging of cell undergoing apoptosis after chemotherapy.

Currently, several anticancer drugs such as doxorubicin, methotrexate and paclitaxel have been formulated with metallic nanoparticles [123-126]. Similarly, Liang *et al.* demonstrated the ability of radionuclide's containing SPIOs to specifically induce cell death in liver cell *in vitro* [127]. In another investigation, Ross *et al.* successfully demonstrated the therapeutics application of SPIOs, when SPIOs were decorated with antibody Herceptin to target the Her2/ neu receptor in early stages of breast cancer [128].

Nowadays, semiconductor nanoparticles called Quantum dots have been increasingly applied as imaging and labeling probe in cancer therapeutics [129-

132]. Major advantages associated with Quantum dots include high quantum yield, resistance to chemical modification and intrinsic fluorescence emission spectra due to which Quantum particles attain the capability of sensing and releasing anticancer drugs at desired site (Fig. **3**).

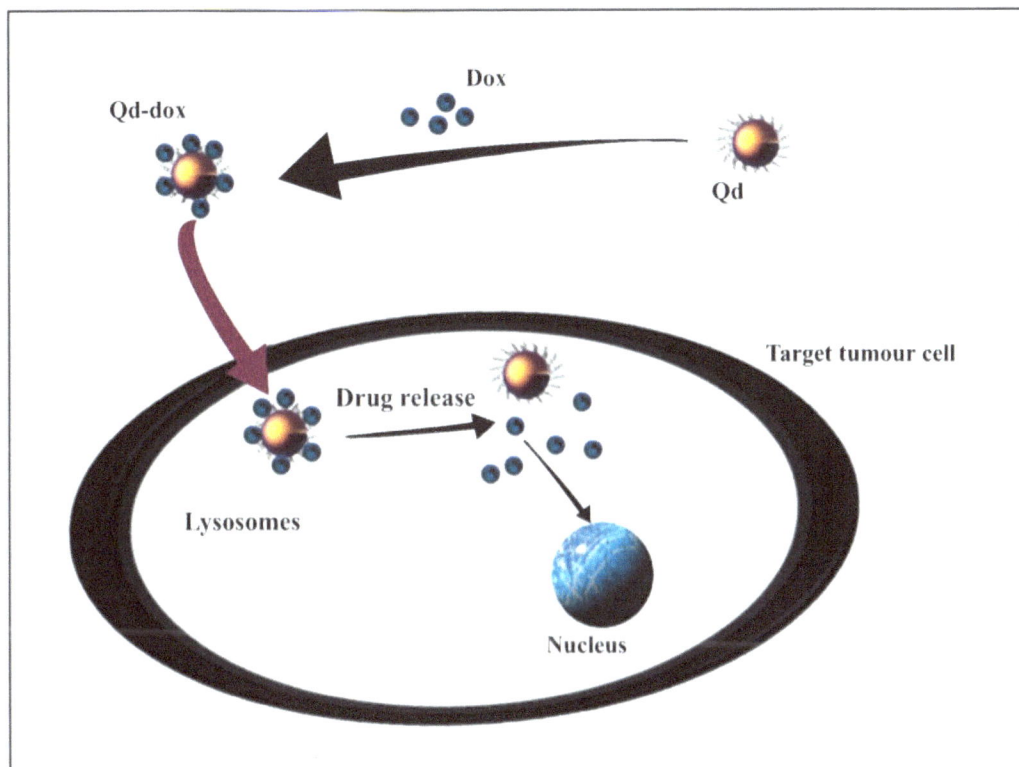

Fig. (3). Illustration of Quantum dots (Qd) - Doxorubicin (Dox) Conjugate as a targeted tumor imaging, sensing and therapy.

Gold nanoparticles have several attractive advantages for diagnostic and therapeutic applications, for example their easy decoration with antibody for tumor specific targeting, biocompatibility and stability [129, 133]. Metallic gold nanoparticles have been extensively studied for their potential application in targeted tumor cell drug delivery [134-140].

Application of gold nanoshells was first reported by Hirish and co-workers in 2003 in hyperthermal therapy of tumor cell [141]. In 2005, Loo *et al.* reported the conjugation of gold nanoshells with hER2 antibody to target breast carcinoma cells [142]. When shape of gold nanoparticles changes from that of nanoparticles to nanorods, their absorption and scattering wavelength also change from visible to near infra red (NIR) region [102], due to which gold nanorods can be used as contrast agents for dual molecular imaging. As follow-up work by Hainfed *et al.* combination of gold nanoparticles followed by X-ray treatment was reported to reduce the size of tumor cell in mice [143]. In one of the investigations, Haung *et al.* reported that cellular uptake of gold nanorods was increased by two fold in malignant cells when gold nanoparticles were conjugated with antibody to target antiepidermal growth factor receptor [144].

Metallic nanoparticles have large impact on cancer treatment. Traditionally, although the diagnosis and treatment were considered as two separate entities in the process of cancer therapy, the marriage of biology, chemistry and physics at nanoscale led to the emergence of metallic nanoparticle technology that blurred the boundary between diagnosis and treatment. Hence, these two (diagnosis and treatment) separate clinical processes were soon merged as a single process that improved the delivery of nanoparticle probe loaded with anticancer agent(s) into cell and cellular compartment. Early diagnosis and targeted drug delivery in cancer therapeutics are the priority research area in which metallic nanoparticles are hoped to play a vital role. Metallic nanoparticles have been gradually developed as new modalities for targeted drug delivery and diagnosis in cancer therapeutics. Despite all these advantages, metallic nanoparticles are still at early stages of development. Some of the great achievements have been attained in this field but many challenges still remain. However, their development is rapid and multidirectional, improved practical potential of metallic nanoparticles highlights their potency as novel tools for future cancer therapeutics modalities. Research activities aimed toward achieving specific and targeted delivery of anticancer agents have expanded tremendously in last 10 years. However, quite less research has been performed on magnetic nanoparticle probes for intracellular molecular imaging. Although significant effort has been devoted to develop a metallic nanoparticles drug delivery system, metallic nano-platforms are still at their infancy stage of development and much more research is required to overcome the problems associated with the nanoparticle properties influencing *in vitro* and *in vivo* toxicity assays.

Toxicity and its Assessment

Apart from the immense importance of nanomaterials in cancer imaging and therapy, their toxic effects are also a major concern especially after chronic administration. Different polymers are associated with various toxicities like complement activation, carcinogenicity, teratogenicity, and immunogenicity. Thus, choosing safe polymers for the design of nanoparticles is itself a major hurdle. Careful evaluation of the potential toxicity of residual solvent, polymer and the developed particle is critically important. Presently, non toxic and biodegradable ingredients are used to design nanoparticles due to which toxicities associated with the carrier molecules as such tend to be mild. However, particular nanoparticles increase the accumulation of drugs in the liver, spleen, and bone marrow, with the chance of increased toxicities to these organs. Many studies have identified liver as the primary organ responsible for reticuloendothelial capture of nanoparticles, often due to phagocytosis by Kupffer cells and this function has been shown to be a main mechanism of hepatic clearance from the blood circulation following the intravenous injection. Among the nanomedicines, metallic nano-carriers have extensively been evaluated for their toxicity and interaction with biological system. Depending on the nature and type of metallic nanoparticles [MNPs], different grades of toxicity have been reported at cells, tissues, organs or at protein levels due to their physiochemical properties (e.g; size, shape, electric charge on the surface, chemical composition, surface structure, surface reactivity, surface group, inorganic or organic coatings, solubility and aggregation behavior). The mechanisms of toxicity induced by MNPs are the combination of different events such as direct destruction of cellular components like DNA, RNA and proteins due to free radical conversion. Moreover, increased oxidative stress plays its key role as well [145]. Metallic nanoparticles influence the reproductive organs as it was found that particles may reduce spermatogonial cell proliferation [145, 146]. Free radical generation and induction of inflammatory mediator are considered as the factors for such effect [147]. Besides their effect on male reproductive organ, Browning *et al. also* reported the effect of MNPs over female reproductive system in an animal experiment [148]. They confirmed that gold nanoparticles can diffuse into the embryo and lead to teratogenic deformities [149]. Increased surface activity due to reduction in particle size (increase in surface area: volume ratio) influences the interaction of MNPs to the biological system [103]. This correlation gets strengthened from the report of De and co-workers that illustrated that colloidal gold nanoparticles with smaller size (10-50 nm) cause more toxicity in comparison to the larger particles (100-200 nm) [150]. Moreover, Chen *et al.* studied the oral toxicity of copper nanoparticles that was in corroboration with the above finding and indicated that with the decrease in particle size, LD_{50} value of copper nanoparticles increases sharply [151]. In another report, it was pointed out that gold nanoparticles with the size of 2.8 to 38 nm were more toxic and induced immunological response [152]. Size dependent adverse effect of silver nanoparticles was found in *in vitro* study on hepatocytes indicating the decreased mitochondrial functions, LDG leakage and abnormal cell morphologies [153]. Influence of the surface charge on the metallic nanoparticles was also addressed in the literature. Recently, dose dependent deteriorating viability and capacity of nerve cells were seen in case of anionic MNPs [154]. However, *in vivo* findings on MNPs toxicity were also reported but majority of the data on the toxicity of MNPs were the outcome of *in vitro* testing. Therefore, more and more *in vivo* models for biological interaction and toxicity testing are needed to be carried out. It is promising to look that various efforts are being taken for lessening the uptake of nanoparticles by MPs cells and to increase their accumulation in the active site through surface modification and/or incorporating targeting ligands to the polymers/nanoparticles [155, 156]. For example, a clinical study conducted on Doxil (PEG-liposome loaded with doxorubicin) showed a reduction in cardiotoxicity over that of doxorubicin [157]. Similarly, Abraxane (albumin nanoparticles loaded with paclitaxel) was found to show an increased therapeutic efficacy as compared to free paclitaxel. On the basis of reports, diagrammatically, the toxic effects of nanomedicines on different body organs are exemplified in Fig. (**4**).

In formulation development of nanomedicine, PEGylation is the most common technique used to prolong the nano-carrier circulation. Moreover, plenty of published papers on this subject indicate that such hydrophilic polymer coating reduces the nanoparticles associated toxicity. Regardless of the prevalent use of PEGylation for prolonging the circulation of nanomedicine, its mechanism for such action and interaction with biological system in systemic circulation is not entirely clear. In fact, PEG has been shown to form a brush border over the

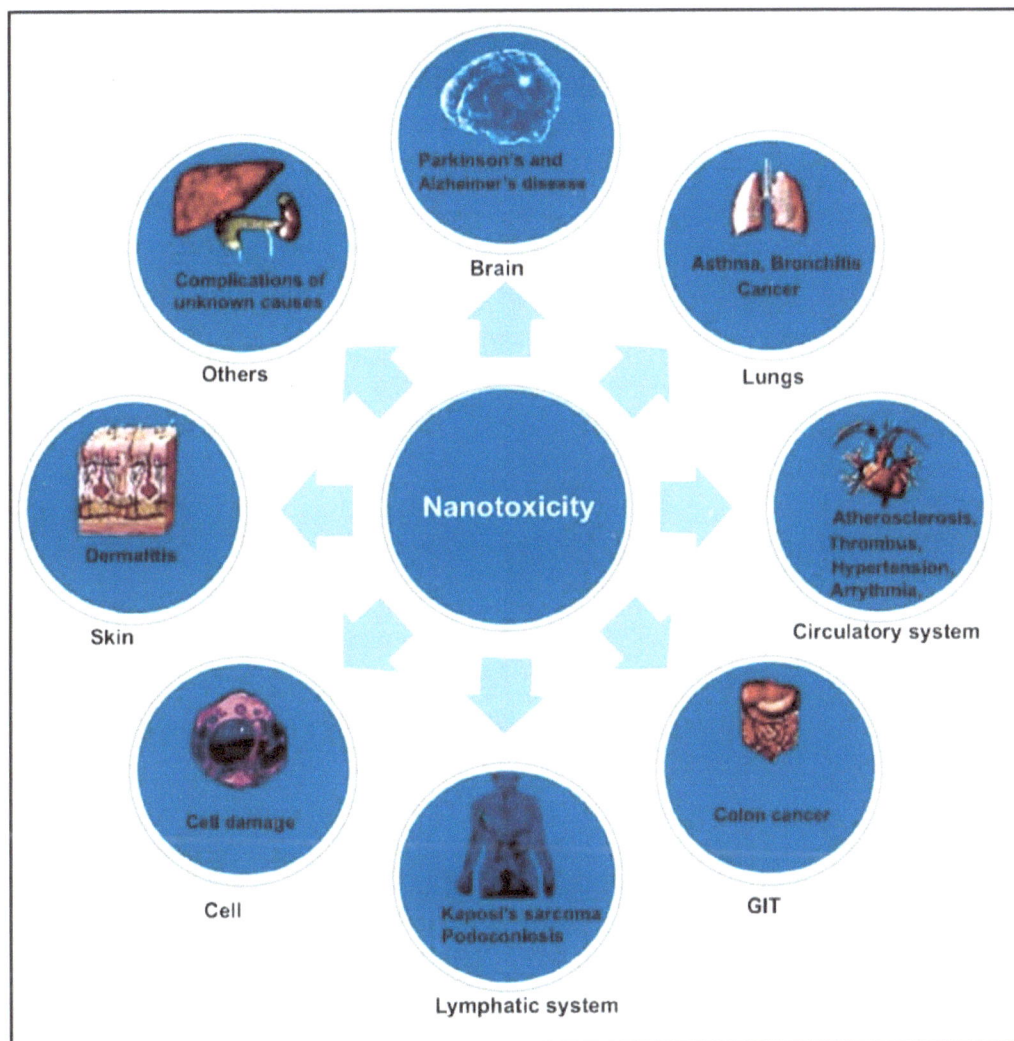

Fig. (4): Highlighting the different body organs that may be affected under the influence of MNPs [166].

nanomedicine surface that leads to nonspecific impermeable hindrance and sterically prevents access of tissue proteins [158]. Chain length, density, conformational freedom and flexibility of PEG would be critical in making the nanomedicine surface free from interaction [159]. Although such kind of coating provides nonspecific shielding but it was found that in case of PEGylated hexadecyl cyanoacrylate nanoparticles, PEG was able to reduce the adsorption of ApoC and immunoglobulins, but not with the other proteins [160]. Similarly, with uncharged liposome (made up of phosphatidylcholine and cholesterol) and liposome with negative charge (made up of phosphatidic acid), coating with PEG-DSPE 2000 does not provide shielding from protein adsorption [160]. Even with significant prolongation of nanomedicine circulation time and clearance half-life by PEGylation, some issues are still need to be addressed. Recently, several reports have been published that indicate the quick clearance of PEGylated liposomes [161]. This effect is attributed to the formation of PEG-specific antibodies that prompt complement absorption [160]. Besides this, folic acid stabilized metallic nanoparticles resulting receptor mediated endocytosis and tumor specific delivery of theranostic agent in a more significant way. Mironava *et al.* observed preferential penetration of folic acid coated nanoparticles into keratinocytes and mammary breast cancer cells with significantly low IC$_{50}$ value compared to normal cells [162]. In another study, Wei *et al.* found that iron oxide (Fe$_3$O$_4$) nanoparticles coated with WSG peptides resulted in good cellular compatibility in cell viability assay and could more easily be assembled into the cancer cell [163]. Thus, the WSG-coated Fe$_3$O$_4$ nanoparticles could be promising in cancer diagnosis and treatment due to tumor cells targeting peptides. Therefore, it should be noted that expression of specific antibodies to the particles or coating material may affect the pharmacokinetics, efficacy and the safety of nanomedicines.

In Vitro Cells and Gene Based Toxicity

To generate the information on toxicity, studies at different levels (*in vitro*, *in vivo* and biochemical) must be carried out. Although, *in vitro* studies may overcome the animal based experiment and animal studies complexities, they may also decrease accuracy and *in vitro-in vivo* correlation. However, they allow for a level of control well suited for elucidating toxic effects and their mechanism at molecular level which is extremely difficult to interpret in *in vivo* studies. A gene based approach (DNA strand breaks, chromosome damages and gene mutations *etc.*) has the advantage of assessing toxicity at low dose level and may express carcinogenic effect which may not be monitored through cytotoxicity studies. The nature and mechanism of interaction between nanoparticles and molecular and cellular targets can be elucidated by TEM, SEM or X-ray based microscopy. This ongoing advancement looks forward to solve the concerns like adsorption, absorption and associated processes such as diffusion and endocytosis *etc.*

Oxidative Stress and Reactive Oxygen Species (ROS)

Reduction of size at nanoscale leads to conversion of normal particle to a highly active charged particle, which on interaction with cellular components and biological process generates ROS and oxidant injury. This paradigm may be used to evaluate the toxic potential of nanoparticles [103]. Oxidative stress occurs when ROS production exceeds the defense capacity of the system and in such circumstances damage of biomolecules like lipid, DNA, RNA, mitochondria and proteins *etc.* results in excess cell proliferation, apoptosis, lipid peroxidation and mutation. Metallic and inorganic nanoparticles are known to induce oxidative stress through ROS generation during redox reaction by interruption of the electronic flux, perturbation of the permeability transition and diminution of protective cellular component like glutathione [164, 165]. ROS production can be monitored through ESR or with the use of fluorescent spectroscopy with or without quenchers such as furfuryl alcohol and superoxide dismutase. Furthermore, within a living cell this activity can be monitored through fluorescence microscope or confocal microscopy with the use of fluorescent dye such as dichlorofluorescein diacetate or FITC. In addition, change in intracellular free calcium, mitochondrial function and structural integrity also serve as the tool to study the ROS production and associated oxidative stress.

REGULATORY APPREHENSION

Viewing positive impact on the impaired quality of life in life threatening diseases like cancer, current market and progressive result of clinical trials in nanomedicines is well evident. However, involvement of these R & D outcomes to the clinical practice still needs to be rationalized and carefully controlled in terms of risk to benefit ratio. These steps and clinical practice are carefully overseen by regulatory authorities such as FDA, MHRA and EMEA, *etc.* to ensure that the new medicines, diagnostic agents and devices are safe for clinical practice in terms of the risk-benefit ratio. For any such products, the agencies have a set of protocols that basically work for the assessment of three parameters:

quality, safety and efficacy. Production of nanomedicines is already in clinical practice and some of these nanomedicines are now in the phase of generic development. Both generic manufacturers and regulatory agencies are struggling to finalize the studies that are required to demonstrate the bio-equivalency of nanometric generic medicines compared to the innovator and the developed generic nanomedicines and whether they have the same physicochemical properties and are safe and effective. This setback was clearly visualized with several unproductive efforts in the generic development of nab-paclitaxel formulation. The claimed bio-similar of nab-paclitaxel, when evaluated, did not fit to reproduce particle size, stability, potency and other physicochemical attributes of nab-paclitaxel. Moreover, unlike nab-paclitaxel, the reconstituted nanomedicines exhibited poor stability when evaluated for accelerated stability testing and formed aggregates even within 24 h of study period. Pharmaceutical/chemical properties and/or bioequivalence may not sufficiently symbolize the function of the nanomedicines at the site of action, as assumed for standard preparations. In addition, several liposomal formulations available in market those containing amphotericin B and doxorubicin have recently gone off patent. The lack of critical information regarding composition, dimensional configuration of components and critical parameters that are essential for function of nanomedicines, raises the concern of risk that "generic" may be approved based on the guidelines compiled with conventional manufacturing and bioequivalence standards for generic drug approvals but which may result in substandard products in the market. This exemplifies that how generic nanomedicine manufacturers and regulatory authorities are going to face troubles in their development and approval. So, it is crucial that a comprehensive physicochemical based understanding of nanomedicine and recognition of critical parameters that affect their functions be conducted early in development stage to put down a defined rule for such generics in near future. Indeed, FDA has recently begun to consider relevant approval standards for generic copies of nanomedicines. Recently issued guideline in case of doxorubicin loaded liposome (Doxil®) is an example which is reliable with this approach. Current scenario illustrates that ample of nanomedicines have defined the clinical pharmacokinetics; considering this, there is an imperative need to improve the pharmacokinetic models for such nanometric medicines. Considerations such as pathophysiology, target tissue, ADME, impact of their size and surface characteristics on organ, tissue and cellular localization and better understanding of PK-PD correlations need to be addressed in experimental models. Moreover, quantitative techniques need to be strengthened for biodistribution study of polymers and metals. In the context of polymeric and metallic nanomedicine therapeutics, new carrier systems are being developed with newer complex architectures (*e.g.* dendrimers, quantum dots, SPIONs and theranostic gold nanomaterials, *etc.*) and such carrier systems may be given by different routes such as pulmonary, i.v and organ directed injection. With the increased complexity of the architecture, induction of multifunctionality in single carrier system frequently falls into a gap between medicines to medical devices regulation. It is noted that biological and medical devices assessment guidelines are based on general and nonspecific standards. Still the standard validation specifications for nanomedicines are lacking in current formats of regulatory guidelines and such complications will probably push the introduction of completely new set of regulatory guidelines. Moreover, a regulatory guideline addressing new nanometric devices and different categories of medicines harmonized for the global regulatory will be highly productive.

CONCLUSIONS

MNPs with theranostic applications in oncology are presently a research based glossary on cancer nanotechnology in which drug/diagnostic probe can successfully be fabricated with organ/tissue targeting and controlled release behavior. It will reduce the chemotherapy associated predictable toxic effects and the cost of the therapy due to dose reduction. In conclusion, the reports assure the far reaching theranostic/therapeutic applications of MNPs in oncology. In the near future, to establish these nanocarriers as nanomedicines for successful clinical use, following developmental/safety issues have to be resolved:

➢ The fabrication of MNPs is more complicated than the conventional dosage form.

➢ Formulation stability, control of drug release and insertion of targeting nature in MNPS are some onerous tasks.

➤   Large scale manufacturing and scale-up.

➤   With the change in physicochemical properties of nanomaterials due to reduced size in nanoscale, they have the potential to induce toxicity to the DNA, proteins, cellular components, tissues and other organs. Furthermore, MNPs may cause behavioral, physiological and metabolic alteration.

➤   Challenges exist in toxicity assessment presenting meager *in vivo* findings and poor *in vitro-in vivo* correlation due to lack of appropriate technique/tools to directly interrogate MNPs in complex biological system. Moreover, a regulatory guideline addressing new nanometric devices for the global regulatory will decidedly be industrious.

ACKNOWLEDGEMENTS

Declared none.

CONFLICT OF INTEREST

The authors confirm that this chapter contents have no conflict of interest.

REFERENCES

[1]   Feng SS, Chien S. Chemotherapeutic engineering: Application and further development of chemical engineering principles for chemotherapy of cancer and other diseases. Chem Eng Sci 2003; 58: 4087-14.
[2]   Brannon PL, Blanchette JO. Nanoparticle and targeted systems for cancer therapy. Adv Drug Deliv Rev 2004; 56: 1649-59.
[3]   Pellequer Y, Lamprecht A. Nanoscale canger Therapeutics. In Alf Lamprecht, Eds. Nanotherapeutics: Drug delivery concepts in nannoscience. Pan Stanford Publishing 2009; pp. 93-124.
[4]   Brigger I, Dubernet C, Couvreur P. Nanoparticles in cancer therapy and diagnosis. Adv Drug Deliv Rev 2002; 54: 631-51.
[5]   Torchilin VP. Targeted polymeric micelles for delivery of poorly soluble drugs. Cell Mol Life Sci 2004; 61: 2549-59.
[6]   Alisar SZ, Michael VP. In: de Villiers MM, PornanongA, Glen SK, Eds Nanotechnology in drug delivery. New York: Springer, AAPS Press, 2009; pp. 491-518.
[7]   Allen TM. Ligand-targeted therapeutics in anticancer therapy. *Nature* 2002; 2: 750-63.
[8]   Kim CK, Lim SJ. Recent progress in drug delivery systems for anticancer agents. Archives of Pharmacal Research 2002; 25: 229-39.

[9]   Kingsley JD, Dou H, Morehead J, Rabinow B, Gendelman HE, Destache CJ. Nanotechnology: A focus on nanoparticles as a drug delivery system. *J Neuro Pharmacol* 2006; 1: 1340-50.

[10]   Salata OV. Applications of nanoparticles in biology and medicine. *J Nanotechnol* 2004; 2: 3-8.

[11]   Moghimi SM, Hunter AC, Murray JC. Long-circulating and target-specific nanoparticles: Theory to practice. *Pharmacol Rev* 2001; 53: 283-18.

[12]   Ferrari M. Cancer nanotechnology: opportunities and challenges. *Nat Rev Cancer* 2005; 5: 161-71.

[13]   James DB, Tania B, Lisa BP. Active targeting schemes for nanoparticle systems in cancer therapeutics. *Adv Drug Deliv Rev* 2008; 60: 1615-26.

[14]   An-Hui L, Salabas EL, Ferdi S. Magnetic nanoparticles: Synthesis, protection, functionalization, and application. Angew Chem Int Ed 2007; 46: 1222-44.

[15]   Woodle MC. Controlling liposome blood clearance by surface grafted polymers. Adv Drug Deliv Rev 1998; 32: 139-52.

[16]   Papisov MI. Theoretical considerations of RES-avoiding liposomes: Molecular mechanisms and chemistry of liposome interactions. Adv Drug Deliv Rev 1998; 32: 119-38.

[17]   Moghimi SM, Patel HM. Serum-mediated recognition of liposomes by phagocytic cells of the reticuloendothelial system-the concept of tissue specificity. Adv Drug Deliv Rev 1998; 32: 45-60.

[18]   Kreuter J, Tauber U, Illi V. Distribution and elimination of poly(methyl-2-14C-methacrylate) nanoparticle radioactivity after injection in rats and mice. J Pharm Sci 1979; 68: 1443-47.

[19]   Maruyama K, Ishida O, Takizawa T, Moribe K. Possibility of active targeting to tumor tissues with liposomes. Adv Drug Deliv Rev 1999; 40: 89-102.

[20]   Nafayasu A, Uchiyama K, Kiwada H. The size of liposomes: A factor, which affects their targeting efficiency to tumors and therapeutic activity of liposomal antitumor drugs. Adv Drug Deliv Rev 1999; 40: 75-87.

[21]   Giulio FP, Lawrence T. In Deepak T, Michel D, Yaswant P. Eds, Nanoparticulate drug delivery systems. New York: Informa Healthcare 2007; 141-58.

[22]   Yvonne P, Thomas R. Site-directed drug targeting. Fast track: Pharmaceutics-drug delivery and targeting. London: Pharmaceutical press 2010; 141-60.

[23]   Moghimi SM, Patel HM. Altered tissue specific opsonic activities and opsonophagocytosis of liposomes in tumor bearing rats. Biochem Biophys Acta 1996; 1179: 157-65.

[24]   Moghimi SM, Hunter AC, Murray JC. Nanomedicine: Curent ststus and future prospect. *FASEB J* 2005; 19: 311-30.

[25]   Absolom D. Opsonins and dysopsonins: An overview. Methods Enzymol 1986; 132: 281-18.

[26]   Petrak K. Essential properties of drug-targeting delivery system. Drug Disc Today 2005, 23:1667-73.

[27]   Chonn A, Cullis PR, Devine DV. The role of surface charge in the activation of the classic and alternative pathways of complement activation by liposomes. J Immunol 1991; 146: 4234-41.

[28]   Moghimi SM. Recent development in polymeric nanoparticle engineering and their application in experimental and clinical oncology. Anticancer Agents Med Chem. 2006; 6: 553-61.

[29]   Moghimi SM, Islam H. In: Melgardt M. de Villiers, Pornanong Aramwit, Glen S. Kwon Eds, Nanotechnology in drug delivery. New York: Springer, AAPS Press. 2009; 267-82.

[30]   Serra MV, Mannu F, Mater A, Turrini F, Arese P. Enhanced IgG and complement-independent phagocytosis of sulfatide-enriched human erythrocytes by human monocytes. FEBS Lett 1992; 311: 67-70.

[31]   Chonn A, Semple SC, Cullis PR. Association of blood proteins with large unilamellar liposomes *in vivo*. Relation to circulation lifetimes. J Biol Chem 1992; 267: 18759-65.

[32]   Moghimi SM, Hunter AC. Recognition by macrophages and liver cells of opsonized phospholipids vesicles and phospholipids head groups. Pharm Res 2001; 18: 1-8.

[33]   Moghimi SM, Szebeni J. Stealth liposomes and long circulating nanoparticles: Critical issues in pharmacokinetics, opsonization and proteinbinding properties. Prog Lipid Res 2003; 42: 463-78.

[34]   Abul KA. Disease of immunity. Robbins and Cotran Pathologic Basis Of Disease. Philadelphia: Elsevier Saunders. 2007; pp. 152-65

[35]   Moghimi SM, Patel HM. Tissue specific opsonins for phagocytic cells and their different affinity for cholesterol-rich liposomes. *FEBS Letters* 1988, 233: 143-47.

[36]   Ulrich F, Zilversmit DB. Release from alveolar macrophages of an inhibitor of phagocytosis. Ameri J Physio 1970; 218: 1118-27

[37]   Fredika MR, Mauro F. In: Amiji MM Eds, Nanotechnology for cancer therapy. Boca Raton: CRC press 2007; 3-10.

[38]   Mohammed JM, Pankaj P, Ya-Ping S. In: De Villiers MM, Pornanong A, Glen SK Eds, Nanotechnology in drug delivery. New York: Springer, AAPS Press 2009; 69-104.

[39]   Schiffelers RM, Ansari A, Xu J, *et al.* Cancer siRNA therapy by tumor selective delivery with ligand-targeted sterically stabilized nanoparticles. Nucl Acids Res 2004; 32: e149.

[40]   Abra RM, Bosworth ME, Hunt CA. Liposome disposition *in vivo*: Effect of pre-dosing with liposomes. Res Commun Chem Pathol Pharmacol 1980; 29: 349-60.

[41]   Woodle MC, Scaria P, Ganesh S, *et al.* Sterically stabilized polyplex: Ligand-mediated activity. J Control Release 2001; 74: 309-11.

[42]   Moghimi SM, Davis SS. Innovations in avoiding particle clearance from the blood by Kupffer cells: Cause for reflection. Crit Rev Ther Drug Carrier Syst 1994; 11: 31-59.

[43]   Yuan F, Leunig M, Huang SK, Berk DA, Papahadjopoulos D, Jain RK. Microvascular permeability and interstitial penetration of sterically stabilized (stealth) liposomes in a human tumour xenograft. Can Res 1994; 54: 3352-56.

[44]   Dagar S, Krishnadas A, Rubinstein I, Blend MJ, Nyuksel HO. VIP grafted sterically stabilized liposomes for targeted imaging of breast cancer: *In vivo* studies. J Control Release 2003; 91: 123-133.

[45]   Maeda H, Sawa T, Konno T. Mechanism of tumor-targeted delivery of macromolecular drugs, including the EPR effect in solid tumor and clinical overview of the prototype polymeric drug SMANCS. J Control Release 2001; 74: 47-61.

[46]   Matsumura Y, Maeda H. A new concept for macromolecular therapeutics in cancer chemotherapy: Mechanism of tumour itropic accumulation of proteins and the antitumor agent Smancs. Cancer Res 1986, 46: 6387-92.

[47]   Upasna G, Sanjeeb KS, Tapas KD, Prahlad CG, Amarnath M, Ghosh PK. Biodistribution of fluorosceinated dextran using novel nanoparticle evading reticuloendothelial system. Int J pharm 2000; 202: 1-10.

[48]   Moghimi SM, Porter CJH, Muir IS, Illum L, Davis SS. Non-phagocytic uptake of intravenously injected microspheres in the rat spleen: Influence of particle size and hydrophilic coating. Biochem Biophys Res Commun 1991; 177: 861-66.

[49]   Campbell RB, Fukumura D, Brown EB, *et al*. Cationic charge determines the distribution of liposomes between the vascular and extravascular compartments of tumors. Cancer Res 2002; 62: 6831-36.

[50]   Gabizon A, Horowitz AT, Goren D, Tzemach D, Shmeeda H, Zalipsky S. *in vivo* Fate of folate-targeted polyethylene-glycol liposomes in tumor-bearing mice. Clin Cancer Res 2003; 9: 6551-59.

[51]   Campbell RB, Balasubramanian SV, Straubinger RM. Influence of cationic lipids on the stability and membrane properties of paclitaxel-containing liposomes. J Pharm Sci 2001; 90: 1091-05.

[52]   Pan X, Lee RJ. Tumour-selective drug delivery *via* folate receptor-targeted liposomes. Expert Opin Drug Deliv 2004; 1: 7-17.

[53]   Gabizon A, Shmeeda H, Horowitz AT, Zalipsky S. Tumor cell targeting of liposome entrapped drugs with phospholipid-anchored folic acid-PEG conjugates. Adv Drug Deliv Rev 2004; 56: 1177-92.

[54]   Mornet S, Vasseur S, Grasset F, *et al*. Magnetic nanoparticle design for medical applications. Prog Solid State Chem 2006; 34: 237-47.

[55]   Jones A, Harris AL. New developments in angiogenesis: A major mechanism for tumor growth and target for therapy. Cancer J Sci Am 1998; 4: 209-17.

[56]   Baban DF, Seymour LW. Control of tumour vascular permeability. Adv Drug Deliv Rev 1998, 34: 109-19.

[57]   Folkman J, Merler E, Abernathy C, Williams G. Isolation of a tumour factor responsible for angiogenesis. J Exp Med 1971; 133: 275-88.

[58]   Rubin P, Casarett G. Microcirculation of tumors. II. The supervascularized state of irradiated regressing tumors. Clin Radiol 1966; 17: 346-55.

[59]   Hobbs SK, Monsky WL, Yuan F, *et al*. Regulation of transport pathways in tumor vessels: Role of tumour type and microenvironment. Proc Natl Acad Sci USA 1998; 95: 4607-12.

[60]   Shubik P. Vascularization of tumors: A review. J Cancer Res Clin Oncol 1982; 103: 211-26.

[61]   Maeda H, Wu J, Sawa T, Matsumura Y, Hori K. Tumour vascular permeability and the EPR effect in macromolecular therapeutics: A review. J Control Release 2000; 65: 271-84.

[62]   Maeda P. The enhanced permeability and retention (EPR) effect in tumor vasculature: The key role of tumor-selective macromolecular drug targeting, Adv Enz Regu 2001, 41: 189-207.

[63]   Stolnik SIL, Davis SS. Long circulating microparticulate drug carriers. Adv Drug Deliv Rev 1995; 16: 195-14.

[64]   Weissleder P, Bogdanov A, Papisov M. Drug targeting in magnetic resonance imaging. Mag Res Quar 1992; 8: 55-63.

[65]   Sinha R, Kim GJ, Nie SM, Shin DM. Nanotechnology in cancer therapeutics: Bioconjugated nanoparticles for drug delivery. Mole Canc Therapeut 2006; 5: 1909-17.

[66] Zhang Y, Kohler N, Zhang MQ. Surface modification of superparamagnetic magnetite nanoparticles and their intracellular uptake. *Biomaterials* 2002; 23: 1553-61.

[67] Yigit MV, Mazumdar D, Kim HK, Lee JH, Odintsov B, Lu Y. Smart "turn-on" magnetic resonance contrast agents based on aptamer-functionalized superparamagnetic iron oxide nanoparticles. Chem BioChem 2007; 8: 1675-78.

[68] Herr JK, Smith JE, Medley CD, Shangguan D, Tan W. Aptamer-conjugated nanoparticles for selective collection and detection of cancer cells. Anal Chem 2006; 78: 2918-24.

[69] Kresse M, Wagner S, Pfefferer D, Lawaczeck R, Elste V, Semmler W. Targeting of ultrasmall superparamagnetic iron oxide (USPIO) particles to tumor cells *in vivo* by using transferrin receptor pathways. Magn Reson Med Sci 1998; 40: 236-42.

[70] Hatakeyama H, Akita H, Ishida E, *et al.* Tumor targeting of doxorubicin by anti-MT1-MMP antibody-modified PEG liposomes. Int J Pharm 2007; 342: 194-200.

[71] Wunderbaldinger P, Josephson L, Weissleder R. Tat peptide directs enhanced clearance and hepatic permeability of magnetic nanoparticles. Bioconj Chemi 2002; 13: 264-68.

[72] Yoo HS, Park TG. Folate receptor targeted biodegradable polymeric doxorubicin micelles. J Control Release 2004; 96: 273-83.

[73] Cirstoiu-Hapca A, Bossy-Nobs L, Buchegger F, Gurny R, Delie F. Differential tumor cell targeting of anti-HER2 (Herceptin (R) and anti-CD20 (Mabthera (R) coupled nanoparticles. Inter J Pharm 2007; 331: 190-96.

[74] Funovics MA, Kapeller B, Hoeller C, Su HS, Kunstfeld R, Puig S, *et al.* MR imaging of the her2/neu and 9.2.27 tumor antigens using immunospecific contrast agents. Mag Res Imag 2004; 22: 843-50

[75] Mirkin CA, Letsinger RL, Mucic RC, Storhoff JJ. A DNA based method for rationally assembling nanoparticles into macroscopic materials. Nature 1996; 382: 607-09

[76] McNeil SE. Nanotechnology for the biologist. J Leukoc Biol 2005; 78: 585-94.

[77] Zhao M, Beauregard DA, Loizou L, Davletov B, Brindle KM. Non-invasive detection of apoptosis using magnetic resonance imaging and a targeted contrast agent. Nat Med 2001; 7: 1241-44.

[78] Pouliquen D, Lucet I, Chouly C, Perdrisot R, Le Jeune JJ, Jallet P. Liver-directed superparamagnetic iron oxide: Quantitation of T_2 relaxation effects. Mag Reso Imaging 1993; 2: 219-28.

[79] Stark D, Weissleder R, Elizondo G, *et al.* Neuroblastoma: Diagnostic imaging and staging. Radiology 1988; 168: 201-97.

[80] Weissleder R. Liver MR imaging with iron oxides: toward consensus and clinical practice. Radiology 1994; 193: 593-95.

[81] Remsen LG, McCormick CI, Roman-Goldstein S, *et al.* MR of carcinoma-specific monoclonal antibody conjugated to monocrystalline iron oxide nanoparticles: The potential for noninvasive diagnosis. Am J Neuroradiol 1996; 17: 411-18.

[82] Dmitri A, Noriko M, Baasil O, Zaver MB. MR molecular imaging of the Her-2/*neu* receptor in breast cancer cells using targeted iron oxide nanoparticles. Magn Reson Med 2003; 49: 403-48.

[83] Grimm J, Perez JM, Josephson RW. Novel nanosensors for rapid analysis of telomerase activity. Cancer Res 2004; 64: 639-43.

[84] Perez JM, Josephson L, Loughlin TO, Hogemann D, Weissleder R. Magnetic relaxation switches capable of sensing molecular interactions. Nat Biotechnol 2002; 20: 816-20.

[85]   Jason RM, Ralph W. Multifunctional magnetic nanoparticle for targeted imaging and therapy. Adv Drug Deliv Rev 2008; 60: 1241-51.

[86]   Reddy GR, Bhojani MS, McConville P, *et al.* Vascular targeted nanoparticles for imaging and treatment of brain tumours. Clin Cancer Res 2006; 12: 6677-86.

[87]   Berry CC, Curtis ASG. Functionalization of magnetic nanoparticle for application in biomedicine. J Phys Appl phys 2003; 36: R198-R206.

[88]   Hu FQ, Wei L, Zhou Z, Ran YL, Li Z, Gao MY. Preparation of biocompatible magnetite nanocrystals for *in vivo* magnetic resonance detection of cancer. Adv Mater 2006; 18: 2553-56.

[89]   Harisinghani MG, Barentsz J, Hahn PF, *et al.* Noninvasive detection of clinically occult lymph-node metastases in prostate cancer. N Engl J Med 2003; 348: 2491-99.

[90]   Alexiou C, Arnold W, Klein RJ, *et al.* Locoregional cancer treatment with magnetic drug targeting. Cancer Res 2000; 60: 6641-48.

[91]   Alexiou C, Jurgons R, Schmid R, *et al. in vitro* and *in vivo* Investigations of targeted chemotherapy with magnetic nanoparticles. J Magn Magn Mater 2005; 293: 389-93.

[92]   Farrer NJ, Salassa L, Sadler PJ. Photoactivated chemotherapy (PACT): The potential of excited-state d-block metals in medicine. Dalton Trans 2009; 48: 10690-701.

[93]   Rinat OE. Radiation and nanoparticles for enhancement of drug delivery in solid tumours.US6165440; 2000.

[94]   Nicholas AK. Bioconjugates of nanoparticle as radiopharmaceuticals. US6689338; 2004.

[95]   Huachang L, Guangshun Y, Depu C, Lianghong G, Jing C. Fluorescent magnetic nanoparticles and process of preparation. EP 1651957, 2011.

[96]   Penades S, Martin-Lomas M, Martines De La Fuente J, Rademacher TW. Magnetic nanoparticles linked to a ligand. EP 2277548, 2013.

[97]   Fernandez C, Litran R, Rojas R, Sanchez L, Hernando G, Sampedro R. Magnetic nanoparticles of noble metals. EP 1746610, 2012.

[98]   Maurice PB. Bioconjugated nanoparticles. US3177868; 2008.

[99]   Levy L, Germain M, Devaux, C. Magnetic nanoparticles compositions and uses thereof. EP 2010152, 2011.

[100] Bahr M, Berkov D, Buske N, *et al.* Magnetic nanoparticles having biochemical activity, method for the production thereof and their use. US6767635; 2004.

[101] Suwa T, Ozawa S, Ueda M, Ando N, Kitajima M. Magnetic resonance imaging of esophageal squamous cell carcinoma using magnetite particles coated with anti-epidermal growth factor receptor antibody. Int J Cancer 1998; 75: 626-34.

[102] Shen TT, Bogdanov AJr, Bogdanova A, Poss K, Brady TJ, Weissleder R. Magnetically labeled secretin retains receptor affinity to pancreas acinar cells. Bioconjug Chem 1996; 7: 311-16.

[103] Reimer P, Weissleder R, Shen T, Knoefel WT, Brady TJ. Pancreatic receptors: Initial feasibility studies with a targeted contrast agent for MR imaging. Radiology 1994; 193: 527-31.

[104] Liong M, Lu J, Kovochich M, Xia T, Ruehm SG, Nel AE, *et al.* Multifunctional inorganic nanoparticles for imaging, targeting, and drug delivery. ACS Nano 2008; 2: 889-96.

[105] Kohler N, Sun C, Fichtenholtz A, Gunn J, Fang C, Zhang M. Methotrexate-immobilized poly (ethylene glycol) magnetic nanoparticles for MR imaging and drug delivery. Small 2006; 2: 785-92.

[106] Jain TK, Richey J, Strand M, Leslie-Pelecky DL, Flask CA, Labhasetwar V. Magnetic nanoparticles with dual functional properties: Drug delivery and magnetic resonance imaging. Biomaterials 2008; 29: 4012-21.

[107] Hu SH, Tsai CH, Liao CF, Liu DM, Chen SY. Controlled rupture of magnetic polyelectrolyte microcapsules for drug delivery. Langmuir 2008, 24: 11811-18.

[108] Liang S, Wang YX, Yu JF, Zhang CF, Xia JY, Yin DZ. Surface modified superparamagnetic iron oxide nanoparticles: As a new carrier for biomagnetically targeted therapy. J Mat Sci: Materials in Medicine 2007; 18: 2297-302.

[109] Ross JS, Fletcher JA, Bloom KJ, Linette GP, Stec V, Symmans WF. Targeted therapy in breast cancer: The HER-2/neu gene and protein. *Mol Cell Proteomics* 2004, 3:379-398.

[110] Kyeongsoon P, Seulki L, Eunah K, Kwangmeyung K, Kuiwon C, Ick CK. New generation of multifunctional nanoparticles for cancer imaging and therapy. Adv Funct Mater 2009; 19: 1553-66.

[111] Seydel C. Quantum dots get wet. Science 2003; 300: 80-91.

[112] Bruchez M, Jr, Moronne M, Gin P, Weiss SA. Semiconductor nanocrystals as fluorescent biological labels. Science 1998; 25: 2013-16.

[113] Gao X, Cui Y, Levenson RM, Chung LW, Nie S. *in vivo* Cancer targeting and imaging with semiconductor quantum dots. Nat Biotechnol 2004; 22: 969-76.

[114] Elghanian R, Storhoff JJ, Mucic RC, Letsinger RL, Mirkin CA. Selective colorimetric detection of polynucleotides based on the distance-dependent optical properties of gold nanoparticles. Science 1997; 277: 1078-81.

[115] Hirsch LR, Jackson JB, Lee A, Halas NJ, West JL. A whole blood immunoassay using gold nanoshells. Anal Chem 2003; 75: 2377-81.

[116] Thanh NT, Rosenzweig Z. Development of an aggregation-based immunoassay for anti-protein A using gold nanoparticles. Anal Chem 2002; 74: 1624-28.

[117] Nam JM, Thaxton CS, Mirkin CA. Nanoparticle-based bio-bar codes for the ultrasensitive detection of proteins. Science 2003; 301: 1884-86.

[118] Daniel MC, Astruc D. Gold nanoparticles: Assembly, supramolecular chemistry, quantum-size-related properties, and applications toward biology, catalysis, and nanotechnology. Chem Rev 2004; 104: 246-93.

[119] Love JC, Estroff LA, Kriebel JK, Nuzzo RG, Whitesides GM. Self-assembled monolayers of thiolates on metals as a form of nanotechnology. Chem Rev 2005; 105: 1103-69.

[120] Hirsch LR, Stafford RJ, Bankson JA, *et al.* Nanoshell-mediated near-infrared thermal therapy of tumors under magnetic resonance guidance. Proc Natl Acad Sci USA 2003, 100; 13549-54.

[121] Loo C, Lowery A, Halas N, West J, Drezek R. Immunotargeted nanoshells for integrated cancer imaging and therapy. Nano Lett 2005; 5: 709-11.

[122] Hainfeld J, Slatkin DN, Smilowitz HM. The use of gold nanoparticles to enhance radiotherapy in mice. Phys Med Biol 2004; 49: N309-15.

[123] Huang X, El-Sayed IH, Qian W, El-Sayed MA. Cancer cell imaging and photothermal therapy in the near-infrared region by using gold nanorods. J Am Chem Soc 2006; 128: 2115-20.

[124] Kwon J, Hwang S, Jin H, *et al.* M.H. Body distribution of inhaled fluorescent magnetic nanoparticles in the mice. J Occup Health 2008; 50: 1-6.

[125] Komatsu T, Tabata M, Kubo-Irie M, *et al.* The effects of nanoparticles on mouse testis Leydig cells *in vitro*. Toxicol *in vitro* 2008; 22: 1825-31.

[126] Braydich SL, Hussain SM, Schlager J, Hofmann MC. *In vitro* cytotoxicity of nanoparticles in mammalian germline stem cells. Toxicol Sci 2005; 88: 412-19.

[127] Browning LM, Lee KJ, Huang T, Nallathamby PD, Lowman JE, Xu XH. Random walk of single gold nanoparticles in zebrafish embryos leading to stochastic toxic effects on embryonic developments. Nanoscale 2009; 1: 138-52.

[128] De JWH, Borm P. Drug delivery and nanoparticles: applications and hazards. Int J Nanomed 2008; 3: 133-49.

[129] Chen HW, Su SF, Chien CT, Lin WH, Chen JJW, Pan CY. Titanium dioxide nanoparticles induce emphysema-like lung injury in mice. FASEB 2006; 20: 2393-95.

[130] Yen HJ, Hsu SH, Tsai CL. Cytotoxicity and immunological response of gold and silver nanoparticles of different sizes. Small 2009; 5: 1553-61.

[131] Hussain SM, Hess KL, Gearhart JM, Geiss, KT, Schlager JJ. *In vitro* toxicity of nanoparticles in BRL 3A rat liver cells. Toxicol *in vitro* 2005; 19: 975-83.

[132] Pisanic TR, Blackwell JD, Shubayev VI, Fiñones RR, Jin S. Nanotoxicity of iron oxide nanoparticle internalization in growing neurons. Biomaterials 2007; 28: 2572-81.

[133] Kirpotin DB. Drummond DC, Shao Y, *et al*. Antibody targeting of long-circulating lipidic nanoparticles does not increase tumor localization but does increase internalization in animal models. Cancer Res 2006; 66: 6732-40.

[134] Clift MJ, Rothen-Rutishauser B, Brown DM, *et al*. The impact of different nanoparticle surface chemistry and size on uptake and toxicity in a murine macrophage cell line. Toxicol Appl Pharmacol 2008; 232; 418-27.

[135] Rahman AM, Yusuf SW, Ewer MS. Anthracycline-induced cardiotoxicity and the cardiac-sparing effect of liposomal formulation. Int J Nanomedicine 2007; 2: 567-83.

[136] Romberg B, Hennink WE, Storm G. Sheddable coatings for long-circulating nanoparticles. Pharm Res 2008; 25: 55-71.

[137] Dos Santos N, Allen C, Doppen AM, *et al*. Influence of poly(ethylene glycol) grafting density and polymer length on liposomes: relating plasma circulation lifetimes to protein binding. Biochim Biophys Acta. 2007; 1768: 1367-77.

[138] Karmali PP, Simberg D. Interactions of nanoparticles with plasma proteins: implication on clearance and toxicity of drug delivery systems. Expert Opin Drug Deliv 2011; 8: 343-57.

[139] Ishida T, Atobe K, Wang X, Kiwada H. Accelerated blood clearance of PEGylated liposomes upon repeated injections: effect ofdoxorubicin-encapsulation and high-dose first injection. J Control Release. 2006; 115; 251-58.

[140] Limbach LK, Wick P, Manser P, Grass RN, Bruinink A, Stark WJ. Exposure of engineered nanoparticles to human lung epithelial cells: influence of chemical composition and catalytic activity on oxidative stress. Env Sci Technol 2007, 41: 4158-63.

[141] Xia T, Kovochich M, Brant J, *et al*. Comparison of the abilities of ambient and manufactured nanoparticles to induce cellular toxicity according to an oxidative stress paradigm. Nano Letters 2006; 6: 1794-807.

[142] Pasqualini R, Koivunen E, Kain R, *et al*., Amino peptidase N is a receptor for tumor-homing peptides and a target for inhibiting angiogenesis. Cancer Res 2000; 60: 722-27.

[143] Oh P, Borgstrom P, Witkiewicz H, *et al*. Live dynamic imaging of caveolae pumping targeted antibody rapidly and speci fically across endothelium in the lung. Nat Biotechnol 2007; 25: 327-37.

[144] Borisch B, Semac I, Soltermann A, Palomba C, Hoessli DC. Anti-CD20 treatments and the lymphocyte membrane: pathology for therapy. Verh Dtsch Ges Pathol 2001; 85: 161-6.

[145] Graham J, Muhsin M, Kirkpatrick P. Cetuximab. Nat Rev Drug Discov 2004; 3: 549 -50.

[146] Fonsatti E, Nicolay HJ, Altomonte M, Covre A, Maio M. Targeting cancer vasculature *via* endoglin/CD105: a novel antibody-based diagnostic and therapeutic strategy in solid tumors. Cardiovasc Res 2010, 86: 12-19.

[147] Ferguson LR, Philpott M. Cancer prevention by dietary bioactive components that target the immune response. Curr Cancer Drug Targets 2007; 7: 459-64.

[148] Singh RP, Agarwal R. Tumor angiogenesis: a potential target in cancer control by phytochemicals Curr Cancer Drug Targets 2003; 3: 205-17.

[149] Desnick RJ, Schuchman EH. Enzyme replacement and enhancement therapies: lessons from lysosomal disorders. Nat Rev Genet 2002; 3: 954-56.

[150] LeBowitz JH, Grubb JH, Maga JA, Schmiel DH, Vogler C, Sly WS. Glycosylation-independent targeting enhances enzyme delivery to lysosomes and decreases storage in mucopolysaccharidosis type VII mice. Proc Natl Acad Sci USA 2004; 101: 3083-88.

[151] Brekken RA, Overholser JP, Stastny VA, Waltenberger J, Minna JD, Thorpe PE. Selective inhibition of vascular endothelial growth factor (VEGF) receptor 2 (KDR/Flk-1) activity by a monoclonal anti-VEGF antibody blocks tumor growth in mice. Cancer Res 2000; 60: 5117-24.

[152] Binetruy-Tour naire R, Demangel C, Malavaud B, *et al*. Identification of a peptide blocking vascular endothelial growth factor (VEG F)-mediated angiogenesis. EMBO J 2000; 19: 1525-33.

[153] Ren J, Agata N, Chen D, *et al*. Human MUC1 carcinoma-associated protein confers resistance to genotoxic antic ancer agents. Cancer Cell 2004; 5: 163-75.

[154] Ming X. Cellular delivery of siRNA and antisense oligonucleotides *via* receptor-mediated endocytosis. Expert Opin Drug Deliv 2011; 8: 435-49.

[155] Ladewig K, Xu ZP, Lu GQ. Layered double hydroxide nanoparticles in gene and drug delivery. Expert Opin Drug Deliv 2009: 6: 907-22.

[156] Agus DB, Sweeney CJ, Morris MJ, *et al*. Efficacy and safety of single-agent pertuzumab (rhuMAb 2C4), a human epidermal growth factor receptor dimerization inhibitor, in castration-resistant prostate cancer after progression from taxane-based therapy. J Clin Oncol 2007; 25: 675-81.

[157] Biao-xue R, Xi-guang C, Shuan-ying Y, Wei L, Zong-juan M. EphA2-dependent molecular targeting therapy for malignant tumors. Curr Cancer Drug Targets 2011; 11: 1082-97.

[158] Zha J, Lackner MR. Targeting the insulin-like growth factor receptor-1R pathway for cancer therapy. Clin Cancer Res 2010: 16: 2512-17.

[159] Wang Y, Sun Y. Insulin-like growth factor receptor-1 as an anti-cancer target: blocking transformation andinducing apoptosis. Curr Cancer Drug Targets 2002; 2: 191-207.

[160] van der Veeken J, Oliveira S, Schiffelers RM, *et al*. Crosstalk between epidermal growth factor receptor- and insulin-like growth factor-1 receptorsignaling: implications for cancer therapy. Curr Cancer Drug Targets 2009; 9: 748-60.

[161] Akhter S, Ahmad MZ, Ahmad FJ, Storm G, Kok RJ. Gold nanoparticles in theranostic oncology: current state-of-the-art. Expert Opin Drug Deliv 2012; 9: 1225-43.

[162] Mironava T, Simon M, Rafailovich MH, Rigas B. Platinum folate nanoparticles toxicity: cancer *vs* normal cells. Toxicol *In Vitro*. 2013; 27: 882-9.

[163] Wei Y, Yin G, Ma C, Huang Z, Chen X, Liao X, Yao Y, Yin H. Synthesis and cellular compatibility of biomineralized Fe_3O_4 nanoparticles in tumor cells targeting peptides. Colloids Surf B Biointerfaces. 2013; 107: 180-8.

[164]   Limbach LK, Wick P, Manser P, Grass RN, Bruinink A, Stark WJ. Exposure of engineered nanoparticles to human lung epithelial cells: influence of chemical composition and catalytic activity on oxidative stress. Environ Sci Technol. 2007, 41: 4158-63.

[165]   Xia T, Kovochich M, Brant J, Hotze M, Sempf J, Oberley T, Sioutas C, Yeh JI, Wiesner MR, Nel AE. Comparison of the abilities of ambient and manufactured nanoparticles to induce cellular toxicity according to an oxidative stress paradigm. Nano Letters 2006, 6: 1794-97.

[166]   Akhter S, Ahmad I, Ahmad M Z, Ramazani F, Sing A, Rahman Z, Kok RJ. Nanomedicines as Cancer Therapeutics: Current Status. Current cancer drug targets. 2013, 13: 362-78.

INDEX

A

ABC transporters   111, 123, 127-9, 131, 134

ABCB1   11, 109-11, 120, 123-7, 128, 129-37
  cancer cells overexpressing   130

ABCG2   11, 120, 124-5, 128, 134

Abnormal karyotype   37

Acetyl-CoA   159-60

Aclarubicin   14, 16, 20

Activation   14, 17, 61-2, 68, 71, 74, 111, 113, 115, 136, 152, 157, 163, 210, 223-4
  constitutional   207, 210
  mutational   74, 202
  oncogene   154-6, 159-60, 162, 167

Activity   5, 9-11, 17-18, 21-2, 24, 45, 56, 71, 76-7, 112, 129-30, 156-7, 159-60, 163-4, 204
  biochemical   271
  transcriptional   56, 91, 115-16, 118, 164

Acute myeloid leukemia (AML)   16-17, 19, 32-3, 36, 40, 43, 46, 60, 122, 128-9, 222-3

Acute promyelocytic leukemia (APL)   223

Adenocarcinomas   203, 207, 214-15

Adjuvant therapy   191

ADP   57-8, 159

Agents   10-11, 13, 16-19, 21, 23-4, 32, 80, 130-1, 134, 201, 205
  antitumor   238-9
  microtubule stabilizing   133, 135
  targeted   90, 118, 203, 205
  therapeutic   234, 243, 264-5, 269

Akt   59, 62, 80-1, 122, 176, 210, 219

ALK1   61-2, 71, 87, 89

ALK5   61-2, 71, 89

N

T

W